"I used the first edition, *An In* undergraduates multiple times, ond edition is updated with va̲ ̲...at̲ion and remains just as clear, careful, and compassionate. The focus on human dignity, human flourishing, and justice provides a normative basis. Principles and criteria for various issues help students to develop their own capacity for moral discernment. Each chapter stimulates discussion with intriguing cases. The book invites critical thinking by offering consideration of various perspectives. The new chapter on health care reform opens up important macro-issues, competing under-standings of justice, and the need for reform. This excellent text is recommended for anyone who realizes that sooner or later they will need to be engaged in the serious and loving work of health care decision making."

—Marie J. Giblin, PhD, Xavier University, Cincinnati

HEALTH CARE ETHICS

Theological Foundations, Contemporary Issues,
and Controversial Cases

REVISED and EXPANDED

Michael R. Panicola, David M. Belde, John Paul Slosar, Mark F. Repenshek

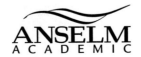

ANSELM
ACADEMIC

Created by the publishing team of Anselm Academic.

Cover image royalty free from istockphoto.com

Printed in the United States of America

7034

ISBN 978-1-59982-103-0

In gratitude we dedicate this book to:

Dr. Ronald P. Hamel
Friend, Mentor, Colleague, Scholar

ACKNOWLEDGMENTS

Our thanks to the following individuals who advised the publishing team or reviewed this work in progress:

Dr. Debra Bennett-Woods
Regis University, Denver, Colorado

Dr. Janine Idziak
Loras College, Dubuque, Iowa

Dr. Karen Elliott, CPPS
Mercy College of Northwest Ohio, Toledo, Ohio

Dr. Ron Hamel
Catholic Health Association, Saint Louis, Missouri

Rev. Steven O'Hala
Saint Vincent de Paul Regional Seminary, Boynton Beach, Florida

Dr. Tim McFarland
Saint Joseph's College, Rensselaer, Indiana

CONTENTS

PREFACE

This book is intended as a theologically inspired introductory text in health care ethics geared primarily toward college students but also appropriate for medical, nursing, and other students in health care-related fields, as well as health care practitioners. Our goal in writing this book is to encourage moral reflection and moral discourse on ethical issues in health care rather than resorting to ready-made and prescriptive answers to concrete dilemmas. This book examines real-life concerns and issues that confront real people every day. It is an applied ethics textbook written by theological ethicists working in health care.

We believe this book offers three elements that set it apart from similar texts. First, this book does not assume extensive knowledge of theology, ethics, or medicine on the part of readers. Second, this book includes case studies that we have confronted in our work, giving real-life relevance to the text. These cases are intended to show how particular circumstances have an effect on ethical decision making. Finally, each chapter provides a list of further readings and multimedia aids, such as documentaries and movies, that touch on the core themes of the chapter and that, with the case studies, can be incorporated easily into creative teaching and learning strategies.

As with the first edition, this revised and expanded edition of the text has two main parts, beginning with theological and ethical foundations (chapters 1–3), followed by concrete ethical issues in health care (chapters 4–12). The foundations lay the groundwork for the discussion of ethical issues that follows in subsequent chapters through, among other ways, outlining a normative basis that provides a backdrop or point of reference against which we can evaluate the ethical issues. In our experience as college teachers and ethicists within health care institutions, we have learned that it is pointless to discuss controversial issues without some kind of normative basis.

Lacking such a basis, ethical discussion inevitably degenerates into individual relativism.

Two things should be noted up front about our normative basis. First, though it is grounded in some values and concepts that are central to the Catholic moral tradition and Catholic social teaching—such as human dignity, justice, and human flourishing—our normative basis is not exclusively Catholic, and this book is not intended as a textbook on Catholic health care ethics. Second, our normative basis is not a moral method per se. That is, it does not provide a methodological process for ethical decision making. Instead, it presents a picture of who we ought to become as persons living among others in the context of community. The central concern of our normative approach is human flourishing and right relationships. Although principles and virtues provide some objective basis for ethical decision making, our normative approach is rooted in a holistic view of the person and principally concerned with the role of discernment in attaining human flourishing.

All the chapters that remain from the first edition have been updated with new material, cases, and suggested readings and multimedia aids. Some of these chapters will look slightly different from the first edition because new and emerging topics have been added. For instance, in chapter 5, we now include a discussion about the considerations of costs when assessing treatment options for critically ill newborns; in chapter 9, we have added a section on pharmaceutical and device manufacturers' involvement in clinical research, and the conflicts of interest that can arise for investigators or institutions; in chapter 10, we have added a discussion on the 2009 revision to the *Ethical and Religious Directives for Catholic Health Care Services* and the implications for treatment decisions related to artificial nutrition and hydration; and in chapter 11, we have added a section on advance care planning and the critical role it plays in ensuring patients approaching the end of life receive care that conforms to their personal values and wishes.

In addition to this updated material, we have condensed the four foundations chapters from the first edition into two and added a new chapter to the foundations section on professionalism and the patient-professional relationship. We felt this was important for two primary reasons, namely, (1) the first edition lacked a sustained discussion on this topic, and several health care professionals who read our book noted this absence, and (2) health care ethics unfolds most immediately in the privacy of the patient–professional relationship, and ethics can provide balance to the inherent unevenness in this relationship by critically shaping how we understand the nature of the relationship itself. Coupled with the condensed foundations chapters from the first edition, this discussion of professionalism and the patient–professional relationship adds depth to the ethical analysis of the issues that follows in subsequent chapters.

Also new in this edition is chapter 12, which deals with health care reform. Given the significant ethical concerns that have been raised about the American health care system in recent years—concerns over access, limited resources, high costs, racial disparities, quality, and safety—we simply had to confront this issue in this revised and expanded edition. Though we do not delve into any great detail on the recently passed Patient Protection and Affordable Care Act, we do consider the issue of health care reform from an ethical perspective, a perspective that has been sorely lacking in the current American debate.

We must note one last thing. As with the first edition, this book is the product of four authors. Consequently, you will once again encounter four different voices and writing styles. Though we all work from the same foundations, there are differences in how extensively and explicitly we apply the normative basis to the issues discussed. Similarities will exist across the chapters in terms of content and structure, but subtle differences will be perceptible, as well, given the collaborative nature of this text.

—*Michael Panicola and David Belde*

CHAPTER 1

Understanding Ethics and How We Approach Ethical Decisions

Michael Panicola

Understanding Ethics

Each of us encounters ethics every day, whether or not we are aware of it. We cannot avoid situations in which we must make ethical decisions because "there are virtually no ethical-free zones of life, only differences of ethical importance."[1] Yet despite such daily encounters, ethics remains a difficult concept to define. Think about it for a minute. How would you define *ethics*? What descriptive words or phrases would you use?

The Scope and Task of Ethics

Most people, when asked to define *ethics*, mention right and wrong actions and highlight sources of morality or ethics that guide them in concrete situations, like personal values, religious beliefs, rules, laws, customs, traditions, or feelings. How we act in particular situations and which sources of morality guide our decisions are definitely a part of ethics, but ethics is much more. So before we start talking about health care ethics and its complex issues, we need to get a sense of what *ethics* is generally and what it requires. This will better prepare us for what lies ahead in this book and hopefully in life. To get us pointed in the right direction, consider the following hypothetical cases:

Case 1A

After work, you drive to the shopping center to buy a few items. Upon leaving, you back your car out from your narrow parking space and inadvertently catch your front bumper on the rear quarter-panel of the car next to you. You get out to assess the damage and find only a small scratch on the other car and nothing on your own. No one has witnessed the incident. *What would you do in this situation?*

Case 1B

One of your closest friends tells you he has been having an affair for nearly a year. He is distraught and seeks comfort from you. You are the first person he has told, and just telling you gives him relief. During your discussion, he begs you not to say anything to anyone. Several weeks later his significant other, who is also your close friend, confides in you that she thinks her partner is cheating on her. As she talks, she is clearly tormented, unsure if she is just being paranoid or if there is truth to her suspicions. She asks what you think and what she should do. *What would you do in this situation?*

Case 1C

You are a midlevel executive in a large, fast-moving organization. You value your job and know it would be difficult finding another like it with the same salary in your town. You value your job for other reasons as well, not least of which is you need the income to pay costly school loan payments and a hefty monthly rent for an apartment you love. One unpleasant aspect of your job is that your supervisor seems less talented than his staff and is prone to violent outbursts with some of the lower-ranking employees. Recently, he publicly berated his administrative assistant for not completing a report on time, even though he had given her the data to complete it at the last minute. It was obvious to everyone that he was attempting to blame someone else for his

cont.

Case 1C *cont.*

---

poor work habits. You want to do something about his behavior, perhaps report him to one of his superiors. However, due largely to his ability to bring in big accounts, he has gained the favor of the company's president. Consequently, no one else is willing to stand up to him, and you will have to go it alone. You are unsure how your accusations will be handled. You fear that you will be seen as a "problem" and could even lose your job. *What would you do in this situation?*

Setting aside for now the question of what we should do in these situations, let us instead use these cases as a backdrop to explore the scope of ethics, what ethics is and what it involves in practice. Simply stated, ethics concerns any behavior or decision that affects human well-being (dignity, character, quality of life) and the good of the community. Each of the above cases in some way deals with ethics. Whether we decide to wait for the person whose car we hit, maintain our friend's confidence, or stand up to our boss, our decisions will affect the well-being of those involved, including ourselves, and community life as a whole. We mentioned above that there are virtually no ethical-free zones in life, only differences of ethical importance. Thus the scope of ethics is large, and its basic task is to ask and seek answers to two related questions: "Who ought we to become as persons?" (BEING) and "How ought we to act in relation to others (people, God, and creation)?" (DOING) (see figure 1A).

In addressing these questions, ethics considers such things as

- *the goal(s) of human life* and what our lives should ultimately be directed toward (e.g., love of God, right relationships, just social order)
- the *virtues*, or character traits, attitudes, feelings, and dispositions, that should define us as people and shape how we act in relation to others (e.g., love, compassion, honesty)

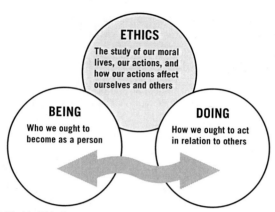

FIGURE 1A What Is Ethics?

- the **principles** that should guide our decision making, conscience formation, and discernment in concrete situations (e.g., human dignity, justice, solidarity)
- the **circumstances**, including the facts surrounding a situation and the possible consequences of our actions, that should influence our decisions

Understanding ethics in this way avoids the common misconception that ethics deals only with how we act. Admittedly, the focus of ethics is on our actions, which is why in health care ethics, for example, we tend to debate issues such as abortion, physician-assisted suicide, stem cell research, and genetic testing, all of which center on what we do in specific situations. But this focus tends to overshadow something that Socrates, Plato, Aristotle, Aquinas, and other philosophers took great pains to clarify: our actions not only say something about who we are but also help determine who we ultimately become. We may not always act in ways consistent with who we are or ought to become, and though no single action may completely define us as a person, we cannot escape that who we are affects how we act, and how we act affects who we are becoming as persons in relation to other people, God, and creation.

Perhaps an example, using one of the cases above, will help to clarify this. If you wait for the person whose car you hit and tell the truth about what happened rather than sneaking off and not facing the consequences, and you consistently tell the truth in similar situations where it would be easier to lie, your actions would suggest that you value honesty and either already are or are on your way toward becoming an honest person. The same is true in reverse. If you continuously lie when in tough spots, your actions would suggest that you either already are or are on your way toward becoming a dishonest person—a liar. How could you claim otherwise? The connection between *doing* and *being* is essential to properly understanding ethics, because ethics is not only about what we do but also, and simultaneously, about who we are becoming through our actions.

Requirements for Ethics

As a human endeavor concerned with who we ought to become and how we ought to act, ethics requires freedom and knowledge, reasoning and discernment, and a normative basis. Each of these elements constitutes a vital part of ethics; without any one, it would be impossible to do ethics.

    A. Freedom and Knowledge. In ethics, freedom is divided into two aspects: freedom of choice and freedom of self-determination. Freedom of choice relates to *doing;* it is simply our ability to choose this or that. For example, it is the freedom we have to either go out with friends or study, or to shop at Target as opposed to Walmart. Freedom of self-determination is the freedom to shape our lives and become the person we want and are called to be. Some people argue that our freedom of self-determination is weakened, even crippled, by original sin, social forces, physical characteristics, or other factors. There is some truth to this; we are not totally free because of spiritual, social, biological, and other factors that at times limit our choices and our ability to make good decisions. Yet despite such limitations, at the core of our being we are each free (barring extreme incapacity) to choose the type of person we want to become through our actions, even in the most challenging circumstances. Viktor Frankl, a survivor of the Holocaust, provides proof of this:

> We who lived in concentration camps can remember
> the men who walked through the huts comforting

others, giving away their last piece of bread. They may have been few in number, but they offer sufficient proof that everything can be taken away from a man but one thing: the last of the human freedoms—to choose one's attitude in any given set of circumstances, to choose one's own way.[2]

In addition to freedom, ethics requires that we have knowledge. Knowledge in ethics refers to the information we have at our disposal to make decisions in concrete situations. This knowledge can be personal, moral, or circumstantial. Personal knowledge has to do with the level of insight we have into ourselves in terms of who we are and are called to become as persons. Moral knowledge derives from the sources of morality or ethics that guide us in making decisions. Circumstantial knowledge encompasses the facts surrounding the decisions with which we are faced. Obtaining the knowledge necessary to make an ethical decision may not be easy: we may not know where to look nor have the time and energy to pursue the requisite knowledge. Nevertheless, if we have the capacity, we must seek to acquire the knowledge necessary to adequately inform our conscience.

With freedom and knowledge come responsibility. Ethics presupposes that we have choices in shaping our own lives through our actions in specific situations and as such are responsible for the types of individuals we become and for the consequences of our actions on others. When we act with freedom and knowledge, we are held morally or ethically accountable. Because our freedom or knowledge may be constrained at times, our moral responsibility can be diminished proportionately (i.e., in equal measure to our lack of freedom or knowledge). In real-life situations, limiting factors may require us to assess our own or another's accountability differently than we might otherwise. We see this necessity all the time in law, and it is no less true in ethics. When a child, with incomplete knowledge about the consequences of her actions, commits a crime, she is judged differently from an adult, who should know better. When a man is caught stealing food from a grocery store to feed his starving family, his offense is considered less than if he were acting without this constraint.

One caution is in order: by describing how our moral responsibility can be diminished due to a lack of freedom or knowledge, we do not wish to create a loophole in ethics. We simply wish to call attention to the brokenness of human life and the limitations we all experience as humans. Living morally or ethically is not easy; at times it is painfully difficult. Nevertheless, we cannot use this as an excuse for making bad decisions that hurt ourselves or others. We must take responsibility for who we are and strive, in any given situation, to make truly ethical decisions. This is what is required of us as moral beings living out our lives within communities.

B. **Reasoning and Discernment.** Ethics also requires the ability to reason through a situation and discern which action, among various options, best reflects who we are called to become morally as persons and best promotes the well-being of others. Reasoning and discernment are not simply following orders from an authority figure, blindly applying well-known rules or principles to a case, or succumbing to desires or feelings. Rather, they involve self-reflection, in which we consider our hopes, motivations, intentions, and desires; contextual analysis and investigation, in which we consult the sources of ethics and consider the morally relevant circumstances of a situation; and critical evaluation, in which we consider different courses of action against some well-established moral criteria. We will say more about this in chapter 2; for now it is sufficient to say we cannot do ethics without the ability to reason and discern, and we cannot reason and discern without a normative basis.

C. **Normative Basis.** This may be an unfamiliar term, but the concept is something you know well. We all have a normative basis, though most of us never give it much thought. If we did not have a normative basis, we would never be able to say, "I really need to be a better listener" or "You really are a good person" or "I should not have yelled at him like that" or "That was nice what you did for that woman." These statements indicate that you have a sense, no matter how unformed, of who we should be as individuals and how we should act toward others. This is a normative basis: a framework, point of reference, or backdrop against which we judge individuals, actions, and the effect of actions on others. A normative basis gives us insight into the goals of human life, the virtues and characteristics that should define us as persons, and the principles that should guide our actions in concrete situations.

Despite the differences we may have when it comes to specific issues or decisions (e.g., whether physician-assisted suicide is acceptable), most of us share many common thoughts about the elements that fill out a normative basis. We can say many things about human life and people from a normative perspective that transcend religious, cultural, ethnic, political, geographic, and other boundaries. For instance, most of us would agree with Aristotle and Aquinas that the goal of life is to flourish as individuals and communities. What *flourishing* means to a particular person at a particular time may differ, but one cannot deny that this is a basic goal of life.

This elemental consistency is also true of the virtues or characteristics that people should strive to acquire and that mark a person who is considered good. Who could deny that being a loving, compassionate, and courageous person is better than being a hateful, apathetic, and cowardly person? This is true also of moral principles; although here we are approaching the concrete level of ethics where disagreements occur more frequently. Nonetheless, it is hard to oppose the principle that says "do not harm others" (the principle of nonmaleficence) or "promote the good of others" (the principle of beneficence). It would be equally hard to oppose the principle that says "people should be free to choose their own way in life" (autonomy) or "we should treat others fairly" (justice). What *harm, good, freedom,* and *justice* mean in different cultures or contexts might be debatable, but not that we should promote the good of others, that we should not harm others, that we should be free to direct our own lives, and that we should act justly in relation to others.

These are just a few examples of commonly held, normative views. There are countless others. Yet in recent years some have questioned whether there is even an objective normative basis against which we can judge individuals and their actions. Some claim everything is relative and the only value things (or people) have is what someone attributes to them. This is a serious matter: without some objective normative basis, we could never say that someone acted ethically or unethically or was a good or bad person, and as a result moral responsibility would be destroyed. Think about the implications for ethics, for life. How could we judge or hold someone accountable for stealing, being unfaithful to a spouse, cheating on an exam, or even killing someone? On what basis could we oppose these actions?

To put this into perspective, consider the attacks of 9-11. If there were no objective normative basis, how could we say the perpetrators were wrong? On what basis could we make such a claim? One could argue that innocent civilians were attacked, or that those killed never agreed to be killed, or that the attacks disrupted the social order. But isn't this saying something on a normative level? Why can't we kill innocent people, or take someone's life without their consent, or disrupt society? These things should not matter, if, as some suggest, there is no objective normative basis and everything is relative. But they do matter. They matter precisely because we know through our shared human experience that people are of value, that we have a responsibility to treat others with respect, and that there should be peace and stability in society because holding to these ideals aids us in our attempt to flourish as human beings and communities.

We may not all agree on the specifics of a normative basis, but at minimum we can agree that we need a normative basis, and we can begin to sketch some of the general elements of what it would contain—as we do in chapter 2. Here we simply observe that without a normative basis we cannot do ethics because ethics is not simply about *describing* how we live as persons and how we act toward others but about *determining* how we ought to live and act as persons in relation to others.[3] This is the task of ethics, whether done personally in the context of everyday living or analytically in the context of a classroom.

In summary,

1. Ethics deals with any behavior or decision that affects human well-being (dignity, character, quality of life) and the good of the community.

2. The fundamental task of ethics is to address two related questions: "Who ought we to become as persons?" (BEING) and "How ought we to act in relation to others (people, God, and creation)?" (DOING).

3. To do ethics and begin to answer these questions, we need a normative basis that lends insight into the goals of human life, the virtues and characteristics that should define us as persons, and the principles that should guide our actions in specific situations.

Understanding Health Care Ethics

A Field of Ethical Inquiry

Now that we have defined what ethics is generally, we can move on to health care ethics (HCE). Before we offer a definition of HCE and outline the various ethical issues that arise in health care, it is important to understand why we study the ethics of health care. What is so special about health care that people dedicate their lives to studying its ethical dimensions? Why is HCE a fixture in course catalogs at colleges and universities? Why do we have strict ethical codes for nurses, physicians, and other health care professionals? In short, why is health care a field of ethical inquiry? There are three main reasons.

First, health care is a basic need we all have and supports perhaps the most basic of all human goods: physical health and mental well-being. Without these it would be difficult if not impossible to pursue life's other important goods, such as friendship, education, family, work, recreation, and religion. As the adage goes, "Without our health, we have nothing." This separates health care from other fields of ethical inquiry. Although business, journalism, education, and other fields all have ethical dimensions, the goods they promote are not as basic as the good promoted by health care.

Second, patients tend to be vulnerable in relation to their caregivers. From a moral perspective, vulnerability means that one is at risk of not being seen as a person deserving of respect and loving concern. One could argue that we are always vulnerable, no matter what the situation, because theoretically someone could always treat us poorly and not value us as people. Nevertheless, in health care situations our vulnerability is much higher than in other settings because there is far more at stake and a real imbalance in the patient–caregiver relationship.

For one thing, patients are seeking services related to their physical health and mental well-being, which is certainly more important than services related to mere material goods. Because they often know less about their condition than their caregivers, patients are usually completely dependent on caregivers to provide the necessary services and must trust that their caregivers have the proper training and seek to promote their patients' best interests. Furthermore, patients often have to divulge sensitive personal information that could be embarrassing or even incriminating. Perhaps most importantly, patients may be sick, frightened, and uncertain about the future and may have to expose themselves physically and emotionally to people they do not know well. Customers in a grocery store, readers of a newspaper, or students in a classroom do not experience this same degree of vulnerability. Patients need ethical safeguards to ensure that their dignity and well-being will be protected.

Finally, health care is a profoundly social endeavor. The decisions we make in health care—whether on the policy-making, organizational, or clinical level—affect not only those directly involved but also society at large. Consider the following case.

Case 1D

John is in a serious car accident and is transported by helicopter to the nearest trauma center. After extensive testing, he is diagnosed with a severe head injury and sent to the intensive care unit (ICU) for close observation and treatment. Two months later John remains in a coma, and there has been no improvement in his condition despite round-the-clock intensive care and rehabilitation therapy. The physicians, knowing from evidence and experience that John has virtually no chance of recovering consciousness after so long in a coma, suggest to John's wife that

cont.

Case 1D *cont.*

they cease certain invasive and ineffective technologies, including the breathing machine, which they feel are merely prolonging John's death. The physicians also suggest moving John from
the ICU to a nursing floor where he will receive care from nurses
and physicians specially trained to tend to the needs of dying
patients. John's wife refuses and demands that everything be
done to prolong his life. The physicians protest but, fearing a
lawsuit, ultimately comply with her wishes.

Though this case focuses on decisions that unfold at the bedside
of an individual patient, it highlights the social implications of health
care. For one thing, continuing to treat John aggressively in the ICU
could negatively affect other patients. The resources (health care
professionals, ICU bed, equipment, money) used to sustain John's life
may not be available for other patients who may actually benefit from
them. This is not a theoretical problem. As we learned in discussions
about emergency preparedness during the H1N1 pandemic in 2009,
hospitals do not have breathing machines for every patient, ICUs
have only a certain number of beds and trained staff, and emergency
departments sometimes must close their doors to new patients
because they cannot move their current patients to certain parts of
the hospital due to the lack of available beds.

In America we tend to think of health care resources as unlimited. In reality there are only so many resources to go around. Some
people object to this situation because they assume that as a nation
we could simply spend more money on health care. But experience
shows that this would require much to be sacrificed in other areas,
and even then there remains a breaking point. The situation is similar
to our personal finances. Every day we decide about what we can and
cannot afford, because we have only a limited amount of funds. We
could obtain credit and go into debt buying things we want, but this
would limit us in other areas and would eventually catch up to us.
This is reality for most people, and it is the same reality we experience in health care.

Second, continuing to treat John aggressively in the ICU could affect the lives of those caring for him. The physicians have already expressed their concerns about further aggressive treatment. Will their integrity be compromised because they complied with John's wife's demands against their better judgment? Will this decision change the way they think of medicine and the role of patients and families in decision making? What about the nurses and other health care professionals? They must now continue to provide intensive treatment to John and manage the complications that will inevitably arise. What about their feelings? It may be emotionally difficult to stop treatment for a dying patient, but it can be equally hard to continue to provide aggressive treatment for a patient who will likely suffer longer because of it. Frontline caregivers, such as nurses, often feel this emotional entanglement most because of their frequent contact with patients and families.

The hospital and John's health insurance plan, assuming he is insured, could also be affected. Hospitals receive only a certain amount of money for the services they provide, and sometimes the costs exceed the reimbursement. Is it fair to hospitals to provide care that is not benefiting a patient when they have to absorb the costs? What if this limits their ability to care for other patients and to provide just wages and cost-of-living salary increases to their employees? Would it be right for other members of John's health insurance plan to have to pay higher premiums because of the costs associated with his care? An additional four dollars a month may not be a lot to some, but to others it can make the difference between being insured or uninsured.

Third, continuing to treat John aggressively in the ICU could drive up overall health care costs and affect society at large. Though John's is an isolated case that might not break the bank, in the United States the reality is we spend a considerable amount of money on unnecessary and ineffective care, with a significant portion of this coming at the end of life for patients, like John, who do not benefit meaningfully from the care. This is a significant problem that we have to get a handle on, especially when you consider that in the United States in 2009 we spent $2.5 trillion on health care (more than $8,000 per person), and conservative estimates suggest this number will rise to more than $4 trillion by 2017, which will represent at least 20 percent of our overall spending as a nation (often referred to as the gross domestic product or GDP).[4] This means that for every dollar we spend as a nation, 20 cents or more will go to health care. Although this may seem justifiable because health is a basic and essential good, it limits our ability to spend money in other areas that are also important for personal and community development, such as education, defense and homeland security, highway and road improvements, agriculture, and alternative energy sources. We should also keep in mind that health care insurance is getting more and more costly, and the number of uninsured in the United States as of 2010 is at roughly 50 million. Though health care reform legislation signed into law by President Barack Obama on March 23, 2010, is designed to lower the number of uninsured in America by some 30 million, health care costs will continue to be a problem, especially in the absence of significant health care delivery and payment reform, and could get worse as the population ages. Costs, limited resources, and the effect of our individual health care decisions on others are often overlooked in our individualistic society, but they constitute vital reasons why health care is a field of ethical inquiry.

Definition and Description

We can now explain what HCE is. HCE, a subspecialty of ethics, is the study of how health care, in its structure, organization, delivery, relationships, and means, affects human well-being (dignity, character, quality of life) and the good of the community. Like ethics generally, HCE is done against the backdrop of a normative basis.

Though ethical issues in health care seem rather common nowadays, HCE is a relatively new phenomenon. It only became a distinct discipline and formal area of study in the 1960s. This somewhat misrepresents that concerns about the ethics of health care (or medicine) surfaced thousands of years ago, as evidenced by the Hippocratic oath (c. fourth century BCE) and that Christian theologians dating back to the early church have dealt with problems we tend to group under HCE (e.g., abortion, contraception, sterilization, and euthanasia).

Several factors led to the recent rise of HCE as a formal discipline, but none more so than advances in science and medical technology. Ethical issues have always been present in health care, but as medicine became more advanced and developed technologies capable of diagnosing complex conditions, doing elaborate surgeries, and, particularly, sustaining life, the number and complexity of ethical issues increased considerably. Not surprisingly, one of the most prominent health care ethics cases to date, that of Karen Ann Quinlan, arose in the 1970s and concerned the question of sustaining life. As health care obtains more technological might, new ethical issues and concerns are quick to follow.

There are other factors, as well. Significant change has occurred in the patient–physician relationship and in the structure and delivery of health care. Traditionally, physicians have made decisions for patients; they have not only had the technical expertise but also assumed responsibility for deciding what was best for their patients and promoted their well-being. This approach is called *paternalism* because it is similar to how parents assume almost complete decision-making responsibility for their minor children. Strange as it may seem today, in the past physicians knew their patients quite well, often having cared for them from birth until death. In such a context, paternalism tended to work relatively well, as the physician could adopt a course of treatment that accurately represented the views of the patient and family. As health care itself changed—from family physicians who came into the home to complex delivery networks involving multiple structures (hospitals, clinics, insurance companies, government payers) and caregivers (not just physicians) who often know little about their patients—the close relationship between patient and physician began to break down. People in developed countries started to want to make their own decisions. These factors led to a new model of the patient–physician relationship, one that is driven by patient autonomy as opposed to physician paternalism. This new model, though beneficial to a point, has led to greater conflict in health care decision making.

Of other important milestones that gave rise to HCE, perhaps the three most important are the Nuremberg Tribunal, the Tuskegee syphilis study, and the use of dialysis committees: At the Nuremberg Tribunal, several Nazi physicians were tried for performing unethical, harmful, and sometimes fatal experiments on concentration camp prisoners during World War II. What came out of Nuremberg was a commitment that all research subjects must be adequately informed about the benefits and risks of participating in medical research and must give their free and informed consent before anything is done to them.

The Tuskegee syphilis study was conducted by the U.S. Public Health Service and began around 1930 during the Great Depression and lasted until 1972. The study was conducted on poor, uneducated African American men who lived in Tuskegee, Alabama, where a relatively high number of people suffered from syphilis. The researchers at Tuskegee lied to the men about the nature of the study and the extent of their disease. In addition, they did not tell some men who acquired the disease while in the study that they were sick and deceived study participants into thinking they were receiving the best treatment for their condition. What is worse, after penicillin began to be used to effectively treat syphilis in 1946, the government blocked these men from receiving it. This outrage was exposed by an Associated Press reporter, whose investigation was first printed on July 26, 1972, and later appeared on the front pages of most national newspapers. The story and the subsequent congressional hearings on Tuskegee opened the eyes of the American public to the danger of ethical abuses in medical research and practice.

Dialysis committees were fixtures in sophisticated acute care hospitals in the 1960s and early 1970s before federal legislation authorizing the End Stage Renal Disease Program under Medicare. They were charged with determining which patients with severe kidney disease would receive dialysis, a treatment that essentially does the work of the kidneys outside the body by artificially filtering the blood and reintroducing the filtered blood back into the body. At the time, dialysis machines were not readily available, so hospitals could not provide dialysis to all patients with severe kidney disease. The dialysis committees "played God" by deciding who would receive dialysis and who would not—and consequently would most likely live or die. This obviously raised ethical questions, and people began to wonder how these committees made their decisions and what criteria they used.

Advances in science and technology, changes in the patient–professional relationship and in health care generally, and ethical health care milestones, such as Nuremberg, Tuskegee, and dialysis committees, all contributed to the rise of HCE as a formal discipline

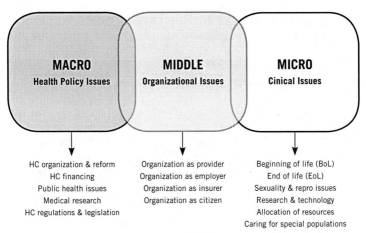

MACRO	MIDDLE	MICRO
Health Policy Issues	Organizational Issues	Cinical Issues

HC organization & reform	Organization as provider	Beginning of life (BoL)
HC financing	Organization as employer	End of life (EoL)
Public health issues	Organization as insurer	Sexuality & repro issues
Medical research	Organization as citizen	Research & technology
HC regulations & legislation		Allocation of resources
		Caring for special populations

FIGURE 1B Three Levels of HCE

of study. The ethical challenges these developments posed could not be ignored and as a result, people began studying the ethical dimensions of health care in earnest. At first, such study was largely restricted to the clinical level (i.e., issues related to patient care). However, it quickly became clear that HCE encompasses three interrelated levels: the macro level (health policy issues), the middle level (organizational issues), and the micro level (clinical issues). Decisions made at one level affect the other levels. We have already seen how decisions at the bedside might affect the other levels (refer to Case 1D). This can also go the other way. For example, when the government started reimbursing hospitals for dialysis through Medicare, committees no longer had to make difficult decisions as to who would receive treatment (middle or organizational level); more patients were allowed access to the treatment and as a result, more patients lived longer (micro or clinical level) (see figure 1B).

Following, we list the major ethical issues that arise in health care. As we proceed in this book, we will focus primarily on issues at the micro (clinical) level but will keep an eye on how decisions at this level affect our relationship to others, our communities, and society at large. This is necessary because ethics is not only about who we are and how we act as individuals but also, and more profoundly, who we are becoming in community and how our actions affect others.

Major Ethical Issues at the Three Levels of Health Care

Macro Level (Health Policy Issues)

1. **Health care organization and reform**
   - Creating a just system, ensuring access to care, defining public or private coverage and setting limits, allocating societal resources for health care, responding to the needs of the underinsured and uninsured, and establishing adequate structures for delivering care

2. **Health care financing**
   - Reimbursement, controlling costs, balancing societal values, and payment mechanisms (who pays and how best to structure payment: employer, government, insurers, out-of-pocket)

3. **Public health concerns**
   - Immunizations, infectious disease control, disparities in health care, safety programs, health infrastructure (lead paint, toxic substances, sanitation, water supply), health promotion, and disease prevention

4. **Medical research**
   - Protecting research subjects, allocation of public funds, Human Genome Project, and stem cell research

5. **Health care regulation and legislation**
   - Insurance, government-sponsored programs, patient privacy (HIPAA, the Health Insurance Portability and Accountability Act), patient-dumping (EMTALA, the Emergency Medical Treatment and Active Labor Act), physician-assisted suicide, embryonic and fetal research, and regulation of other research applications

Middle Level (Organizational Issues)[5]

1. Health care organization as provider

- Physician relationships, staffing levels, patient safety, health care service lines offered (e.g., cardiac care, cancer care, maternal-fetal care, orthopedics), vendor relationships, planning, budgeting, staffing, capital allocation, clinicians and conflicts of interest, patient rights and responsibilities, admissions (especially for high-cost specialty services, medical records, billing procedures, discounted and charity care, provider shortages, and requests for futile or nonbeneficial treatments)

2. Health care organization as employer

- Employee strikes, union activity, justice and responsibility in hiring practices, just wages, downsizing, diversity and affirmative action, whistle-blowing, sexual harassment, and executive compensation

3. Health care organization as insurer

- Setting health benefits for a plan, reviewing appeals for denied coverage in a plan, coverage exceptions for contractually excluded benefits, prescription drug plans, covering disenfranchised populations, paying for investigational interventions for life-threatening conditions, and balancing commitment to individual enrollees with overall plan

4. Health care organization as citizen

- Hospital closures/sales, community needs assessment, fairness in selection of vendors, responsible advertising, environmental responsibility, community-serving mergers and acquisitions, socially responsible investing (investment screens, proxy voting, and community investing), advocacy and lobbying activities, social responsibility

Micro Level (Clinical Issues)

1. **Allocation of scarce resources**
   - Life-sustaining treatments, organ transplants, intensive medical care, genetic technologies, and goals and limits of medicine

2. **Providing care to patients unable to pay**
   - Addressing the needs of the underinsured and uninsured, charity care, and cost-shifting

3. **Nature of the patient–professional relationship**
   - Rights and responsibilities, conflict of ethical principles (e.g., autonomy, beneficence, nonmaleficence), advance directives, informed consent, patient competency, disparities in health care, and clinicians and conflicts of interest

4. **Treatment of people living with HIV/AIDS**
   - Vaccinations, treatments, pastoral care, partner involvement in treatment decisions, and aiding developing nations ravaged by the disease

5. **Treatment of people living with mental illness**
   - Access issues, stigmatization, and patient rights

6. **Definition of death**
   - Heart-lung versus brain-death criteria

7. **Withholding and withdrawing treatment at the end of life**
   - Treatment criteria, who decides, case conflict, questions about futility, professional integrity, patient rights, and cost concerns

8. **Euthanasia and physician-assisted suicide**
   - Personal liberty versus societal restraints, and compassion versus killing

cont.

9. **Care of dying patients**
   - Pain management, palliative care, hospice, and recognizing limits of life and medicine

10. **Care of critically ill newborns**
    - Pushing limits of viability, treatment criteria, parental authority in decision making, and cost concerns

11. **Organ and tissue transplantation**
    - Dead versus live donors, donation after cardiac death, artificial and animal organs, cloning for organs or tissues, transplants for questionable populations, and cost concerns

12. **Reproduction and reproductive technologies**
    - Personal rights, societal limits, abortion, maternal-fetal conflicts, fetal surgery, assisted reproduction, embryo adoption, and human cloning

13. **Genetics, genetic testing, and gene therapy**
    - Access, confidentiality, insurance and employment discrimination, goals and limits of medicine, and safety and efficacy

14. **Stem cell research**
    - Allocation of federal dollars, access, moral status of embryos, and goals and limits of medicine

15. **Research and experimentation on humans**
    - Informed consent, progress versus limits, protecting vulnerable populations (children, prisoners, mentally ill), and research across borders

Before moving on to the next section, we would like you to consider again Cases 1A–1C. This time, however, we want you to decide what you would do in each case. While you are deciding, reflect on what factors are important to you as you make your decisions. For example, would you decide to wait for the person whose car you hit because you strive to be an honest person or because legally you are required to do so? Would you divulge the truth to your friend about the affair her significant other is having because you cannot support lying and deceptive behavior or because you feel she has a right to know? Would you refuse to stand up to your supervisor because you do not want to lose your job or because you have always been told to obey your superiors? This exercise will help you prepare for the next section, where we will look more deeply at how we approach ethical situations; specifically, what factors we consider to be most important when making ethical decisions.

How We Approach Ethical Decisions

Common Approaches to Ethics

How do we make ethical decisions? Better yet, what factors do we consider to be most important when making ethical decisions? Once again, to get us started, let's consider a case.

Case 1E

Noah, a 22-year-old college student, visits his physician for a checkup and an HIV test. The checkup goes fine, and he seems to be in good health. However, the results of the HIV test will take several days to come back. After the physician's office receives Noah's negative test results, the hospital secretary faxes them to the number Noah left. Inadvertently, the results get faxed to a law firm the hospital often uses. One of the lawyers informs the physician office of the blunder. The physician alerts the hospital of the mix-up, and at an

cont.

Case 1E *cont.*
_____

ad hoc meeting of top hospital officials, the discussion centers on whether to disclose to Noah that the results were seen
by others. The chief legal counsel argues not to inform Noah
because everything turned out fine for him and if they do,
he will probably sue the hospital and there will be a lot of
bad publicity. Noah's physician, however, argues that she has
a duty to disclose the truth to her patient, no matter what
the costs. The hospital president also thinks Noah should
be informed but for slightly different reasons: he believes it
is a matter of personal and institutional integrity and argues
against concealing the truth.

This challenging case does not lend itself to easy answers. All of
the hospital representatives make good, compelling arguments. Our
purpose here, however, is not to evaluate their arguments and decide
which is best morally. Rather, we wish to point out that they are all
reasoning and coming to their decisions in different ways, ways that
reflect classic ethical theories or traditional approaches to ethical
decision making.

Classic Ethical Theories

Discussion of theories of ethical decision making may sound a bit
abstract and removed from reality. However, classic ethical theories are nothing more than descriptions of common ways we make
and justify decisions every day. These descriptions were not simply
invented, as if those who first mentioned them made them up
through their own ingenuity and innovation. Rather, they are tied
to human experience and depict how we tend to approach complex
ethical matters. This will become clearer later in the chapter, when
we ask you to think through some tough case scenarios, an exercise
that may help you to see how we commonly and routinely draw on
these ethical theories.

The best way to grasp classic ethical theories is to first consider
what ethics is. Remember that ethics is about who we ought to

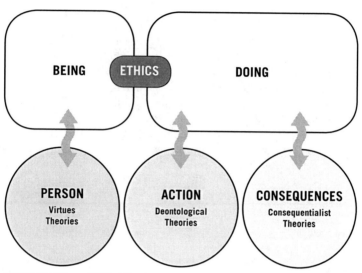

FIGURE 1C Ethics and Ethical Theories

become as persons (BEING) and how we ought to act in relation to others (DOING). Ethical theories tend to focus on either *being* or *doing*—though you can never truly focus on only one. Some ethical theories focus more on the question of *being* and draw our attention to who the person is becoming (virtue theories). Others focus more on the question of *doing* and draw our attention to either (1) the action itself and the laws, principles, rules, or duties that should guide our actions (deontological theories) or (2) the consequences of our actions for ourselves and others (consequentialist theories) (see figure 1C).

Before describing classic ethical theories, it is important to note they do not provide a complete picture of how we make ethical decisions. They do, however, reflect more common ways we approach ethical situations. Ethical decisions are made by using both our head and our heart: we draw on our reason and intelligence, as well as our faith, feelings, experiences, relationships, intuition, and imagination. The classic ethical theories, though less so in virture theories, tend to give the impression that we use only "head-related" elements in ethical decision making. This is not the case, as we will explain in chapter 2. For now, let us examine the theories.

A. Virtue Theories (VTs)

Virtue theories are rooted in ancient philosophy. Both Plato and Aristotle, for example, constructed what we now call virtue theories to describe how we ought to live and act in relation to others. In various works, Aristotle outlined numerous virtues, including temperance, justice, courage, dignity, generosity, love, truthfulness, and others that he said had no name. No matter which virtues are emphasized, though, all VTs focus on who the person is and who the person is becoming in light of a particular notion of the ideal human person and the moral (or good) life. Principles and consequences, which are both linked with actions, maintain some relevance but are secondary to virtues and a focus on the person.

It bears mentioning that VTs are not relativistic and should not be confused with ethical theories that determine right and wrong solely on the basis of an individual's feelings or intuitions. Rather, VTs are rooted in virtues that we recognize (through shared human experience) as necessary to be a good person and live a moral life in relation to others. Though we may not all agree on an exact list of virtues, some are simply indispensable for living morally. Take Aristotle's virtue of love, for instance. No one can deny that love is a virtue and something we should strive to achieve and live out in concrete circumstances. This is not relative; we ought to love others. What is relative, however, is how virtues are expressed by different people in different times and cultures. What love looks like in the context of real-life ethical situations may not be the same at all times and for all people. Nonetheless, love we must.

The underlying premise of VTs is that who one is (BEING) largely determines how one acts morally (DOING). In other words, we do what we are. If we are virtuous, then we will do good things. If we are vicious, then we will do bad things. It would seem Jesus had something like this in mind when he said, "In the same way, every good tree bears good fruit, but the bad tree bears bad fruit. A good tree cannot bear bad fruit, nor can a bad tree bear good fruit" (Mt 7:17–18). If a child is taught and shown how to be kind, respectful, and compassionate, and this becomes ingrained in the child's character as she matures, then she will most likely act in these ways when faced with challenging ethical situations. On the contrary, if mean-spiritedness, hate, and rage are impressed on this child, then she will most likely act out these qualities.

Virtue can be described as what we do when no one is watching, because it is who we are. For example, there are rules against cheating in school, which students generally follow, especially when a teacher is present and attentive and the consequences for cheating are severe. Most students even follow these rules when the teacher is not present and there is little chance of getting caught. This suggests virtue: doing good for its own sake because that is the sort of person we are. Some students, however, seize an opportunity to cheat, especially when it is unlikely they will be caught and punished. Such students do not exhibit the characteristics of a virtuous person. They tend to do good not for its own sake but because cheating could have bad consequences.

We have said a lot about virtues without saying what they are. Hopefully, from what we have outlined above you understand that virtues are not just ideas or principles imposed on us by others. In a real way, virtues become a part of us. Virtues are habits, character traits, feelings, and intuitions that comprise who we are and are necessary for being a good person and living a moral life. As we acquire virtues and cultivate them in ourselves, they become second nature to us. So much so that to act against them feels awkward, like a right-handed person trying to write a letter or throw a ball with his left hand. Because virtues ultimately comprise who we are, they are personal, much more so than laws, principles, rules, or duties. Who we are (our identity) is bound up with virtues and is directly related to how closely we live them in concrete ethical situations (our integrity).

Fortunately, there has been a resurgence of interest in VTs; people are once again realizing that ethics is not just about what we do but also, and perhaps even more, about who we are becoming as individuals and as communities. But VTs are not without their challenges. VTs must contend with some difficult questions: Which virtues are necessary to be a good person and live a moral (or good) life? Who decides what these virtues are and on what basis? How do we acquire these virtues and integrate them into our character? How do we determine whether one is acting virtuously in specific situations? These questions are not easily answered, which is likely one reason the *doing* dimension of ethics tends to get the most attention. Focusing on actions and consequences is much easier than defining and defending some notion of the ideal person and the moral (or good) life.

Hopefully, you now have a strong grasp of the perspective of VTs. To deepen this understanding, let's return to Case 1E. Of the three hospital representatives, which one argues primarily from a virtue perspective? Based on our brief overview of virtue theory, you can see that the hospital president speaks mostly from this perspective. His words indicate someone who is operating from a virtue perspective. Someone who invokes integrity, as he does when he argues that this case "is a matter of personal and institutional integrity," is usually basing an ethical decision on virtue. Other words or phrases that point to a virtue perspective are *moral character, values, personal qualities/characteristics, compromising/violating self, true to self, promoting the good of self and others, who I ought to become, living a good/moral life*, and, of course, *virtue*. The key question for the hospital president is "Am I promoting in this situation the virtues necessary for living a moral life?" He does not refer to laws, principles, rules, duties, or even potentially bad consequences for the hospital. Instead, telling the truth to the patient, Noah, is directly related to who the president is and wants to become as a person and what he believes the hospital should be or should become as an institution.

B. Deontological Theories (DTs)

DTs can be traced back to the legal traditions of Judaic and later Roman thought. Philo of Alexandria and the Roman jurist Cicero are two of deontology's oldest supporters. In modern times, deontology has been linked mostly with the work of Immanuel Kant. DTs focus mainly on our actions, what we choose to do as the means to an end. What we do matters much more in DTs than who we are becoming or what we hope the results will be (ends). As such, virtues, intentions, extenuating circumstances, and consequences have little to no relevance. The premise of most DTs is that some actions are right *in themselves* and therefore should be done always and everywhere, whereas other actions are always and everywhere wrong and therefore should never be done. For DTs the ends can never justify the means.

In DTs the question of whether our actions are right or wrong is reduced to our obedience or disobedience to a given code of laws, principles, rules, or duties derived from an authority figure, such as God (divine law such as the Ten Commandments), nature (natural law), a ruler or government (civil law), or ourselves (autonomous law). Unlike VTs, which are more inductive in reasoning (meaning we derive a sense of virtues from our shared experience in a community with others), DTs use deductive reasoning. So, for example, if we are following divine law as articulated in the Ten Commandments, we are forbidden from stealing in all instances no matter what the circumstances. Even if you needed to steal bread to feed your starving family, you could not do so morally under DTs that strictly prohibit stealing. Likewise, many governments have laws against torturing suspected criminals and prisoners of war. The famed character from the FOX television hit *24*, Jack Bauer, would be a frequent violator of such laws for his aggressive tactics in obtaining information from suspected terrorists, despite that his intentions are good and his actions often result in saving innocent human lives.

In DTs, moral creativity comes from trying to figure out which laws, rules, principles, and duties apply to concrete situations. Difficulties arise for DTs when laws, rules, principles, or duties are in conflict with one another. Here deontologists must determine which of the conflicting deontological factors take precedence. Another example may help. In health care ethics are three well-known principles: beneficence (do good for another), nonmaleficence (don't harm another), and autonomy (respect a person's wishes). As we saw in Case 1D, sometimes patients or their family members request treatment that physicians, nurses, and others believe will be harmful. What is a physician to do when a patient asks to receive a treatment that the physician knows or suspects will actually cause the patient more suffering? Respecting the patient's wishes (autonomy) in such cases may cause the physician to violate other principles to which she is bound. How does the physician determine which principle trumps or outweighs the others?

In addition, how do we know which set of laws, principles, rules, or duties to follow when these often compete with one another? Do we follow those handed down by God, the government, a specific religion, or ourselves? What if we cannot trust an authority figure? Are we then free to break from the rules? Is there room for our conscience, or must we always follow the law? What if following strict principles results in greater harm to oneself or others? These questions highlight the limitations of DTs. Still, laws, principles, rules, and duties in ethics have their place, as we shall see later in this chapter.

With that said, let's go back to Case 1E for a moment and apply what we have learned so far about DTs. Of the three hospital representatives, which one argues primarily from a deontological perspective? In this case the physician most exemplifies deontological theories. A telltale sign was her reference to duty when she spoke of "a duty to disclose the truth." Other words or phrases that identify the deontologist include *obligations, beliefs, convictions, rights, responsibilities, principles, right and wrong, have to, always/never, bound by, requirement,* and *absolute.* For this physician, the key question is "Does my action in this situation conform to the relevant laws, principles, rules, or duties to which I am bound?" What weighs most heavily on her is not so much virtue and certainly not the consequences of her action ("no matter what the costs"). Rather, it is the duty she has to her patient. For her, living morally is equated with fulfilling her duties.

C. Consequentialist Theories (CTs)

CTs find their fullest expression in modern thought, especially in the British utilitarians Jeremy Bentham, John Stuart Mill, and Henry Sidgwick. Though there are various versions of CTs, all focus on the consequences of our actions, in light of the good we are trying to promote through our actions. In CTs, the outcome of our actions (the ends) matters much more than who we are becoming or what we are doing (the means). As such, virtues and deontological factors such as laws and principles are seen as morally relevant only when they guide us to do that which results in the best outcome; failing that, there is no moral obligation to attend to them. The premise of CTs is that some goods should be promoted regardless of the means used. In contrast to DTs, the ends justify the means for consequentialists.

The rightness or wrongness of our actions in CTs is determined by the consequences of our actions as they relate to the good we want to promote. "Good" in this sense is usually defined in broad terms, such as happiness (understood as pleasure and the absence of pain), preference satisfaction, or social utility; it is the end for which we are striving and that we want to promote in each and every action. In essence, the morality of our actions within CTs is deduced through a cost-benefit analysis, in which we add up positive and negative consequences and choose the action with the best overall result for the good we seek. According to one CT, known as utilitarianism, maximizing positive consequences consists in doing that which results in the greatest good for the greatest number of people (sometimes referred to as the "happiness principle"). So, for instance, while *24*'s Jack Bauer would often be condemned by deontologists, his actions would be considered morally acceptable under CTs because he aims to promote the greatest good for the greatest number. His aggressive interrogation tactics and violation of government protocols often save lives in the end.

It should be noted that when we must choose between two or more negative outcomes, CTs say that we ought to do that which minimizes bad consequences; that is, we ought to choose the course of action that results in the lesser evil. This is a common way of thinking through such situations. We see it frequently on television and, less often, in real life. To use another *24* example, in Season 3 Jack Bauer was placed in an impossible situation. Terrorists demanded that Jack kill his superior, with whom he had worked for years, or else they would immediately release a lethal virus in a populated area. Jack chose the former, which he perceived as the lesser evil—the killing of one person to save hundreds of thousands. In a similar way, this consequentialist viewpoint of the lesser evil has implicitly provided the moral context for government decisions on military interventions and even for the practice of medicine in some settings where goods or values collide. A good example of a "lesser evil" in medicine is a surgical procedure that results in the death of a pre-viable fetus (less than 23 weeks' gestation) when the pregnancy threatens the life of the mother and both will die if the procedure is not immediately performed. For consequentialists, this is a classic case of choosing the lesser evil: rather than doing nothing, which will result in the death of both mother and fetus (greater evil), you perform the procedure and save the one life that can be saved (lesser evil).

For policy making, as well as personal decision making, no one can deny the usefulness and popularity of CTs. Despite this, CTs have limitations, as do the other ethical theories. For example, How do we identify the good for which we should strive and against which we should weigh consequences? If it is happiness, as some CTs hold, how should happiness be defined, and who gets to define it? More practically, what do we do when it is unclear which action will result in the best overall results or consequences? What if we cannot accurately predict the consequences? And do the ends always justify the means? Are there limits to this rule, or can we do absolutely anything so long as we bring about the good? Like VTs and DTs, CTs raise difficult questions for which there are no easy answers. We hope to address some of these concerns later in this chapter and throughout the foundational sections of this book.

To conclude this section, let's apply what we have learned about CTs to Case 1E. Of the three hospital representatives, you have no doubt surmised that the chief legal counsel argues primarily from a consequentialist perspective. As he puts it, we don't have to inform the patient "because everything turned out fine for him," and if we do, "he will probably sue the hospital and there will be a lot of bad publicity." He may not use telling consequentialist words and phrases—such as *outcomes, results, consequences, interests, goods, greater good, lesser evil, balance, weigh, exception because, ends justify the means*—but his rationale focuses on the negative consequences that will result from disclosing the truth. For him, the key question is, does my action bring about the best (or the least bad) consequences in light of the good I am trying to achieve? He understands the good as protecting the hospital's interests and, to a lesser extent, the well-being of the patient. He is not driven by virtue or deontological factors but rather by averting potentially negative effects for the hospital.

Ethical Theories in Personal Decision Making

We have spent a good amount of time describing classic ethical theories. Now we would like you to consider which theory or theories you most often use when reasoning through ethical situations. Listed below are several scenarios that address ethical issues.[6] Each scenario is followed by three statements representing each of the classic ethical theories supporting the position the scenario directs you to take. You may not agree with either the position or the statements, but we would like you to choose the statement that best fits how you would decide the issue. This exercise is not meant to shape your viewpoints on these issues but rather to provide insight regarding which factors you most take into account when making ethical decisions. There are no right or wrong answers; simply respond truthfully.

1. The question of embryonic stem cell research (ESCR) has been a hot topic lately. While out with your friends one evening, the topic comes up. When asked your opinion, you argue for ESCR using embryos left over from in vitro fertilization because

   a) the medical profession has an obligation to promote the best interests of sick patients by pursuing potential cures for deadly diseases.

   b) you can't imagine why anyone wouldn't support the research given that the embryos will be destroyed and discarded anyway, and the economy will benefit greatly from the money brought in through research dollars and future therapies.

   c) it could remove obstacles to good health that currently impede people from pursuing goods related to human flourishing.

2. You overhear your friend, with whom you have been close for more than 10 years, lying to his spouse while on the phone. This is not the first time, either, and you worry that it is becoming a pattern with your friend. You confront your friend about this and other lies by saying,

   a) "It is not right to lie to anyone, especially to those closest to you."

   b) "This is not the type of person I know you to be and certainly not the type of person you want to become."

   c) "This is probably not something you want to do routinely. If you get caught, you know your spouse will leave you and you will most likely lose all of your shared possessions."

3. You are watching late-night television and see a commercial for a human-subject research trial for a new HIV vaccine. You call

the number given and find out you can make more than $1,000 for allowing yourself to be injected with an inactive HIV strain that is reported to have low risks associated with it. You decide to do it because

a) although this is medical research and may not yield any tangible benefits, you feel being true to yourself requires that you do what you can to help those living with HIV/AIDS. From a very young age, it has been ingrained in you to promote the overall good of others whenever possible and as such you feel that you would not be true to yourself if you did not participate.

b) you would be doing a really good thing for others and at the same earn a lot of much-needed money.

c) you consider it the right thing to do to help those in need.

4. You and a friend are watching the nightly national news, and the story of a man who has been unconscious for more than 10 years and kept alive only by a feeding tube comes on. Your friend asks what you would want done if you were in that condition. You answer that you would want the tube removed because

a) it would make no sense to continue treatment when there is no chance of recovery and it would only cause pain, suffering, and needless expense to your family.

b) God does not require you or others to preserve life at all costs.

c) even though the use of a feeding tube could keep you alive for some time, you would no longer be yourself in your truest form.

5. A local man who was convicted several years ago for a series of murders is scheduled to be executed. Your teacher brings up the case in your philosophy class and asks your opinion. You answer that you are opposed to capital punishment because

a) killing, except in self-defense, is always wrong.

b) it is not consistent with the goals of a democratic society and weakens the moral character of those who take part directly and indirectly.

c) it has been proven that capital punishment is not a deterrent to crime, is not fairly and justly applied across the system, and actually costs taxpayers more than imprisoning criminals for life.

6. The U.S. military recently captured several leaders of an international terrorist cell. Newspapers have reported abusive and harmful interrogation tactics being employed by members of the military and counterterrorist task force units. Your friend argues that such tactics are acceptable, but you disagree because

   a) it is a strongly held belief in your faith tradition that all people have inherent dignity and should not be subjected to cruel and unusual punishment.

   b) even though we should do our best to keep the American people safe, this type of behavior will ultimately result in anti-American sentiment and make it more difficult to secure the cooperation of other countries and the United Nations.

   c) it undermines the trustworthiness of the government and is not consistent with how you want your government to represent the American people.

7. Six weeks after you and your boyfriend went to the college dance, you inform him that you got pregnant that night. He wants you to have an abortion, but you object because

   a) you pride yourself on being the type of person who owns up to your actions and accepts responsibility for the consequences of those actions.

   b) all human life, at every stage of development, is sacred and should never be destroyed.

   c) you do not want to lose the respect and affection of your parents, who will be disappointed when they find out you are pregnant but would be devastated were you to have an abortion.

8. For various reasons, your parents have stopped paying your tuition for college. Though you obtain school loans, you are

still short and cannot pay the balance. You see an ad in the local paper requesting sperm and egg donation for an infertile couple. You inquire and discover that if you donate, you can get enough money to cover the balance of your tuition and then some. You decide to donate because

a) no one will find out what you did, you could help the couple achieve an important dream, and you stand to make a good sum of money.

b) you live by the rule that life is about helping others.

c) concern for others and helping people in need are traits you consider important, especially in yourself.

9. Your father is terminally ill with ALS (amyotrophic lateral sclerosis, i.e., Lou Gehrig's disease) and is rapidly declining. He has lost most of his physical capacities and can no longer feed himself. One day, he asks you to mix almost a full bottle of sedatives with his mashed potatoes, with the intent of ending his misery and killing him. You refuse because

a) your faith tradition forbids you from taking the life of another.

b) you love your father and want to be someone who finds more effective ways to care for him and ease his suffering rather than someone who shortens his life.

c) you could not live with the guilt of killing your father. You are also afraid that someone would find out and you would be charged with homicide.

10. You have just had a baby who was born 15 weeks prematurely and weighs just over 2 pounds. The doctors tell you there is a chance they could save the baby, but even if they do the baby might be severely disabled and need a considerable amount of medical attention. This will require a lot of money and care on your part, which will mean little to no time for other activities. You decide to pursue aggressive treatment because

a) you are the type of person who makes sacrifices for the good of others, especially your own family members.

b) there is still a chance that your baby will defy the odds, not suffer from any severe disability, and be able to live a normal life.

c) you believe that the sanctity of life obligates you to use any available means to protect and preserve life.

Now we need to tally up your responses and see how often you responded from a virtue, deontology, or consequentialist perspective. Although this is not a scientific test, it should give you some idea of how you tend to approach ethical situations. As we describe each statement under each case scenario in terms of the theory it represents, note how you answered the particular scenario and place a check in the appropriate column in the table below. After we have finished going through all ten scenarios, total up your numbers, noting how many times you responded from each perspective.

Scenario 1

a) Deontology: the focus is on the *obligation* medical professionals have

b) Consequentialism: the focus is on *outcomes* (what will become of frozen embryos and the overall benefits of pursuing embryonic stem cell research)

c) Virtue: the focus is on the *overall good* of society and individual patients

Scenario 2

a) Deontology: the statement articulates a *principle* (you can never lie to anyone)

b) Virtue: the focus is on who your friend is *becoming* as a person

c) Consequentialism: the focus is on the *negative consequences* (such as getting caught)

Scenario 3

a) Virtue: the focus is on promoting the *overall good* of others because of *who you are* as a person

b) Consequentialism: the focus is on the *benefits* to others as well as yourself

c) Deontology: the focus is on the *means,* stated as the *right thing to do*

Scenario 4

a) Consequentialism: the focus is on *results* (what will happen if the feeding tube is continued)

b) Deontology: the focus is on the *rule* (what God requires of you)

c) Virtue: the focus is on the *characteristics* that define you as a person

Scenario 5

a) Deontology: the focus is on the *law* or *principle* against killing

b) Virtue: the focus is on the *goals* of society (what society ought to become) and the *moral fabric* of those who take part in executions

c) Consequentialism: the focus is on the *negative effects* or *consequences* of capital punishment

Scenario 6

a) Deontology: the focus is on a strongly held *belief* (the inherent dignity of human beings)

b) Consequentialism: the focus is on *outcomes* (what will happen if the United States resorts to torturing)

c) Virtue: the focus is on *characteristics* (such as trustworthiness and what you think the United States should be as a nation)

Scenario 7

a) Virtue: the focus is on the *type of person* you are

b) Deontology: the focus is on an *absolute prohibition* (against taking life)

c) Consequentialism: the focus is on the *effects* aborting the baby will have on your parents and your relationship with them

Scenario 8

a) Consequentialism: the focus is on the *outcomes* and the *benefits* of donation

b) Deontology: the focus is on a *rule* (one should help others)

c) Virtue: the focus is on *traits* you consider important for yourself and others

Scenario 9

a) Deontology: the focus is on a *prohibition* (against taking life)

b) Virtue: the focus is on the *type of person* you want to be or become in relation to others (in this case, your father)

c) Consequentialism: the focus is on the *effects* of your actions (how you will feel and what might happen to you if you help your father to die)

Scenario 10

a) Virtue: the focus is on the *characteristics* that define you as a person

b) Consequentialism: the focus is on *possibilities* and potential good consequences

c) Deontology: the focus is on a *principle* (the sanctity of life) and your *obligation* to follow it

Scenario	Virtue	Deontology	Consequentialism
1.			
2.			
3.			
4.			
5.			
6.			
7.			
8.			
9.			
10.			
Total			

It does not matter how you scored in this exercise. All three of these classic, common approaches to ethical decision making are acceptable; no one approach is necessarily better than any other because no single theory is perfect from a normative perspective. Therefore, you do not have to worry whether you had more virtue responses or deontology responses or consequentialist responses. This exercise is intended to give you some idea of how you tend to approach ethical situations and to do two other things as well.

First, reviewing your answers should help you to become more familiar with the classic ethical theories. This contributes to your own understanding and also helps as you engage in dialogue on ethical issues. When talking about ethical issues with friends or family, there may have been times when you did not understand where they were coming from or the grounds on which they based their arguments. Perhaps you even became frustrated because you could not fathom how they could think in such a way. By understanding classic ethical theories better and recognizing some of the key words and phrases of each, you are now better positioned to understand the reasoning behind many ethical arguments and to engage more effectively in ethical dialogue. Now, when someone argues for embryonic stem cell research on the grounds that the frozen embryos that would be used for the research will be destroyed anyway, you will be able to see this is a consequentialist argument, as opposed to, for example, a deontological one ("it is never acceptable to destroy a human embryo"). Recognizing this will provide you with greater insight into ethical arguments and may allow you to respond more effectively, perhaps even from the same perspective as the ones with whom you are debating.

Second, by forcing you to choose one statement representative of one ethical theory for each scenario, the exercise challenges you to accept one way of thinking through the ethical issue, to the exclusion of other approaches. For many people this is difficult because they do not like being confined to one theory or perspective. Rather, they feel more comfortable considering the issue from two, perhaps even all three, perspectives, and then arguing on the basis of whichever perspective provides the most compelling reasons either for or against. This is one reason why you probably did not answer all 10 case scenarios from the same perspective. Intuitively, you know that virtues, principles, and consequences are all important factors to be considered when analyzing ethical issues and making ethical decisions in concrete situations.

This highlights one of the major weaknesses of contemporary approaches to health care ethics, many of which are grounded in only one of the classic ethical theories: they tend to be too narrowly focused. By concentrating predominantly on one aspect, often to the exclusion of other morally relevant features, they limit their usefulness and applicability. We cannot do justice to the complex nature of ethical issues in health care by looking just at virtues or just at principles or just at consequences. It makes no sense, for instance, to consider only virtues to the exclusion of principles. Principles can support virtues by specifying what it means generally to be an honest or just or compassionate person. In fact, without principles (or action guides), virtues remain a little abstract and unclear. Likewise, it makes no sense to consider only principles to the exclusion of consequences. Consequences need to be incorporated with principles because sometimes principles must yield to the concrete realities of the situation. Generally, we should not steal or be overly aggressive with suspected terrorists, but there may be particular instances when the consequences dictate that we set aside a given principle. In the same vein, it makes no sense to consider only consequences to the exclusion of virtues. If we always do that which brings about the best consequences without weighing who we are becoming as individuals and communities, we may, on further reflection, come to feel that our actions were wrong.

Conclusion

This chapter suggests that the best approach to ethics is one that looks at all aspects of morality: the person and the virtues that ought to define us as people; the laws, principles, rules, and duties that should guide our actions; and the short- and long-term consequences of our actions for ourselves and others. For these to have any meaning, though, they must be considered against the backdrop of a normative basis that describes, at least in general terms, what is the ultimate goal of human life, who we should become as individuals, and how we should act in relation to others (people, God, creation).

This will be part of the focus of the next chapter, as we consider the bases of our decisions.

SUGGESTED READINGS

Ashley, Benedict M., Jean deBlois, and Kevin D. O'Rourke. *Health Care Ethics: A Catholic Theological Analysis*. 5th ed. Washington, DC: Georgetown University Press, 2006.

Beauchamp, Tom L., and James F. Childress. *Principles of Biomedical Ethics*. 5th ed. New York: Oxford University Press, 2001.

Devettere, Raymond J. *Introduction to Virtue Ethics: Insights of the Ancient Greeks*. Washington, DC: Georgetown University Press, 2002.

Devettere, Raymond J. *Practical Decision Making in Health Care Ethics: Cases and Concepts*. 3rd ed. Washington, DC: Georgetown University Press, 2010.

Jonsen, Albert R. *Birth of Bioethics*. New York: Oxford University Press, 1998.

Jonsen, Albert R., Mark Siegler, and William J. Winslade. *Clinical Ethics: A Practical Approach to Ethical Decisions in Clinical Medicine*. 6th ed. New York: McGraw-Hill, 2006.

Lammers, Stephen E., and Allen Verhey, eds. *On Moral Medicine: Theological Perspectives in Medical Ethics*. 2nd ed. Grand Rapids, MI: Eerdmans, 1998.

Munson, Ronald. *Intervention and Reflection: Basic Issues in Medical Ethics*. 9th ed. New York: Wadsworth (forthcoming).

O'Toole, Brian. "Four Ways People Approach Ethics." *Health Progress* 79 (November–December, 1998): 38–41, 43.

Solomon, W. David. "Normative Ethical Theories." In *Encyclopedia of Bioethics*, edited by Warren T. Reich. New York: Macmillan, 1995.

Walter, James J., and Thomas A. Shannon. *Contemporary Issues in Bioethics: A Catholic Perspective*. Lanham, MD: Rowman and Littlefield, 2005.

MULTIMEDIA AIDS FOR TEACHERS

Numerous movies can be used to show what different ethical theories look like in practice. These movies can help students understand the theories and see how they have a role in everyday decisions. What follows is a select list of movies, with comments as to what theory or theories they depict. All are available on DVD through retailers.

A Man for All Seasons. Directed by Fred Zinnemann. Starring Paul Scofield. Rated G. 1966. This movie provides examples of virtue.

Avatar. Directed by James Cameron. Starring Sam Worthington. Rated PG-13. 2010. Examples of all three ethical theories are presented.

Braveheart. Directed by Mel Gibson. Starring Mel Gibson. Rated R. 1995. This movie illustrates virtue in Mel Gibson's character, as well as deontology in the soldiers and consequentialism in the so-called nobles.

Dad. Directed by Gary David Goldberg. Starring Jack Lemmon. Rated PG. 1989. Deontology is modeled by the doctor and the hospital administrator, and the path toward virtue is displayed by the son, Ted Danson.

Gladiator. Directed by Ridley Scott. Starring Russell Crowe. Rated R. 2000. This movie supplies examples of virtue.

Good Night, and Good Luck. Directed by George Clooney. Starring David Strathairn. Rated PG. 2005. This movie portrays instances of virtue.

Insomnia. Directed by Christopher Nolan. Starring Al Pacino. Rated R. 2002. This movie provides examples of consequentialism and at the end implicitly teaches the importance of virtue.

Life Is Beautiful. Directed by Roberto Benigni. Starring Roberto Benigni. Rated PG-13. 1998. This movie depicts examples of virtue.

Saving Private Ryan. Directed by Steven Spielberg. Starring Tom Hanks. Rated R. 1999. Examples of deontology are offered throughout; elements of virtue are also depicted, especially in the end.

Scent of a Woman. Directed by Martin Brest. Starring Al Pacino. Rated R. 1992. This movie provides examples of virtue, especially in Chris O'Donnell's character.

Tears of the Sun. Directed by Antoine Fugua. Starring Bruce Willis. Rated R. 2003. Examples of all three ethical theories are found in this movie, especially in the Bruce Willis character, who alternates from one to the other based on the circumstances.

The Man from Elysian Fields. Directed by George Hickenlooper. Starring Andy Garcia. Rated R. 2001. This movie shows examples of consequentialism.

The Pianist. Directed by Roman Polanski. Starring Adrien Brody. Rated R. 2002. Characters in this movie depict virtue, especially in the German officer who allows Adrien Brody's character to go undetected at the end of the movie.

The Twilight Saga: Eclipse. Directed by David Slade. Starring Kristen Stewart. Rated PG-13. 2010. This movie provides examples of all three ethical theories, with virtue exhibited particularly by the main characters.

Training Day. Directed by Antoine Fugua. Starring Denzel Washington. Rated R. 2001. Examples of deontology are offered in the character of Ethan Hawke (especially in the early parts) and consequentialism, in the character of Denzel Washington.

ENDNOTES

1. John W. Glaser, "Hospital Ethics Committees: One of Many Centers of Responsibility," *Theoretical Medicine* 10 (1989): 275–88, at 278.

2. Viktor Frankl, *Man's Search for Meaning*, trans. Ilse Lasch, rev. ed. (New York: Simon and Schuster, 1962), 65.

3. Raymond J. Devettere describes this well in his book *Practical Decision Making in Health Care Ethics: Cases and Concepts*, 3rd ed. (Washington, DC: Georgetown University Press, 2010), 4–6.

4. For up-to-date information on U.S. health care expenditure data and other important health care information, see the Centers for Medicare and Medicaid Services (CMS) at *http://www.cms.hhs.gov/*, the Henry J. Kaiser Family Foundation at *http://www.kff.org/*, the Commonwealth Fund at *http://www.commonwealthfund.org/*, and the Dartmouth Atlas of Health Care at *http://www.dartmouthatlas.org/*.

5. These issues are revised and expanded from Leonard Weber, *Business Ethics in Health Care: Beyond Compliance* (Bloomington: Indiana University Press, 2001).

6. The idea for this exercise was adapted from Brian O'Toole, "Four Ways People Approach Ethics," *Health Progress* 79 (November–December, 1998): 38–41, 43. Although the structure and format are similar, the scenarios and statements are our own.

CHAPTER 2

The Bases for Our Decisions and the Role of Discernment

Michael Panicola

A Proposed Normative Basis

So far we have defined what ethics is generally, described what health care ethics is specifically, and considered how we tend to approach ethical situations. Now we will ask, on what do we base our decisions? Whether we tend toward virtues, principles, consequences, or some combination of the three, underlying our decisions is a *normative basis*. Without a normative basis, we could not determine what virtues we should seek to develop, or what principles apply, or what consequences are most desirable. In short, there would be no ethics because there would be no criteria for making ethical decisions. So in this chapter we take the next, critical step and outline a normative basis that will shape how we view all moral matters. Sketching a normative basis is a tall task, and there may be disagreements when we get down to particulars—after all, we are attempting to articulate the goals of human life, the virtues and characteristics that ought to define us as persons, and the principles that should guide our actions in concrete situations. Yet we know that we need a normative basis and that we share many common normative beliefs.

Describing a Normative Basis

A normative basis is something that gives us insight into who we should become as persons (BEING) and how we should act in relation to others, namely, people, God, and creation (DOING). A normative basis is a framework, point of reference, or backdrop against which we make ethical decisions and evaluate who we are as persons, the morality of our actions, and the effect of our actions on others. It may help to think of a normative basis in terms of something familiar, like basketball. Basketball referees call fouls on players. Although not every foul called may be warranted, fouls are called nonetheless based on some idea of how basketball players should conduct themselves while on the court. Over the years this idea of how the game should be played has evolved and been codified in a rulebook that referees use to distinguish between appropriate and inappropriate behavior. In essence, this rulebook is a normative basis. A normative basis need not be as detailed or as rigid as a basketball rulebook to serve as our blueprint for living morally. Human experience, revelation, community life, and other sources have afforded us some idea of who we should become as persons and how we should act in relation to others. Ethics is nothing more than making ethical decisions and judgments in light of this idea, this normative basis.

The Goal of Human Life

As we pointed out in chapter 1, we all make use of some normative basis, whether we know it or not. In fact, most everything we do socially or interpersonally is guided by a normative basis. Nevertheless, we do not all lead good, moral lives or act ethically in every situation. How can this be if we all have and use a normative basis? There are many reasons for this. Experience and personal reflection tell us that we are imperfect people, beset by physical, intellectual, psychological, moral, and spiritual limitations, who live within a social context that is at once good but also sinful. Because of this, like Saint Paul, we sometimes lack the moral strength and courage to do the good we desire and instead do the bad that we know we should not (see Rom 7:19–20).

Practical reasons also account for our not acting ethically all the time. Sometimes we do not know what is the truly right or good thing to do, other times we may lack the capacity or energy to inform our conscience adequately to make the best ethical decision. Another reason, ever-present in our impatient world, is our tendency to be shortsighted about matters of ethics or morality, our failure to consider the big picture and to link our more immediate goals with the ultimate goals for which we are striving. Some people call this "moral myopia."

Every action we perform in life is directed toward particular goals. We brush our teeth to avoid cavities and to eliminate bad breath; we take classes in college to fulfill the requirements for graduation and to get a good job; we sleep to rejuvenate ourselves and to avoid getting sick; we work to have the means necessary to live a decent life and to develop our talents; we eat to be nourished and sustained physically; we see movies to be entertained and to escape from everyday life; we vote in democratic elections to help shape social structures and to ensure that our rights are protected.

Our moral actions especially are directed toward goals. From an ethical perspective, however, it is important to recognize that beyond our more immediate goals is an even more basic or underlying goal that ought to provide the overall direction for our lives and guide our decisions. The first step in constructing a normative basis is to discern what this goal is, the goal for which we are ultimately striving as human beings. Individuals and communities have struggled with this question for thousands of years. People often say that the ultimate goal of human life is to have fun, to be successful, to be smart, to be compassionate, or to love others. These are indeed good goals for which we should be striving. Without these, life would not be nearly as meaningful. However, all these goals in various ways point to an even more fundamental goal, that of human flourishing. Ethically speaking, human flourishing supersedes all other goals, it is the goal to which all others should be directed. Think about it: we do not want to be successful just so we can feel good about ourselves and receive accolades; we do not want to be smart just to impress people or score high on an IQ test; we do not seek to be compassionate so people will say how kind we are. Rather, we pursue these goals because they offer us the possibility of living a good life, a life in which we flourish as individuals in relation to other people, God, and creation.

We encounter problems in our moral lives when we make ethical decisions without attending to the goal of human flourishing. When this happens our ultimate goal as human beings becomes subordinated to some other, more immediate goal, and our pursuit of human flourishing is often undermined as a result. Take, for example, Case 1C in chapter 1 involving the abusive supervisor. If we focus on the more immediate goals, we might not report him to a higher-ranking executive, although it is probably the right or good thing to do. Think about it: you value your job, make decent money, have bills to pay, enjoy the lifestyle to which you have grown accustomed, and would have difficulty finding another job. If your goals are limited to these issues and do not include human flourishing, your choice would be clear. However, when we compare these against the goal of promoting our own well-being (dignity, character, quality of life) and that of others, as well as the good of the community, these immediate goals probably would take a backseat to doing the hard but ultimately right thing.

This is how a normative basis functions in ethics and acts as a corrective to moral myopia: it helps us "zoom out" so we see the bigger picture and make ethical decisions accordingly. It is like the Google map feature that many of us use for driving directions. While the map can zoom in to show us the street and particular area we want to find, it can also zoom out to give us a sense of where we are and where we are headed. To live a good moral life in relation to others, it is critical that we "zoom out" by considering our more immediate goals against the backdrop of human flourishing and other morally relevant features.

Understanding Human Flourishing

It is pretty hard to deny that human flourishing is the overarching goal of human life, as we pointed out in chapter 1. What is debatable is what it means to flourish as human beings. This is where we run into challenges, because people can and do have different conceptions of human flourishing. Many of the ancient Greek philosophers who considered this question spoke of human flourishing in terms of *eudaemonia*—what we might call happiness. They believed that happiness is the only goal we seek for itself alone and never for the sake of something else.[1] The term *happiness* could easily be misconstrued to refer to having our desires fulfilled or achieving pleasure in every situation. This is not what the Greeks had in mind. Happiness for them was generally understood as having a well-formed character that allows one to live a life of virtue.

Think about what human flourishing means to you and what you think you need to flourish as a person. In the space provided below, list ten things that you feel are necessary for living a good life, a life of flourishing. These could be such things as money, a big house, health, sports, music, people or love, friendships, community, peace, religion—the choice is yours.

_____   _____

_____   _____

_____   _____

_____   _____

_____   _____

If you were forced to live without five of the ten items you selected above, which five would be most important for human flourishing? List them here.

_____   _____

_____   _____

_____

Now go one step further and consider which two of the five remaining items are most important for human flourishing. Write them below.

_____   _____

This can be quite a difficult exercise because it is hard enough limiting the items necessary for human flourishing to a list of ten, let alone two. Interestingly, as we do this exercise with students, health care professionals, and others, the two most common final items are health and relationships (which you may have listed as a specific person, your family, your friends, community, or something equivalent). Health is an obvious choice; without health it becomes difficult to pursue any goals or ends. Relationships, though, are another matter altogether. What makes relationships so essential for flourishing as human beings? This is where the Christian understanding of human flourishing is so instructive.

Although the Greeks equated human flourishing with eudaemonia, translated as best we can in today's terms as "happiness," for Christians human flourishing is understood as love of God. What this means in practical terms is that we live truly rich and full lives when we love God in all that we do, when we direct our lives totally to loving God. Jesus made this clear when responding to the Pharisee who asked him what the first and greatest commandment was. Jesus' simple response was to "love the Lord your God with all your heart, and with all your soul, and with all your mind" (Mt 22:37). The Judeo-Christian tradition tells us that we have been created out of God's unconditional and unyielding love and that we are directed toward God as our ultimate end. Through human life we enter more fully into communion with God by loving God and giving glory to God in how we live our lives.

Admittedly, saying that human flourishing means love of God is vague, especially because ethics is a practical discipline. How do we love God when we do not necessarily encounter God immediately? Jesus' response to the Pharisee provides us with an answer to this question. After saying that we should love God with our whole heart, soul, and mind, Jesus went on to say that there is a second commandment, which is like the first: "You shall love your neighbor as yourself" (Mt 22:39). The second part of Jesus' statement is as important as the first, for in it Jesus draws the link between relationships and human flourishing. Human flourishing, understood as love of God, is pursued most tangibly within the context of relationships. We encounter God primarily through relationships with others, though we can also encounter God in other ways (e.g., prayer, personal reflection, meditation, and within nature). From an ethical perspective we cannot love God and flourish as human beings without loving our neighbor as we love ourselves. Saint John also made this clear in describing how we love God in the context of human life: "Those who say, 'I love

God,' and hate their brothers or sisters, are liars; for those who do not love a brother or sister whom they have seen, cannot love God whom they have not seen" (1 Jn 4:20). Love of God and love of neighbor are thus inextricably bound together in ethics. Significantly, *neighbor* in the Judeo-Christian tradition does not refer to the person living next door to you or on your block. Rather, *neighbor* encompasses all members of the human family and can even be broadened to include all of God's creation.

People who cite relationships as necessary for human flourishing often do not have this in mind when they place it on their list. What we have done here is to put in theological terms what they, and perhaps you, already knew intuitively, that relationships with others (people, God, creation) provide the meaning and substance of human life and contribute significantly to our flourishing as human beings.[2] Relationships, especially those with our fellow humans, provide us with the opportunity to love God and to become more truly and fully human. We are social beings by nature and have difficulty appreciating and grasping the fullness of life outside the context of relationships. This is why Tom Hanks's character, Chuck Noland, in the movie *Castaway*, develops a friendship with a volleyball while stranded on a deserted island for roughly four years. Although this appears ridiculous, it makes sense when you consider the importance of relationships for our well-being and flourishing. Noland's life was not as meaningful when lived in isolation, and so he sought something, anything, that could fill the void. The volleyball, which he called "Wilson," served this purpose—though not sufficiently, as we find out later in the movie when he agonizingly decides not to go after the ball, which had been swept overboard from his makeshift boat, because it would have meant leaving his boat and giving up his only chance to return home to his beloved girlfriend. We see this also in the movie *I Am Legend*, starring Will Smith. Smith's character, Dr. Robert Neville, is the last healthy person living in New York City after an engineered virus mutates into a lethal strain and kills most of humanity. Neville profoundly misses his family and longs for human contact, which explains in part his close connection with his dog, as well as his odd behavior of talking to mannequins at the video store he frequents.

We should point out that when we talk about the link between human flourishing and relationships, we are not talking about just any relationships. We are in lots of relationships, but not all of our relationships are characterized by the love of neighbor of which Jesus speaks. For us to truly flourish and show our love of God through loving our neighbor, we need to be in what we will call "right relationships." This does not mean that we can never be in conflict with others, or that we might not get angry with others at times, or even that we have to like every person with whom we come in contact. What it means is that we need to be in relationships that are grounded in the values of love, respect, dignity, and justice. This we do by becoming virtuous people oriented toward the good and by acting virtuously with the aid of moral principles that foster right relationships.

Becoming Virtuous: The Role of Virtues

From what we have said above it may be seen that virtues—the habits, character traits, feelings, and intuitions that make up who we are as human beings—are essential for right relationships because they are the key to becoming good, virtuous people. If, as experience suggests, the way we act in relation to others is determined largely by who we are, then we must build a strong moral character through the development of virtue so that we are predisposed to do the good. In other words, if "doing the right thing" is predicated largely on "being a good person," then we have to strive to become virtuous, because that is the surest way to act virtuously. It really is not possible to be in right relationships and ultimately flourish as human beings without developing virtues and striving always to become virtuous.

There is no magical formula for becoming virtuous; the only tried-and-true method is practice. Just as it takes practice to learn how to read, ride a bike, drive a car, or eat with a fork, so it is with virtue. We each may have the capacity to act virtuously, but unless we consciously and intentionally do so, day in and day out, virtue will never become a part of who we are as people. The more we practice acts of virtue, the more ingrained it becomes in our character and the easier it is to act virtuously. Unfortunately, as we mentioned in chapter 1, the reverse is also true. We must be careful in the choices we make, because we are essentially making ourselves through our choices.

The path to becoming virtuous is less a race than a journey. It is not as if by performing one hundred acts of kindness, we cross the finish line of virtue once and for all. The journey toward the virtuous life may not have an endpoint; there may not be a time when we actually "get there." If we are honest with ourselves, we have to admit that there is always room for improvement in our moral lives: we can always love more, care better, protest more strongly against injustice. Virtue, especially in Christian ethics, does not call us to live a perfect life, but rather an examined life in which we constantly ask ourselves, "Who am I becoming through this action and is it consistent with who I ought to become in relation to others (people, God, creation)?" Living this type of life, an examined life directed toward virtue, gives us the best chance to love God by loving our neighbor as ourselves in every one of our actions.

When we think of what it means to be virtuous from a Christian perspective, we think of Jesus, who, in addition to being true God, was fully human and immersed in the human condition. For Christians, Jesus is the moral ideal of who we ought to become; he is normative morally speaking in that he perfectly embodied what it means to love God and love neighbor. Through his life, death, and resurrection, Jesus showed us not only who God is but also who we can become as human beings made in God's image and likeness. The Gospels are filled with stories portraying the virtue of Jesus. For example: Jesus showed great restraint in many situations, specifically when he withstood the temptations of the devil while alone in the desert (see Lk 4:1–13); Jesus displayed great courage and fidelity to God throughout his adult life, especially while praying in the garden and contemplating his fate, which he agonizingly knew would lead to the cross (see Mk 14:32–42); Jesus exhibited great compassion to the most vulnerable people in his society, particularly to a leper who was on the fringes of society but was brought back into the human community through Jesus' healing actions (see Mt 8:1–4); and Jesus practiced empathy and forgiveness to many, most notably an adulterous woman, whom Jesus protected from a hypocritical crowd that wanted to stone her to death (see Jn 8:1–11).

Living morally as Jesus did, however, is no easy task, and we all fall short of the ideal. Yet this does not mean that becoming virtuous is unattainable. That this is true is seen in the lives of ordinary people who, despite their own limitations, nonetheless live virtuously. Some of us have been privileged to know such a person, maybe a parent, a friend, or a teacher. Most of us have at least heard of such individuals. Some of the more remarkable examples include Saint Thomas More, who refused to betray his conscience by sanctioning King Henry VIII's divorce and declaring him the head of the Church of England, even though More was imprisoned, separated from his family, and ultimately put to death; Rosa Parks, who stood up to racial discrimination through her simple, yet profound, act of refusing to give up her seat in the "white" section of a segregated bus; Mother Teresa of Calcutta, who spent a lifetime caring for the faceless, nameless poor who were on the fringes of society; Gandhi, who proved that nonviolent demonstration and resistance is a powerful tool against social injustice and the destructive forces of evil; and Martin Luther King Jr., who called us to become more than we imagined we could be by sharing a vision of an utterly just and peaceful society.

Given that we really can become virtuous, as these individuals and numerous other figures have shown, what virtues should we seek to develop and incorporate into our moral character? What habits, character traits, feelings, and intuitions should define us as individuals? There may not be a definitive answer to this question, because any virtue that leads to our moral development as people and allows us to be in right relationships with others could be added to the list. This is why there is no universal agreement on a single list of virtues and why different virtue theorists provide different lists of virtues. Nevertheless, some virtues stand out.

To be human means to be physical and material, psychological and emotional, social and relational, spiritual and intellectual, and morally free and responsible. Despite the differences that account for our uniqueness as individuals, we all participate in these basic dimensions of human life. These dimensions are interconnected and interwoven to form a complex synthesis that makes up who we are as human persons. For each of these dimensions, there are corresponding virtues that ought to define us as persons, because they enable us to be in right relationships and ultimately flourish as human beings.

The main virtue regarding the physical and material dimension of human life is temperance or restraint in our pursuit of earthly and bodily goods such as eating, drinking, and sex. This virtue is essential for maintaining a proper balance among the various goods that contribute to or are instrumental for human flourishing. The main virtues regarding the psychological and emotional dimension of human life are love, empathy, and compassion. These virtues play a crucial role in our close personal relationships. The main virtues regarding the social and relational dimension of human life are justice, honesty, respect, and self-sacrifice. These virtues figure prominently in our broader social relationships and interactions with others. The main virtues regarding the spiritual and intellectual dimension of human life are faith, hope, prudence, and discernment. These virtues have much to do with how we approach human life and respond in concrete moral situations. The main virtues regarding the morally free and responsible dimension of human life are courage, integrity, and righteous indignation. These virtues pertain to how true we are to ourselves as moral beings.

This relatively short list of virtues hardly exhausts all the virtues that build up our moral character and allow us to act virtuously in relation to others. We could have listed others, such as generosity, trustworthiness, gentleness, patience, sympathy, and kindness, all of which are important. However, the virtues we have listed are some of the more important ones pertaining to the various dimensions that make up who we are as human beings in our totality. They encompass more or less what it means to be a good person and what it takes to live in right relationships with others and ultimately flourish as human beings. They also have special relevance for health care ethics because they define what health care professionals should be and give some indication as to how they should act toward their patients. Thus, they will serve us well as we move forward in this book and consider some specific cases in health care ethics.

Acting Virtuously: The Role of Principles

The journey toward becoming virtuous requires moral principles, which are also essential for right relationships because they help us to act virtuously in concrete moral situations. Though virtue theories tend to downplay the significance of principles, they are important for three reasons. First, principles give rise to virtues and pave the way for becoming virtuous. It would be great if we were all born with a strong moral character and acted virtuously without having to consider principles. However, the reality is that we have to learn how to become virtuous, and principles are useful to this end. By acting in accordance with well-established principles that foster right relationships, we learn what virtue means and progress along the path of becoming virtuous.

Second, principles specify what virtue generally demands in concrete moral situations. To say that we should be just, compassionate, and respectful means little without specific principles that articulate what these virtues require in the messiness of real life. Think about how we teach children the virtue of respect. We don't simply say, "Be respectful." Rather, we teach them concrete examples of this virtue through principles such as holding the door for others, cleaning up after themselves, always saying "please" and "thank you," and not talking about others behind their backs. These principles add color and detail to the virtue.

Finally, principles serve as a standard against which we can evaluate our choices. If we think, for example, that the most compassionate response to our dying loved one is to prolong life at all costs, we might consider this action against certain principles like beneficence (which says that we must promote the overall good of another and never harm) or equitable distribution (which says that basic social goods must be shared equitably for the benefit of all). Such reflection may help us to see that the action we thought intuitively was the most virtuous is not really so, all things considered.

It is understandable that virtue theories tend to avoid principles altogether, partly because principles can take on the role of absolute rules that are always binding regardless of the circumstances, at least in some deontological theories. In this way, principles become things we *must* follow, not simply consider, as we evaluate our options. The danger of using principles in this way is that adherence to them in some situations could lead to decisions that actually undermine virtue and fail to promote our well-being and that of others. Take, for example, the case of a pregnant woman who will die unless she undergoes a procedure that will save her life but simultaneously kill her pre-viable fetus (less than 23 weeks' gestation). While terminating a pregnancy is not something we should ordinarily do, given the sanctity and value of human life, there are rare times when this principle might have to yield to what virtue demands in complex circumstances.

Principles are meant to serve people in their pursuit of human flourishing, not the other way around. They need not function in an absolute, uncompromising way. Rather, as we see it, principles should function more as action guides that complement virtue. We should use principles to get a sense of what we may be required to do in a particular situation and to evaluate the choices we are inclined toward based on our moral character and overall orientation in life. However, in the end, principles must be weighed against the total moral picture, which includes consideration of the virtues we ought to be promoting, the morally relevant circumstances surrounding the situation (including consequences), and our ultimate goal of human flourishing. When used in this way, principles offer great help as we attempt to be in right relationships through loving our neighbor as we love ourselves.

While there are numerous moral principles that foster right relationships, they all fall under the headings of two overarching principles. The first is human dignity, which refers to the inherent value and intrinsic worth of human beings. This principle is grounded philosophically in our experience of ourselves and others as basically individuals having value. Theologically, it is grounded in the belief that we are created in the image and likeness of God (see Gn 1:26–27). This alone serves as the basis for our worth as humans. It is not based on functional ability or social utility but on the fact that God loves us and desires to enter into communion with us. We can never lose this basic dignity, because we are irreversibly made in the image of God.

Flowing from the principle of human dignity are a number of other principles, some general and some specific to health care ethics, that outline some of the responsibilities we have to other people because we are inherently valuable. These include the following:

- *sanctity of life:* the awareness that human life is the basis for all we do and must be treated with special care and concern at all stages
- *beneficence:* the responsibility we have to promote the overall good of others and not harm others

- *veracity:* the responsibility we have to be honest and truthful with others
- *autonomy:* the freedom we ought to enjoy to choose our own way in life and to make our own decisions within moral limits
- *informed consent:* the responsibility we have to disclose fully all relevant medical information to patients, ensure they understand the information, and allow them the freedom to make their own informed choices
- *privacy/confidentiality:* the responsibility we have to protect the privacy of patients and maintain the confidentiality of their medical information
- *care for the whole person:* the recognition that human beings are not only physical but also psychological, social, spiritual, and moral, and must be viewed and cared for as such
- *bodily integrity/totality:* the precedence to be given to the overall good of the person over the good of any particular body part or organ
- *proportionate/disproportionate means:* the recognition that the duty to preserve life with medical means is based on a personal moral assessment of the benefits and burdens of treatment relative to the person and taking into account her or his total circumstances
- *principle of double effect:* a methodological principle that helps us determine whether we can proceed ethically with an action that has two effects, one good, the other bad

The second broad category of principles is justice, which refers to what we are due as human beings on the basis of our inherent dignity. Flowing from this principle are others that impose certain responsibilities on us in terms of how we structure society and how we conduct ourselves in relation to others. These include the following:

- *common good:* the various dimensions of social life essential for becoming more truly and fully human and living in right relationships with others; the social structures necessary for pursuing human flourishing, and also, in some contexts, the placing of limits on our individual decisions

- *relationality:* the recognition that, as social beings fundamentally interconnected with others, our personal choices have broader social implications
- *solidarity:* the responsibility we have to stand with our fellow human beings in times of need, for example, when natural catastrophes occur
- *subsidiarity:* the recognition that decisions should be made at the lowest, most appropriate level, by those closest to the situation and with the best understanding of the complexities of the issue (usually applied to social policy decisions, but with implications for personal decision making as well)
- *stewardship:* the responsibility we have to tend to and care for the gifts and goods available to us and to use them responsibly for the benefit of all
- *care for the disadvantaged:* the responsibility we have to ensure that the basic needs of the most vulnerable members of society are satisfied
- *equitable distribution:* the recognition that the basic goods of society should be shared equitably (sometimes based on a person's effort, contribution, or need, but viewed theologically, based on a person's inherent dignity)
- *preferential option for the poor:* the determination to judge social policies and programs first of all (though not only) from the perspective of the poor and marginalized

This somewhat lengthy list of principles completes our normative basis (see figures 2A and 2B), which provides us with the "big picture" view of (1) what we are trying to accomplish ultimately in life (human flourishing, understood as love of God, which is manifested through right relationships/persons understood as love of neighbor); (2) who we should become as persons (virtues necessary for right relationships); and (3) how we should act in relation to others (principles that foster right relationships). These principles apply to all areas of ethics and should be used as a backdrop when evaluating our personal moral decisions, broader ethical issues, and cases that we study in a more academic context.

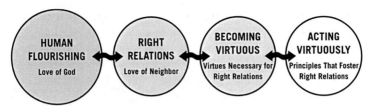

FIGURE 2A Human Flourishing

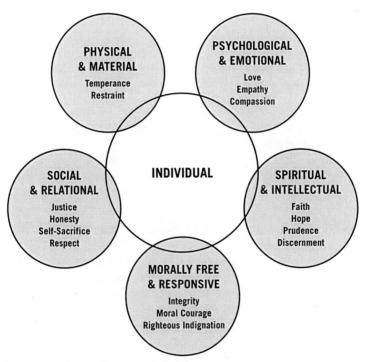

FIGURE 2B A Normative Basis

HUMAN DIGNITY

Sanctity of Life, Beneficence, Veracity, Autonomy, Informed Consent, Privacy/Confidentiality, Care for the Whole Person, Bodily Integrity/Totality, Proportionate/Disproportionate Means

JUSTICE

Common Good, Relationality, Solidarity, Subsidiarity, Stewardship, Care for Disadvantaged, Equitable Distribution, Preferential Option for the Poor

To illustrate how we use our normative basis, consider the following case.

Case 2A

Ms. Hamburg is 86 years old and suffers from advanced metastatic lung cancer (cancer that originated in the lungs but has spread to other parts of her body), as well as profound dementia. Though she has been cared for in the home by family members for several years, she was recently rushed to the hospital in severe respiratory distress (significant difficulty breathing). She was admitted to the intensive care unit of the hospital and placed on a ventilator (breathing machine). After two weeks of aggressive treatment to address her breathing issues and multiple other complications, and of being in a medically induced state of unconsciousness to minimize her pain and anxiety, her doctors suggest to the family that aggressive measures should cease because they are not benefiting Ms. Hamburg and seem to be increasing her suffering. Instead, they recommend focusing mainly on Ms. Hamburg's comfort until she dies. The family is unsure what to do.

Considering the decision to stop aggressive treatment for Ms. Hamburg against the backdrop of our normative basis gives us greater insight into what may be the most ethical response in a situation that is emotionally and ethically challenging for the family. Although we would like Ms. Hamburg to get better, sadly her condition cannot be improved at this point in her illness—she is dying, and medicine has seemingly reached its limits. Moreover, she is so sick that her ability to recognize her surroundings, interact with her loved ones, and pursue other personal goods has been totally eclipsed. Given these and other factors, it no longer makes sense to fight to preserve her physical existence with medical means. After all, we do not live simply so that our vital physiological functions can be maintained; rather, we live so that we can pursue goods bound up with human flourishing, especially human relationships, as well as other personal goods we find important. This view makes sense when we think about what virtues we should be exhibiting in this case and how these virtues are best lived out in light of the particular circumstances. Some of the virtues that come to mind are compassion, empathy, justice, and prudence, which seem best expressed in this case by keeping Ms. Hamburg as comfortable as possible and helping her family cope with their grief and impending loss. Such virtues are not served, however, by treating her aggressively, given her poor prognosis, the additional suffering this seems to be causing her, and the fact that the limited health care resources could be used for patients who might need them more and could truly benefit from them. This view is also supported by the principles that fall under human dignity (beneficence, care for the whole person, and proportionate/disproportionate means), as well as by those that fall under justice (relationality, stewardship, and equitable distribution).

Hopefully, this brief application of the normative basis has shown how it functions in moral decision making. We should mention, though, that the use of this normative basis will not necessarily point to a single ethical response in every case. There is always a subjective dimension in ethics whereby we must account for historical, personal, social, cultural, contextual, and other factors. Moreover, most moral matters are not black and white; in certain situations, there could be a range of good or ethical options available to us, such that different, valid conclusions could be drawn by different people. The key thing for you to remember is that a normative basis does not function like a mathematical formula. We do not punch in variables and always get a single, definitive answer. Rather, it enables us to zoom out and put the moral situation into its total context by reflecting on the primary goal of human flourishing and its relation to our more immediate goals, what virtues we should be living out, how they would best be expressed in the particular situation, and what principles apply. In the next section we will discuss the role of discernment in helping us to make good moral decisions in concrete situations.

The Role of Discernment

Now that we have described a normative basis that gives us insight into what we are striving for in human life, who we ought to become as human beings, and how we ought to act in relation to others, we need to consider in more detail how we bring a normative basis to bear on the decisions we make in concrete moral situations. This leads us to another virtue, one that we have yet to discuss in any detail—discernment. Discernment plays an important role in our moral lives, for it allows us to make good decisions, decisions that promote right relationships and lead ultimately to our flourishing as human beings. Yet what exactly is discernment? How does it work? These questions will be the focus of the remainder of this chapter, in which we will describe discernment and outline a process of discernment for moral decision making that integrates the main features of our normative basis. We should note that our description of discernment and the process that follows is rooted largely in the Christian tradition. However, we will modify the specifically Christian view of discernment to apply it to what we have already discussed.[3]

Discernment as a Virtue

The word *discernment* or variations of it are used often in everyday discussions. Teachers say to students, "You must discern which theory applies to the problem at hand." Counselors say to clients, "You will have to discern how best to reconcile your past with the present." Critics say to authors, "Your analysis of the issue indicates a discerning mind." When used in such ways, discernment means more than simply noticing or seeing something. It goes beyond describing what is happening in a particular situation and engages in evaluative assessments and judgments. Discerning people perceive the subtle nuances and complexity of situations, demonstrate imaginative capacity in bringing together information and formulating responses, differentiate between available alternatives, and maintain flexibility and sensitivity in practical matters.[4] Discernment in this sense refers to the skill or virtue of perceiving and distinguishing degrees of value among diverse factors when making decisions. Traditionally, discernment has not been described in this way. However, like the virtue of prudence, we must develop the capacity to discern well so that we make good moral decisions. Discernment differs somewhat from prudence as classically defined in that discernment seeks integration of all human capacities and does not rely exclusively on our capacity to reason.

Discernment takes on a more particular meaning in ethics. As we have said, the main objective of the moral life is human flourishing understood as love of God, which comes through right relationships understood as loving our neighbor as we love ourselves in every situation. Discernment enables us to pursue these ends in our personal decisions by helping us to differentiate among possible options and come to the most loving and virtuous response in concrete moral situations.[5] As a virtue that we must develop through practice, discernment involves listening attentively to the inner stirrings that arise within us and consulting extensively the objective sources of morality and the accumulated wisdom of others as we face an impending moral decision. In this way, discernment is both a spiritual exercise, whereby we contemplate personal movements or stirrings, and a moral exercise, whereby we consider reasonable choices, past experiences, and other morally relevant factors against the backdrop of our normative basis.

Discernment is as much about figuring out who we ought to become (BEING) as it is about what we ought to do in concrete situations (DOING). In this sense, discernment seeks to get at the heart of our relationship with ourselves, others, and God and to help us determine the moral response most consistent with who we are as persons made in God's image. Discernment goes beyond the typical action-centered questions that tend to dominate ethics to the more person-centered questions that are often overlooked: "Does this action draw me closer to God and others? Will this action contribute to my human flourishing and that of others? What kind of person am I becoming by acting in this way?"[6] In discernment, these person-centered questions precede questions that focus on what we ought to do in concrete situations.

Discernment is based on the belief that various spirits are present in the moral decisions we make every day. In this context, the word *spirits* refers to the various personal stirrings or movements that motivate us to act. These could be our desire to love others, be kind to others, show compassion, be faithful to God, flourish as human beings, and so on. However, they could just as easily be motivating factors that impede our growth as persons and undermine our relationships with others, such as prejudices, disordered desires, self-centeredness, and so on. Discernment seeks to figure out which among the many motivating factors that cause us to act are the driving forces behind our decisions. The task of discernment is to distinguish between the diverse spiritual states that we experience and to choose the course of action that most fully expresses our love for God and our love for neighbor. The goal is always to select from the possible options the action that best promotes right relationships with others and leads us more deeply into communion with God.

As we engage in discernment, the subjective movements or spirits that arise within us are recognized and understood on a deeply personal level. Reason and intelligence play a role in picking up on these interior movements and in helping us make good moral decisions in practical matters, but these skills alone do not lead us to the moral choice that best promotes right relationships and human flourishing. For this we need to engage the whole network of human capacities. This includes the intellect with its power of reason, and also faith, feelings, emotions, intuition, and imagination. Sometimes we tend to overlook these other human capacities as if morality were purely an intellectual endeavor. However, this is not consistent with human experience. The fact is that in most moral matters we are guided by the heart. As the great mathematician and physicist Blaise Pascal put it, "The heart has its reasons which reason knows nothing of."[7] The word *heart* is understood here in the biblical sense as the deepest level of ourselves, where God's Spirit joins our spirit (see Rom 8:16). At this level, we are alone with God, whose voice echoes in our depths.[8]

The heart is the focal point of discernment. "The tradition of discernment maintains that what we want in our heart of hearts will be consistent with whom God is enabling and requiring us to be and with what we are to do."[9] This does not mean that discernment is purely subjective and set against objective sources of morality such as principles, Scripture, moral teachings, and social norms. Discernment unfolds within the boundaries provided by these moral constraints and proceeds from them to concrete moral situations. Discernment builds on objective moral grounding in attending to the situation and its particularities and in determining what is the most loving and virtuous response. It makes judgments based on what we know to be true and good in the deepest part of ourselves.

Understanding who we ought to become and how we ought to act in concrete situations through the virtue of discernment requires an adequate personal foundation. This foundation consists of three interrelated elements. First, we must be committed to growing in our relationship with God. One critical strategy in developing our relationship with God is prayer. Prayer allows us to get in touch with the voice of God and to perceive where God is leading us in our moral lives. Second, we must trust that God is with us in our everyday moral decisions. This trust provides the confidence necessary to follow those inner movements that are consistent with who we ought to become in light of our relationship with God. Third, we must experience a certain degree of freedom from disordered passions so that we can follow the course of action that best promotes our own flourishing and that of others. Without this freedom, we are paralyzed in the face of choices for the good. These foundational elements are crucial for discernment.

Discernment as a Process

Now that we have discussed what discernment is, we turn to how it works in everyday moral decisions. How do we go about discerning what is the most loving and virtuous response in concrete situations? This brings us to the process of discernment, which we outline below and adapt for purposes of studying ethical issues and analyzing cases outside the context of making personal moral decisions. Before we do this, however, we should point out that the process of discerning is not like solving a problem. The practical moral reasoning of discernment is less clear, less certain, and less linear than the experimental model of reasoning designed specifically for problem solving.[10] Discernment does not operate in computer fashion and does not offer certain solutions to moral problems. Rather, discernment gives us an inner sense that we are doing the right thing. Ernest Larkin describes this well:

> [Discernment] does not tell us what to do, since it moves on a different plane from the technical. But it does indicate whether or not we are moving in the right direction on the deepest level of our being, and in this way it enlightens our experiences, reinforces our decisions, and concretizes our desire to find God in all things.[11]

In short, discernment provides us with moral confidence, not scientific certainty, that through our actions we are promoting right relationships and ultimately contributing to our own flourishing and that of others. This may not satisfy those who want black-and-white answers to moral problems. Yet the unsettling fact is that life is messy and many moral situations do not have easy solutions that we can simply deduce or attain by applying principles.

The overall process of discernment consists of three interrelated components: personal reflection, contextual analysis, and critical evaluation. We will discuss these separately below, but keep in mind that they work together in moral decision making.

1. Personal Reflection

Discernment is about distinguishing between the inner movements that motivate us to act so we can make good moral decisions. This requires that we listen to God in prayer and that we attain some degree of knowledge about ourselves. Prayer is an essential feature of discernment because it allows us to get in touch with the deepest level of ourselves, the place where God dwells. The prayer of discernment is not simply reciting formula prayers but, more profoundly, opening ourselves to God's presence so we can get a sense of what is going on inside and outside ourselves.[12] Prayerful openness to God frees us from internal restraints and external pressures that affect our moral vision and our moral judgments. The interior freedom gained from prayer enables God's self-communication to be heard in our hearts and empowers us to respond to God's grace in the present moment. Meditation, contemplation, and centering prayer are just a few types of prayer that can facilitate the openness to God that discernment requires.

Self-knowledge is also a critical feature of discernment because it helps us to understand our beliefs, character, desires, experiences, motives, temperament, values, and so on. The awareness of ourselves that we gain through prayer and other forms of reflection gives us insight into the various forces that motivate us to act in moral situations. In this way, self-knowledge allows us to see the bright side and the dark side of ourselves, the positive possibilities and the limitations. Though the truth that we learn about ourselves may be painful, it is an important part of discernment because it highlights any capacity for false justification or self-deception that we may possess.

Only with this truth can we discern whether our actions promote right relationships and are consistent with who we ought to become as persons made in God's image.

2. Contextual Analysis

Discernment is about making good moral decisions in complex, changing circumstances. We must recognize the morally relevant features of a situation and extensively consult objective sources of morality and the accumulated wisdom of others. Responding in the most loving and virtuous way is difficult if we do not truly understand the situation in which we find ourselves. To uncover the information necessary for moral decision making, we need to ask certain reality-revealing questions, such as, "What?" "Why and how?" "Who?" "When and where?" "Foreseeable effects?" "Viable alternatives?"[13]

"*What?*" centers on the facts and provides an initial picture of the situation ("What is going on?"). This question precedes all others because it supplies the factual information we need to move forward. "*Why?*" and "*How?*" deal with ends and means ("Why am I doing this? How am I doing this?"). Much emphasis is placed on the question "*Why?*" in ethics because it touches that which we hope to accomplish through our action and our intentions in acting (the ends). However, equally important is the question "*How?*" because it forces us to look at what we are doing (the means) to accomplish our end. Sometimes even the noblest end with the purest intention cannot justify the harmful means selected to achieve the end. Many critics of the war in Iraq have used this argument against actions taken by former president George W. Bush's administration. Although removing Saddam Hussein from power was a good end, given his unjust dictatorship and the atrocities committed by his regime, critics argue that the means (i.e., going to war) were not good and the end could have been accomplished in more ethical ways (e.g., diplomatic measures). Whatever your take, the point is that the means matter just as much as the ends.

"*Who?*" focuses not only on the one performing the action but also on those whom the action will affect ("Who is doing this? Who will be affected?"). This question is important in an ethic that seeks to promote right relationships because it helps us recognize the interpersonal nature and social implications of our actions.

"When?" and *"Where?"* locate the event in time and place ("When am I doing this? Where am I doing this?"). These questions may seem irrelevant, but they prove quite weighty in some situations. For example, to scream at church during a quiet moment in the liturgy is different from screaming after a touchdown at a football game. *"Foreseeable effects?"* concentrates on the results or consequences of our actions, both short-term and long-term ("What if I do this?"); this question deals with the ways we and others will be affected by our actions. *"Viable alternatives?"* refers to other options that may be available to us in moral situations ("What else can I do?"). This question requires a good imagination to see alternative courses of action that may not be immediately apparent. Sometimes by asking this question, we come to realize that what we initially thought was the right thing to do is actually not as good as another option.

When engaging in the process of discernment and trying to figure out the moral dimensions of a situation, these reality-revealing questions must be asked. These questions may not offer definitive moral guidance in every situation, but they help us understand the total situation and draw us closer to the action that best promotes right relationships. At any one time, some of these questions may be more important than others. Nonetheless, they must always be taken as a whole. They cannot be separated without sacrificing moral perspective.

Consulting objective sources of morality and the accumulated wisdom of others is also an indispensable feature of the process of discernment. Several religious and nonreligious resources are available to us when facing an impending moral decision. These resources include but are not limited to Scripture, Jesus, Church, community, role models, expert authority, moral principles, and laws. The information supplied by these resources is essential to making good moral decisions that promote our own and others' well-being.

Scripture is a fundamental source of morality. The Judeo-Christian story and the personal witness of the women and men of the Bible are concrete symbols that shed light on who we ought to become and how we ought to act in relation to others. Though we will not find specific answers to many of the ethical issues we face today, Scripture nonetheless gives us insight into, among other things, the values we should be promoting through our actions. *Jesus* is the moral ideal of who we ought to become. As mentioned above, in Jesus we see what it means to be truly and fully human and what it means to act in ways that promote right relationships. *Church* provides the theological foundations necessary for living the gospel message of love through, among other things, mediating God's grace in the sacraments. Church also guides us in moral matters through its formal teachings, as well as through the moral reflections of pastors, theologians, and others. Even though here we have in mind particularly the Roman Catholic Church, we should point out that other religious traditions, Christian or otherwise, can also serve as important moral resources. Moral wisdom is certainly not reserved exclusively for the Catholic Church, and we would not want to give that impression by our comments.

Community is the place where our lives unfold. The communities in which we live shape our moral character and facilitate our moral growth. The collective experience of communities also serves as a source of moral wisdom on which we can draw when making moral decisions. *Role models* give us a life-guiding moral vision. They show us how we can and ought to live morally. *Expert authority* is a critical resource in our highly technical world. Because we cannot know everything there is to know in practical matters, we have to rely on experts to fill in the gaps in our knowledge so we can make informed moral choices. Just as we seek information from the Internet or a sales representative when we buy a cell phone or a car, we often must do the same when making moral decisions. *Moral principles* are excellent sources of morality because they serve as action guides that complement virtue. As noted in the previous section, principles give us a sense of what we may be required to do in a particular situation and help us to evaluate the choices that we are inclined to make based on our moral character and overall orientation in life. *Laws* provide a framework for moral living. They can be helpful as moral guides in identifying personal and social values and in encouraging us to promote such values. However, laws can also fall short of fulfilling the demands of morality.

All of these sources of morality and others play an important role in the process of discernment. Though discernment does not begin and end with an objective analysis of outside sources, discernment relies on the information generated from these sources in helping us arrive at good moral decisions in concrete situations.

3. Critical Evaluation

Discernment is about making good moral choices that truly promote right relationships and lead ultimately to our flourishing and that of others. Because we are imperfect human beings limited in many ways, discernment can end in moral decisions that we wrongly perceive as right. To limit this possibility as much as humanly possible, we need to check our decisions against certain external and internal criteria that help us evaluate whether the course of action we take really contributes to our own well-being and that of others. Just as pilots, machine operators, and electricians have safeguards that seek to eliminate the possibility of error, so should we as moral beings, perhaps even more urgently so, given what is at stake for ourselves and others.

The external criteria for good discernment include Scripture and Church teaching, the community and its values, and moral principles and relevant laws. We look to these criteria to see if our moral decisions in changing circumstances are in harmony or disharmony with these sources of morality. Certain questions help us measure our moral decisions against these criteria: "Is our decision consistent with the substance of Scripture and with Church teaching on the matter? What is the attitude of the community toward our decision or the issue in general? Would the community support us in this decision if it became public? Is our decision consonant with moral principles and laws that apply to this situation?" If we answer yes to these questions, then we can be relatively confident that we are making a good decision. If we answer no to any of these questions, then we need to rethink the matter and try to figure out if we are not in fact proceeding in the wrong direction.

The external criteria have undoubted strength and appeal, but they also have certain limits. First, as we noted above, Scripture does not explicitly address all of the issues that challenge us in our moral lives, and many scriptural texts are ambiguous and open to varied interpretations. Moreover, Church teaching on moral matters is fallible and may not always attend to the complexities of every moral situation. Second, the community can promote certain values and ways of acting that hinder right relationships and actually detract from our pursuit of human flourishing. As such, sometimes it may be necessary to stand against the community so that greater good can be achieved. Third, moral principles can conflict and laws often are reduced to the moral minimum or can even be opposed to morality. These limits suggest that the external criteria of good discernment may not always serve as an adequate check.

To illustrate this, consider the example of slavery in the United States. When slavery was an accepted social institution, people often cited Scripture in its support and used Catholic Church teaching to reinforce their position, which at the time considered slavery permissible. Furthermore, most people in the United States and in individual communities believed slavery was acceptable, at least until the abolitionist movement gained momentum. Moreover, the law permitted the trading and ownership of slaves. Now let's say you lived during this time but opposed slavery. Discernment leads you to believe that slavery is wrong, but when you consider any action against it, you run smack into external criteria supporting it. What do you do? Do you go against your own best judgment because these criteria favor slavery? Absolutely not! The external criteria for good discernment must be complemented and supported by the internal criterion, which is interior harmony and integration (that is, a profound sense of being content).

We look to this criterion to see if our moral decisions in particular situations create agreement or disagreement among the whole network of human capacities—reason, intelligence, faith, feelings, emotions, intuition, and imagination. We measure our moral decisions against the internal criterion by tuning in to the inner movements or spirits that arise within us. On the one hand, when we experience "love, joy, peace, patience, kindness, generosity, faithfulness, gentleness, and self-control" (Gal 5:22–23), we gain confidence that we are acting rightly or virtuously. These inner movements suggest that we are promoting our well-being and that of others through our actions. On the other hand, when we experience hate, discontent, confusion, turmoil, selfishness, callousness, and excess, we lose confidence that this is the case.

Like the external criteria, certain questions can help us measure our moral decisions against the internal criterion: "Do I have a sense of basic inner content with my decision? Is my action consistent with the person I ought to become in terms of the virtues that should shape my character? Do I really believe my action will promote right relationships, contribute to my well-being and that of others, and support the good of the community?" If we answer yes to these questions, then we must stand by the decision we have reached through the process of discernment. This applies even when our decision conflicts with the external criteria, provided we have taken steps to reconcile all the criteria. In these circumstances to do otherwise would be to compromise ourselves and our integrity as moral persons. If we answer no to any of these questions, then we need to rethink the matter and try to figure out if we are not in fact proceeding in the wrong direction.

The internal criterion is given much weight in discernment but, like the external criteria, it has limits.[14] First, identifying and understanding the inner movements that arise within ourselves requires that we be in touch with ourselves and with our relationship with God. Due to our limitations and brokenness, we are not always able to meet this requirement. Second, the ability to distinguish between the inner movements that arise within ourselves requires that we achieve some level of psychological, spiritual, and moral maturity. Human experience shows that not all people ascend to an adequate level in these areas, and those who do are not fixed permanently at that level. Despite these limits our inner peace (or lack of peace) is one of the main safeguards of discernment. However, inner peace is not the exclusive means of discernment; inner peace and content is a vague concept, and the threat of self-deception always lurks in the shadows. Therefore, external and internal criteria must always be used in tandem to evaluate our moral choices critically. In most cases, an honest and thorough discernment process will lead to a decision that is supported by both external and internal criteria.

What we have said about discernment may seem complex, and the process may seem long and cumbersome. In reality, however, we do much of this intuitively when we make personal moral decisions, especially big decisions, even though we may not even be aware of it. We bring our character to bear on decisions, we contemplate who we are or want to become, and we reflect on our motives for acting (personal reflection); we consider factual information, think about our end, intention, and means, consider viable options and alternatives and possible consequences of our actions; we also consult objective sources of morality like moral principles, and seek the wisdom of others such

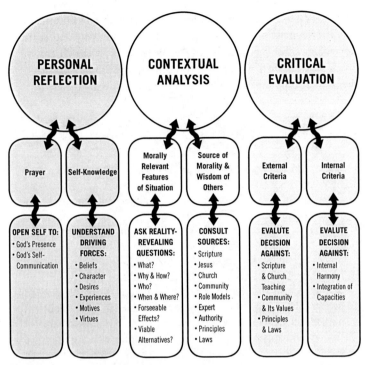

PERSONAL REFLECTION		CONTEXTUAL ANALYSIS		CRITICAL EVALUATION	
Prayer	Self-Knowledge	Morally Relevant Features of Situation	Source of Morality & Wisdom of Others	External Criteria	Internal Criteria
OPEN SELF TO: • God's Presence • God's Self-Communication	**UNDERSTAND DRIVING FORCES:** • Beliefs • Character • Desires • Experiences • Motives • Virtues	**ASK REALITY-REVEALING QUESTIONS:** • What? • Why & How? • Who? • When & Where? • Forseeable Effects? • Viable Alternatives?	**CONSULT SOURCES:** • Scripture • Jesus • Church • Community • Role Models • Expert • Authority • Principles • Laws	**EVALUTE DECISION AGAINST:** • Scripture & Church Teaching • Community & Its Values • Principles & Laws	**EVALUTE DECISION AGAINST:** • Internal Harmony • Integration of Capacities

FIGURE 2C Discernment as a Process

as friends, family, and teachers (contextual analysis); and we weigh the proposed action against external criteria such as what our friends and family might think, our faith, personal and community values, and laws, as well as how we feel about our decision, whether we are at peace or at odds with it (critical evaluation). Discernment is not an abstraction invented for this book. It is a virtue and a process that can help us make good moral decisions in concrete situations, particularly when used in conjunction with a normative basis such as the one outlined in the first section of this chapter (see figure 2C).

Discernment as a virtue and a process comes into play mostly when we make personal moral decisions. These are the most common moral decisions we make in our everyday lives. However, we also make other types of moral decisions, like when we take a stand on an issue such as stem cell research or when we decide how we would act in an ethics case. Although we have talked about discernment in the context of personal moral decision making, we should note that it is just as effective for examining ethical issues and analyzing cases, as we will in subsequent chapters. Many features of the discernment process used when making personal moral decisions also apply to these other types of decisions. Consider the following case.

Case 2B

Ms. J., an 85-year-old woman in relatively good health, comes to Saint Stephens Medical Center for cataract surgery on her left eye. As part of the presurgical routine, the nurse checks the physician order sheet, which states "left-eye cataract surgery" and cross-checks this with the informed consent, which also states "left-eye cataract surgery." However, the paper site-marker, which is supposed to be placed on the spot where the surgery is to be performed and is another step in the process, is placed over the right eye and the surgeon, who is supposed to sign off on the paper site-marker, checking it for accuracy, fails to do so. As a result, Ms. J. undergoes a right-eye cataract surgery. In explaining to Ms. J. and her family why her right eye was operated on, the surgeon points out that the long-range goal was to do both eyes, which is true, and that "when they got into surgery, it was clear that the right eye was worse," which is not true. The surgical nurse overhears the surgeon tell this to the family and is appalled. Consequently, he informs hospital administration. During the administrative council (AC) meeting, several facts are brought up—namely, the surgeon has an outstanding record and brings a lot of "business to Saint Stephens," suspension of the surgeon's privileges could result in her not scheduling procedures at Saint Stephens, and there is a good chance that the family would sue the hospital if the mistake became known. As a member of the AC, how would you handle the surgeon and what would you do about Ms. J. and her family?

This case is typical of those that you will see throughout the rest of this book. How might we use the discernment process with our normative basis to determine what we ought to do or how we ought to respond? Listed below are six steps for decision making that incorporate the key features of discernment and our normative basis. We will go through each of these steps by considering them in light of this case.

1. **Gather all relevant factual information.** This will come from the information provided in the case. We have to work with the information presented to us, with all that is known through the details at our disposal. In most instances, cases do not provide us with all the facts we may want and as such, we are often forced to make the best judgments we can with the information given. In this case we know the following: a mistake was made, the process for ensuring correct surgery broke down, the surgeon had a role in the error, the surgeon concealed the error and lied about why surgery was performed on the wrong eye, the hospital administration is aware of the situation, the hospital could take action against the surgeon and disclose the truth to the patient, the patient may sue the hospital if the truth is disclosed, and the hospital may lose a surgeon who brings in a lot of patients if it chooses to punish the surgeon.

2. **Identify the ethical issues.** Sometimes this may seem pretty obvious, but it is nonetheless a key step because it sets the tone for how we view the case. In describing the ethical issues, it is important to be precise so we know what is at stake. In this case the main ethical issue is whether we should disclose or continue to conceal the truth from the patient, who has already been lied to by the surgeon. There are also secondary ethical issues, such as whether we ought to compensate the patient in some way if we do decide to disclose the truth and how we should handle the surgeon.

3. **Consider what right relationships require and what leads ultimately to human flourishing.** Here we want to tap into the normative basis by asking who we ought to become as persons (or institutions, communities, and so on) in terms of the virtues we should be exhibiting in the present circumstances and how we ought to act in terms of the principles that should guide our action. Recalling our normative basis, we can say that the surgeon should have manifested the virtues of respect, honesty, courage, and integrity. These virtues, in the given circumstances, would

best promote right relationships and contribute to the well-being of the surgeon, the patient, and the hospital. Obviously, the surgeon did not exhibit these virtues. However, the hospital still has a chance to right the situation by showing respect for the patient's dignity, by being honest with the patient, and by acting with courage and integrity through disclosing the truth despite the consequences. With regard to principles, we can see that veracity, which falls under human dignity, and stewardship, which falls under justice, are the main principles that apply to the case. These two principles could conflict because telling the truth to the patient may lead ultimately to a lawsuit that could result in a huge financial loss for the hospital, which has obligations to others (e.g., patients, employees, vendors, and the community). As such, we may have to weigh which principle is more important than the other. Is it worth losing some money if the hospital and its leaders maintain their integrity? From a moral perspective, integrity far exceeds the value of money and so veracity would be the primary principle to consider.

4. **Brainstorm possible options.** This next step involves listing all possible options without regard for what is right or wrong—we will critically evaluate the options later. Some of the options in this case could be (a) maintain the lie by not telling the patient and do nothing to the surgeon; (b) maintain the lie by not telling the patient but reprimand, suspend, or strip the surgeon of her credentials at the hospital; (c) disclose the truth to the patient but do nothing to the surgeon; and (d) disclose the truth to the patient, offer a financial settlement, and reprimand, suspend, or strip the surgeon of her credentials at the hospital. There are probably other options, but these are the main ones and are enough for the purposes of this illustration.

5. **Weigh options and select one.** Now we must weigh the various options by eliminating any that are simply unacceptable in light of the primary virtues and principles necessary for right relationships that we have identified. Once we have done this, we need to consider the remaining options and their consequences and choose the ones that we believe in our heart of hearts truly promotes right relationships and contributes to our flourishing as persons and to the good of the community. Given the virtues

and principles we noted above, options a and b, which keep up the lie by continuing to conceal the truth from the patient, are unacceptable. These options would impair our character as individuals, as well as an institution, and undermine our integrity. Option c, in which we disclose the truth to the patient, might work, but the surgeon would not have to account for her actions. Although we can accept that errors happen and try to correct the steps in the surgical process that went awry, we cannot tolerate lying on the part of our physicians, even those that bring in a lot of money to the hospital. This leaves us with option d, which, all things considered, seems to be the best option morally. Although the patient may not accept our sincere apology and any money we offer her and we could get sued and lose a good surgeon, this option best reflects who we ought to become and upholds an important principle that specifies what respect for human dignity demands.

6. **Evaluate the decision against external and internal criteria.** Here we need to ask whether the option we have selected stands up against the external criteria of Scripture and Church teaching, the community and its values, and moral principles and relevant laws. Although Scripture and Church teaching do not address the issue specifically, the values promoted in each support telling the truth and thereby preserving our integrity, as well as holding the surgeon accountable. Likewise, our decision seems also to be supported by community values, moral principles, and relevant laws, all of which would favor disclosing the truth and addressing the surgeon's action of lying. What about the internal criteria? Although somewhat difficult to evaluate outside of personal moral decisions, it can be reduced to certain questions when analyzing issues or cases: (a) "Who are we becoming as persons (or institutions, communities, and so on) through this action?" (b) "Is our action consistent with who we ought to become?" (c) "Will our action truly promote right relationships and contribute to the overall well-being of ourselves and others as well as the good of the community?" Based on the option we have selected, we can answer all these questions positively and be able to live with the decision we have made, despite its consequences.

Conclusion

This is an illustration of how we use discernment with our normative basis to evaluate cases in ethics. As we move out of the foundations section of this book and into broader issues and other cases in health care ethics, it is important that we consider these issues and cases against the backdrop of our normative basis, using the process of discernment that we have constructed here. This gives us the best chance of identifying ethical concerns, seeing them in their broader context, and making decisions that truly promote right relationships and lead ultimately to our flourishing as human beings.

SUGGESTED READINGS

Devettere, Raymond J. *Introduction to Virtue Ethics: Insights of the Ancient Greeks.* Washington, DC: Georgetown University Press, 2002.

Gula, Richard M. *Moral Discernment.* New York: Paulist Press, 1997.

Gula, Richard M. *The Good Life: Where Morality and Spirituality Converge.* New York: Paulist Press, 1999.

Gustafson, James M. *Christ and the Moral Life.* New York: Harper and Row, 1968.

Harrington, Daniel J., and James F. Keenan. *Jesus and Virtue Ethics: Building Bridges between New Testament Studies and Moral Theology.* Lanham, MD: Sheed & Ward, 2002.

Maguire, Daniel C., and A. Nicholas Fargnoli. *On Moral Grounds: The Art/Science of Ethics.* New York: Crossroad, 1991.

Rahner, Karl. *The Love of Jesus and the Love of Neighbor.* New York: Crossroad, 1983.

Spohn, William C. *Go and Do Likewise: Jesus and Ethics.* New York: Continuum, 1999.

MULTIMEDIA AIDS FOR TEACHERS

Movies can aid students in thinking about a normative basis. Some movies prompt us to ask whether an objective grounding for ethics actually exists. Following is a list of several of the more helpful ones; all are available on DVD through retailers.

North Country. Directed by Niki Caro. Starring Charlize Theron. Rated R. 2005. This movie depicts the horrible actions of male workers against female coworkers in a Minnesota iron mine and can be helpful for examining whether some actions are simply wrong and then exploring the rationale behind this claim.

Rashomon. Directed by Akira Kurosawa. Starring Toshirô Mifune. Not Rated. 1951. The nature of truth is examined in this movie in which four people recount different versions of the story of a man's murder and the rape of his wife. In Japanese with English subtitles, *Rashomon* can be highly effective for exploring the existence of a normative basis.

Schindler's List. Directed by Steven Spielberg. Starring Liam Neeson. Rated R. 1993. The portrayal of atrocities committed by the Nazis against the Jews can be helpful for examining whether some actions are simply wrong because they undermine the value of human life and then for exploring the rationale behind this claim.

Weapons of the Spirit. Directed by Pierre Sauvage. Starring Pierre Sauvage. Not Rated. 1989. This movie depicts the great sacrifices made by the people of the small French community of Le Chambon, who show through their actions what it means to love one's neighbor. At great peril to themselves, they help save hundreds of people, many women and children, from the clutches of Nazis and Nazi sympathizers.

Several movies depict good discernment skills; their characters consider who they ought to become and how they ought to act in relation to others by weighing virtues, principles, consequences, and other factors in light of the circumstances. Two of the best, which are available on DVD through retailers, are listed below.

A Man for All Seasons. Directed by Fred Zinnemann. Starring Paul Scofield. Rated G. 1966. Although this movie is excellent for these purposes, students may not connect with it as much as a more contemporary movie. Still, it is perhaps the best cinematic depiction of discernment in light of a normative basis.

Scent of a Woman. Directed by Martin Brest. Starring Al Pacino. Rated R. 1992. This movie is more current and displays good discernment skills through the eyes of a young character; as such, it should resonate with students.

ENDNOTES

1. For an excellent discussion of the broader moral meaning of happiness, see Raymond J. Devettere, *Practical Decision Making in Health Care Ethics:*

Cases and Concepts, 3rd ed. (Washington, DC: Georgetown University Press, 2010), 20–46.

2. For a discussion of the importance of relationships from a theological perspective, see Richard A. McCormick, "To Save or Let Die: The Dilemma of Modern Medicine," *Journal of the American Medical Association* 229 (July 8, 1974): 172–6, at 174.

3. Much of the discussion of discernment that follows has been adapted from Michael R. Panicola, "Discernment in the Neonatal Context," *Theological Studies* 60 (December 1999): 723–46.

4. For a discussion of the characteristic features of discerning people, see James M. Gustafson, "Moral Discernment in the Christian Life," in *Theology and Christian Ethics*, ed. James M. Gustafson (Philadelphia: Pilgrim Press, 1974), 99–119, at 101–9. This article first appeared in *Norm and Context in Christian Ethics*, ed. Gene Outka and Paul Ramsey (New York: Charles Scribner's Sons, 1968), 17–36.

5. Richard M. Gula, *Reason Informed by Faith: Foundations of Catholic Morality* (New York: Paulist Press, 1989), 315.

6. William C. Spohn, "The Reasoning Heart: An American Approach to Christian Discernment," *Theological Studies* 44 (March 1983), 30–52, at 30.

7. *Pensées and Other Writings*, trans. Honor Levi, introduction and notes by Anthony Levi (Oxford; New York: Oxford University Press, 1995).

8. Vatican Council II, *Gaudium et spes*, no. 16, in *Proclaiming Justice and Peace: Papal Documents from* Rerum Novarum *through* Centesimus Annus, ed. Michael Walsh and Brian Davies (Mystic, CT: Twenty-Third Publications, 1994), 168.

9. Gula, *Reason Informed by Faith*, 321.

10. Richard M. Gula discusses the differences between scientific reasoning and the practical moral reasoning of discernment in his *Moral Discernment* (New York: Paulist Press, 1997), 50–52.

11. Ernest Larkin, *Silent Presence: Discernment as Process and Problem* (Denville, NJ: Dimension Books, 1981), 58.

12. Gula, *Moral Discernment*, 98–9.

13. The reality-revealing questions were first proposed by Daniel C. Maguire, *The Moral Choice* (Garden City, NY: Doubleday, 1978). He further developed these questions in a book he coauthored with A. Nicholas Fargnoli, *On Moral Grounds: The Art/Science of Ethics* (New York: Crossroad, 1991). The presentation of these questions is based on the latter work, pages 49–72.

14. For a review of the limits of Christian discernment, see Gula, *Reason Informed by Faith*, 326–8, and Larkin, *Silent Presence*, 7–8.

CHAPTER 3

Professionalism and the Patient–Physician Relationship

Mark Repenshek

What Does *Professionalism* Mean?

Recall the last time you were at the doctor's office. Regardless of the reason, it is likely you extended a good deal of autonomy to your doctor without question. By autonomy, we mean acceptance of a professional's judgment on matters within his or her expertise.[1] Think again of that doctor's appointment. You likely extended professional autonomy to the physician in at least three areas: (1) determining your specific needs relating to the reason for the appointment, (2) determining the likely outcome of actions that might be taken regarding those needs (e.g., further testing, a prescription, consultation with a specialist, or further intervention), and (3) judging which course of action is most likely to best meet your needs. This is not to say the physician made every decision for you, but she likely made numerous decisions on your behalf within the scope of her expertise, with a high degree of trust extended on your part. This account of a typical office visit to a doctor exemplifies the concept of professionalism.

Some may consider professionalism to derive from an oath or membership in a society or perhaps even from being "called" to serve in a particular manner. Although these are important aspects of professionalism, none fully defines the concept. Each criterion suggests that being a professional is contingent on some personal commitment or admirable characteristic. This narrow focus misses two key aspects of professionalism, however: dialogue between a professional group and the community it serves, and the ethical obligations over and above what "the marketplace" or a contract would demand.

In this chapter we adopt a traditional approach to the term *professional*, which refers not only to specialized expertise but also to particular moral commitments associated with a practice. In the case of the physician, we discuss expertise beyond that derived from time spent in medical school and residency and focus instead on the broader culture and infrastructure supporting medical education. With regard to moral commitments, we discuss both the privileges of the physician and the physician's obligations to those served.

Aspects of Physician Professionalism

In 2002, the American College of Physicians (ACP) and the American Society of Internal Medicine (ASIM) jointly published a charter on physician professionalism. Walter McDonald, then executive vice president and CEO of ACP-ASIM, termed the charter "a call to individual physicians to reaffirm their dedication to the welfare of their patients and to the profession to collectively work to improve health care for all."[2] Of particular interest here is the brevity of its impetus, namely, to combat a tendency in current medical practice that tempts physicians "to abandon their commitment to the primacy of patient welfare."[3] What could have caused this turn in medicine that shifts physicians' focus away from patients? What is competing for physicians' attention? Are there factors other than patient welfare influencing physician behavior? Are physicians obligated as part of their medical training to maintain a contract with society? What is the basis of that contract? Given the specialized knowledge that physicians have, could that knowledge be used for a good other than health and well-being? Will patients be at risk should physicians not reaffirm their "dedication to the welfare of their patients and to the profession to collectively work to improve health care for all"?

Each of these questions concerns a specific aspect of professionalism. We discuss three important aspects of professionalism here: (a) important and exclusive expertise, (b) autonomy in matters of expert practice, and (c) obligations of professions and professionals.

Important and Exclusive Expertise

Medicine is vital to the health and well-being of people. The ultimate reason for the profession of medicine is the complexity of the specialized knowledge the profession controls.[4] Despite Web-MD™, Medline™, or any other Web-based source of medical knowledge, this knowledge is not easily understood by the general public, and consequently the medical profession is given significant control over its use. Thus, the medical profession requires integrity of information, proper application of information, and continued testing and dissemination of information (i.e., clinical trials). Finally, the profession is obligated to transmit medical knowledge to the general public, to patients, and—through teaching and mentoring—to future practitioners.

Medical expertise has two key attributes that qualify it as a profession: it is cognitive and practical. The medical profession depends heavily on those already expert in the field to teach and mentor the next generation of professionals. Given the complexity of medical knowledge and the difficulty in teaching and mentoring its use, those able to perform both tasks well are few. Add to this the responsibility to care for other humans, and the high stakes of physician professionalism become abundantly clear. The following case study will help to illustrate the many pressures unique to the physician in his or her development as a professional.

Case 3A

Early in his medical school education, Jakob knew he was an exemplary student. He was often sought out as a study partner, and many of his classmates turned to him for his knowledge on particular subjects. This continued into his residency at one of the nation's leading academic medical centers in orthopedic surgery. Jakob quickly progressed through his surgery rounds, grabbing the attention of many faculty members with his skill and bedside manner.

During Jakob's second year in his surgery fellowship in orthopedics, he became concerned about a colleague who was

cont.

Case 3A *cont.*

also a good friend. For months Jakob had been concerned about his friend's bedside manner, but recently he had been struck by his colleague's failure to fulfill some of the more advanced technical aspects of certain procedures. Jakob knew that eventually the faculty would need to decide whether his friend was cut out for orthopedics, but he really wanted his friend to progress through with him. In fact, they had often talked about how great it would be to practice in the same city, sharing referrals, knowledge, and new cases.

As things grew worse for Jakob's friend, the friend started using stimulants to stay awake longer to get extra cases and to study harder in areas where he continued to falter. Jakob felt compelled to assist as much as he could but was worried about his friend just getting by. Jakob started to ask himself some troubling questions: Would he ever send a patient to his friend? Would he feel comfortable with his friend's skills were Jakob and he seeing the same patient as partners in a practice? Would Jakob want his friend operating on one of his family members?

As chief resident, Jakob was uncertain as to the next step to take but felt compelled to approach faculty about his friend and the potential risk he posed to future patients. Jakob was also uncertain whether this was appropriate, given the culture of medicine, and was concerned that he would lose his friend as the result of such an inquiry. Jakob had seen colleagues cover for each other many times in far worse situations (involving substance abuse). Also Jakob wondered if this was indeed his responsibility. Shouldn't faculty handle this? Wouldn't they notice his friend failing in skills at the mastery level and decide not to move him on, instead suggesting a different course of surgery? Besides, someone has to be at the bottom of the class, and that person is still considered a doctor.

Ultimately, if Jakob were to see this as a matter for faculty and not for him as chief resident, would Jakob be faithful to the privilege of important and exclusive expertise accorded to the medical profession?

Would Jakob have skirted his responsibility to inform faculty of his observations? Might Jakob's decision during residency become the manner in which he would one day approach such issues in his practice? Does Jakob have an obligation as a matter of professionalism to report his friend who is failing aspects of his fellowship?

Autonomy in Matters of Expert Practice

Along with the privileges accorded to expertise comes a great deal of autonomy in matters of practice.[5] This is not an autonomy that allows the practitioner to do whatever she wants, rather it is an autonomy entrusted to physicians by virtue of their expertise. Others generally accept the professional's judgment when discussing aspects of a case in her field.[6] As an example, think back to a visit with your physician in which you were referred to a specialist (e.g., dermatologist, allergist, cardiologist, oncologist). At least two things occurred with regard to autonomy in practice: (1) your primary physician likely referred you to a particular physician in a specific field, and (2) your primary physician likely had reached her limit of knowledge in the field referred to. It also is likely that you complied with the recommendations offered by the specialist and that this was the only specialist you saw in that field. Let us look at each aspect of this scenario more closely.

Consider your primary care physician's recommendation that you should see a specialist. The first assumption here is that each member of the specialist group possesses the relevant professional expertise to be licensed in the field. With this baseline confidence in the physician's expertise, a high level of autonomy is accorded to her to determine your specific needs, which course of action is most likely to lead to a beneficial outcome for you, and the likely outcome based on your compliance with her recommendations. All of this was likely done with little questioning of the clinical capacity of the physician, the score on her recent exam boards, the residency program from which she graduated, and so on. Because your trusted primary care physician referred you to this specialist, she became the next professional in whom you extended trust to expertly care for your health and well-being.

Although it could be argued that a similar level of trust is placed in a referral to a trusted car mechanic or a heating and cooling contractor, it is often not the case that one seeks only one opinion on the work needed. Often people seek two or three quotes and corresponding references, depending on the level of work needed. Also with a mechanic or heating and cooling contractor, a contract is drafted stipulating the estimated fee for services. Such a contract is not typical of the patient–physician relationship, in which it is presumed that the physician's (professional) primary interest is that of her patient and not the profit margin of the job.[7]

Second, when seeing the medical specialist to whom you were referred, it is likely that you accommodated the physician's schedule by changing your own, even though you were the client. In other words, physicians are granted wide autonomy in what constitutes acceptable daily medical practice, even though that practice depends on seeing patients. In other fields, the marketplace tends to determine the work pattern of the professional; in medicine, physicians largely determine (and society grants their right to determine) the most important day-to-day activities of their practice. Scheduled surgery at a level-I trauma facility is a perfect example of this type of autonomy.[8] Typically, while a surgery schedule may have a full day of patients, the nature of being trauma level-I means any medical emergency that may require the expertise of the scheduled surgeon immediately receives priority, and society grants a level of autonomy to medicine to determine who should receive services sooner and to what extent another can wait. The term describing the process for such determinations is *triage*.[9]

Case 3B

Dr. White was a well-respected oncologist at a community hospital. Dr. White had struggled for years, seeing so many of his patients fall victim to lung cancer as a result of smoking. Despite trying to convince many of his patients that smoking was a leading cause of lung cancer and that, if continued, it would likely lead to their deaths, some of his patients even continued smoking through their chemotherapy and radiation treatments.

cont.

Case 3B *cont.*

While speaking at a conference on the benefits of smoke-free health care campuses, a gentleman from a private venture company approached Dr. White regarding a new product he had developed called "Smoke Stop." This product simulated all the features of smoking in action and nicotine absorption without the smoke by-product. Intrigued by the initial pitch, Dr. White agreed to a follow-up meeting. Over the next couple of months, Dr. White became more convinced of this product and its potential benefit for hundreds of his patients. He agreed to invest in 50-percent ownership of the company. Recognizing the potential benefits of this product, Dr. White was eager to introduce this option to his patients, but he knew it needed to go through proper clinical trials first.

Dr. White approached his colleagues at the hospital, convinced of this new approach to smoking cessation. He eventually was able to present a phase I study to the hospital's institutional review board (IRB). Dr. White was more than willing to disclose his 50-percent ownership in the company, but he insisted on remaining the principal investigator for the study. The IRB eventually approved the study with modifications, and Dr. White began enrolling some of his patients in this phase I study.

Although this clinical trial raises a number of questions for our chapter on human subjects research, we wish to focus on the issues of professionalism here. Is Dr. White using his position of authority and the relative autonomy accorded his profession to access a vulnerable patient population seeking to stop an addictive behavior that is detrimental to their health? Is it fair to ask if Dr. White is looking only to benefit patients or if he has a conflict of interest by owning 50 percent of Smoke Stop? Should a different level of autonomy be accorded a physician researcher versus solely a practitioner? Noting that Dr. White was "more than willing to disclose his 50-percent ownership in the company," has he met the obligations accorded a profession so as not to be potentially influenced by his opportunity to make a profit? Should physicians, by the very nature of the good they serve—namely, human health and well-being—be allowed to invest in technology that can serve this human good? Given his substantial financial interest, will Dr. White be able to resist recommending Smoke Stop to patients should the product *not* show demonstrable benefit over other products? Other than disclosing his investment, are there other matters that professionalism might suggest require Dr. White's attention? These last few questions allude to our final section on the obligations of professions and professionals.

The Obligations of Professions and Professionals

Whereas healing is the goal of the patient–physician relationship, trust is the basis for that relationship—trust that the physician will put the interests of her patient's health and well-being first. Given the vulnerability of a sick person, part of this trust is ensured through the oath physicians take, an oath that establishes the unique relationship society has with physicians. Part of this pledge sets forth the physician's obligations.

The American College of Physicians–American Society of Internal Medicine recently highlighted these obligations as professional responsibilities:[10]

- commitment to professional competence
- commitment to honesty with patients
- commitment to patient confidentiality
- commitment to maintaining appropriate relations with patients
- commitment to improving quality of care
- commitment to improving access to care
- commitment to a just distribution of finite resources
- commitment to scientific knowledge
- commitment to maintaining trust by managing conflicts of interest
- commitment to professional responsibilities

These commitments are derived from the charter's fundamental principles regarding the primacy of patient welfare, patient autonomy, and social justice. These principles begin a conversation between medical professionals and society that seeks to establish how physicians should care for patients and thereby detail the ethics of the profession. In this way, how physicians perform their duties within society becomes normative. That is, persons in need of medical assistance understand what ethical standards apply when they are under a physician's care.

These professional obligations also create ethics for relationships among colleagues. Although not specifically addressed, these professional responsibilities set the stage for how physicians ensure that certain standards are met among themselves. Without clarifying these professional responsibilities, breaches of trust can occur that harm not only a specific patient–physician relationship but also the relationship between society and the profession as a whole. The following case study may help to illustrate this point.

Case 3C

Dr. James Smith was a well-respected anesthesiologist at the University Medical Center. Dr. Smith was fully tenured, with 25 years of experience in the operating room. He was department chair of anesthesiology and was regarded by his peers as one of the best. Having been department chair for three years, Dr. Smith was well accustomed to the administrative matters that many of his peers regarded as meaningless but necessary. This past year, however, Dr. Smith was introduced to a young, aggressive CEO, who was charged with turning the University Medical Center into a world-class health care facility, while doing so on a razor-thin budget. The first few meetings with this CEO were cordial enough, but recently all the department chairs within the division of medicine were convened by the CEO and essentially told they were to provide the same great level of service to which their patients were accustomed but with a 15-percent budget reduction.

Over the next few months, with targets set and unmet time and time again, Dr. Smith became frustrated with administration, disillusioned with medicine, and began to drink more

cont.

Case 3C *cont.*

heavily. Dr. Smith was always one to enjoy a drink, even on days he was on call, but his colleagues began to notice his drinking increase. In fact, this past week, Dr. Smith's colleagues covered for him when he showed up to the hospital noticeably intoxicated and scheduled to conduct surgery. One of his partners sent him home in a taxi and called in the on-call anesthesiologist.

Dr. Smith's partners were becoming very worried. They knew he was not meeting expectations with administration, but he could always fall back on his incredible skills as an anesthesiology and department chair. Only so much slack was going to be allowed, however, especially with this young, aggressive CEO on board. The department was wondering what the next step should be inside the department.

Should the department of anesthesiology go to the chief of staff? What about fellow department chairs? Concerns were also raised as to whether Dr. Smith might be endangering his patients. What about the surgery department and its reputation? Should Dr. Smith be protected if he has not had any clinical mishaps? If no significant adverse events have occurred, should counseling be set as an expectation? Should Dr. Smith be allowed to practice in the interim? Should a report be filed with the state? What about Dr. Smith's future practice and license?

Because no direct harm was caused to a patient, the most significant question was how his physician colleagues, especially his department colleagues, should respond to Dr. Smith's misuse of alcohol. It seems that a variety of commitments are relevant here, but the most relevant professional responsibilities fall into the following areas. As members of a profession, physicians are expected to work among themselves to establish appropriate processes of self-regulation. Only in cases where self-regulation is ineffective should outside disciplines be involved (i.e., law or licensing boards). For Dr. Smith, this includes remediation and discipline for his failure to meet professional standards of conduct with regard to his coming to work intoxicated and his potential to harm patients. The profession should define and organize the education and accountability process for members, as well as the appropriate disciplinary review bodies to accommodate the appropriate appeals or hearings. The profession should also engage in ongoing internal assessment and accept external scrutiny of all aspects of Dr. Smith's work going forward. Just as trust is core to the professional patient–physician relationship, so too is it core to the societal–professional relationship. In cases such as Dr. Smith's, the profession of medicine must ensure the public that the autonomy granted the profession will always be monitored and balanced by its obligation to discipline and dismiss professionals who do not maintain proper standards. Transparency in this process serves to build the integrity of the medical profession.

Conclusion

The role of the physician as a professional has remained unquestioned for nearly 150 years. The modern era, however, has brought unprecedented challenges in virtually all areas of medicine that compete with the primary interests of the patient. As Dennis McDonagh has noted, "Medical professionalism is an ideal toward which we as physicians must always be striving."[11] This ideal is manifest in the professional codes and covenants with patient, society, and colleagues. The price of failure to maintain this ideal would be the loss of medical professionalism and the corresponding trust between patient–physician and society–physician. The ideals to which professionalism binds the physician are competence, high moral standards, and altruism: therein lies the professional healer—the physician.

SUGGESTED READINGS

ACGME (Advancing Education in Medical Professionalism). Toolkit—Wake Forest Physician Trust Scale.

Toolkit—ABIM Scale to Measure Professional Attitudes and Behaviors in Medical Education, 9–10.

Toolkit—Musick 360-degree Assessment, 14–5. Resources found at *http://www.acgme.org/outcome/implement/profm_resource.pdf.*

ACP-ASIM (American College of Physicians–American Society of Internal Medicine). "Medical Professionalism in the New Millennium: A Physician Charter." Project of the American Board of Internal Medicine Foundation, ACP-ASIM Foundation, and the European Federation of Internal Medicine. *Annals of Internal Medicine* 136 (2002): 243–6.

Pellegrino, Edmund D., Robert M. Veatch, and John Langan. *Ethics, Trust, and the Professions: Philosophical and Cultural Aspects.* Washington, DC: Georgetown University Press, 1991, 69–85.

Sox, Harold C. "The Ethical Foundations of Professionalism." *Chest* 131 (2007): 1532–40.

FURTHER CASE STUDIES

Barry, D., E . Cyran, and R. J. Anderson. "Common Issues in Medical Professionalism: Room to Grow." *American Journal of Medicine* 108 (2000): 136–42. Provides the Barry Challenges to Professionalism Questionnaire, with six short case studies and potential responses.

ENDNOTES

1. David Ozar, "Building Awareness of Ethical Standards and Conduct," in *Educating Professionals: Responding to New Expectations for Competence and Accountability,* ed. Lynn Curry and Jon F. Wergin (San Francisco: Jossey-Bass, 1993).

2. Walter McDonald, "ACP-ASIM Pressroom on the New Charter on Medical Professionalism," at *http://www.acponline.org/running_ethics/physicians_charter,* accessed July 19, 2011.

3. Harold Sox, "Medical Professionalism in the New Millennium: A Physician Charter," *Annals of Internal Medicine* 136 (2002): 243–6.

4. Paul Starr, *The Social Transformation of American Medicine* (New York: Basic Books, 1984).

5. Harold Sox, "The Ethical Foundations of Professionalism," *Chest* 131 (2007): 1532–40.

6. E. J. Emmanuel and L. L. Emmanuel, "What Is Accountability in Health Care?" *Annals of Internal Medicine* 124 (1996): 229–39.

7. R. L. Cruess and S. R. Cruess, "Renewing Professionalism: An Opportunity for Medicine," *Academic Medicine* 74 (1999): 878–84; R. L. Cruess,

S. R. Cruess, and S. E. Johnston, "Professionalism: An Ideal to Be Sustained," *Lancet* 356 (2000): 156–9.

8. D. A. Axelrod and S. D. Goold, "Maintaining Trust in the Surgeon–Patient Relationship: Challenges for the New Millennium," *Archives of Surgery* 135 (2000): 55–6.

9. Edmund D. Pellegrino, "Professionalism, Profession, and the Virtues of the Good Physician," *Mount Sinai Journal of Medicine* 69 (2002): 378–84.

10. ACP-ASIM, "Medical Professionalism in the New Millennium: A Physician Charter," project of the ABIM Foundation, ACP-ASIM Foundation, and the European Federation of Internal Medicine, *Annals of Internal Medicine* 136 (2002): 243–6.

11. Dennis McDonagh, "Medical Professionalism," *Northeast Florida Medicine Supplement* (January, 2008): 7.

CHAPTER 4

Abortion and Maternal-Fetal Care

John Paul Slosar

Difficult Questions

Clinical situations involving the termination of a pregnancy are always difficult. Such situations sometimes involve a threat to the life of a pregnant woman, her fetus, or both. In such cases, the woman (or couple) is often faced with a tragic choice between saving her own life or that of her fetus. In other cases, there is no immediate threat to the health of the woman, but there are other factors, such as social pressures or the condition of the unborn baby itself, that may motivate pregnant women to contemplate ending a pregnancy. In contemporary health care ethics, such questions are often resolved by focusing primarily, if not exclusively, on the autonomy of the woman, which basically means the woman has the ultimate right to decide what should be done based on her own values. Following this line of reasoning, the courts in the United States have essentially ruled that such decisions are private ones that the woman alone has the right to make. Resolving the underlying ethical question is more difficult, however, in light of our normative basis, which recognizes the sanctity of human life at all stages of development and seeks to respect and protect both the mother and the fetus. The tension inherent in such situations is illustrated in the following cases.

Case 4A

Bill and Tanya are excited about having their first baby. Eight weeks into the pregnancy, Tanya's obstetrician (OB) recommends that she undergo first trimester screening for Trisomy 21, more commonly known as Down syndrome. Tanya, who is only 28 years old, asks her physician if there is a reason she needs to be concerned, as she thought that test was only recommended for women 35 years or older. Her physician replies that the new standard is to do first trimester screening on all women and then do a confirmatory test if the screen indicates there is a risk. A week later, her obstetrician calls and says the screening came back positive with biochemical markers that indicate it is possible her baby has the extra chromosome that causes Down syndrome. Her physician then recommends Tanya undergo either amniocentesis or chorionic villus sampling (CVS) when she reaches the mid-second trimester. In the meantime, the physician explains to her that, even if the confirmatory test comes back positive, there is still the chance of a false positive, and if indeed the baby does have Down syndrome, there is no way to know how severe the baby's condition will be. "It could be very mild or very significant," the physician explains, "but you should know your options, and in 85 to 95 percent of cases of a positive result, women choose to terminate the pregnancy."

Case 4B

Laura A., a 29-year-old woman who is 20 weeks pregnant, comes to the emergency room because her "water has broken" prematurely (preterm premature rupture of membranes). The baby's heart is still beating, and Laura is not in immediate danger. Still she is admitted to the hospital for observation and bed rest. Her chart notes that she has no children but has lost two previous pregnancies due to miscarriage. On the fourth day in the hospital, Tanya begins running a fever and showing other signs of infection. Her OB physician starts antibiotics right away. Despite the use of intravenous (IV) antibiotics, Laura's infection

cont.

Case 4B *cont.*

continues to worsen. Her physician tells her and her husband, Keith, that she has an infection of the amniotic fluid and chorion (chorioamnionitis) and that Laura could die if they do not induce labor and deliver the baby as soon as possible. The physician also tells them that at this stage in the pregnancy, the baby will inevitably die within hours of being born because its lungs are not fully developed.

Case 4C

Jane, a mother of three children, aged 17 months, two and a half years, and five years, discovered she was pregnant again when she was six weeks along. In the past, she would have been happy about this news, but at the end of her last pregnancy she had acquired a condition known as peripartum cardiomyopathy and had been instructed not to become pregnant again. Cardiomyopathy is a form of heart disease in which the muscle of the heart is weakened and has difficulty pumping adequate levels of blood throughout the body. Pregnancy is contraindicated for patients with cardiomyopathy because the increase in blood volume that occurs naturally in pregnancy can result in cardiac failure and death. At eight weeks of pregnancy, Jane underwent a chemical stress test of her heart to determine whether she could carry the pregnancy to term. The test had to be stopped when only half complete because Jane began experiencing ventricular tachycardia, a potentially lethal abnormal rhythm in the heart. Jane's physician strongly recommended that she terminate the pregnancy because the test showed conclusively that her heart was not strong enough to carry the pregnancy to viability. Jane, a faithful Catholic, resisted, saying she would rather try to carry the pregnancy as close as possible to viability. At 10 weeks, Jane went to the emergency department of the Catholic hospital in town with chest pain and difficulty breathing. She was admitted, and they attempted to manage her arrhythmia medically, but they could not stabilize her. The physicians called an ethics consult because they saw no other option but to terminate the pregnancy using surgical means, thereby, relieving the stress on Jane's heart.

These cases are discussed throughout this chapter as we consider some of the major ethical issues related to abortion, particularly issues that arise in the area of maternal-fetal care when there is a threat to the well-being of the mother, fetus, or both. We begin by setting the clinical, social, and legal context and then move on to a discussion of the ethics of abortion, using as our starting point Catholic teaching in this area. Although our normative basis may lead to a broader ethical analysis of the issues at hand, Catholic teaching on abortion and maternal-fetal care provides a solid basis for shaping our discussion. Catholic teaching on abortion and maternal-fetal care is rooted in centuries of the Catholic moral tradition, as are many of the values and principles that ground our normative basis, most notably human dignity and justice. As you read this chapter, think about the cases above. How would you counsel Laura, who is faced with either losing yet another pregnancy or placing her own life at grave risk? If Tanya's additional test is positive, what is the moral status of a decision to terminate the pregnancy? Is terminating Jane's pregnancy to save her life morally problematic? This chapter is not meant to provide ready-made answers to these questions but to help you consider the ethical questions of such situations against the backdrop of our normative basis.

Setting the Context: Clinical, Social, and Legal Considerations

Induced abortion can be defined as the medical or surgical termination of pregnancy before the time of fetal viability.[1] According to a report published in the medical journal *Lancet* in 2007, an estimated 42 million abortions were performed worldwide in 2003, which is lower than the estimated 46 million that were estimated to have occurred in 1995.[2] In the United States, the abortion rate hit its highest in 1973, remained fairly constant through the 1980s, and has been slowly declining since, with an estimated 1.2 million abortions performed in 2005, approximately 8 percent fewer than in 2000.[3] Approximately 60 percent of abortions are performed within the first 8 weeks of pregnancy, and another 8 percent are performed between 8 and 12 weeks.[4] The method of abortion used depends, in part, on what stage of pregnancy has been reached when the abortion is performed.

Types of Abortion Procedures

In the first 12 weeks (the first trimester), vacuum aspiration (suction curettage) is the most common procedure for terminating pregnancy. This procedure consists of placing a tube (cannula) into the uterus and sucking the amniotic fluid, placenta, and fetus through the cannula.[5] Vacuum aspiration has essentially replaced the procedure known as a dilation and curettage (D&C) because of the high rate of complications associated with D&C procedures. Vacuum aspiration can be performed using either manual vacuum aspiration (MVA) or electric pump aspiration (EPA). In the early stage of the first trimester, MVA is seen as the clinically more effective method over EPA, because in the vast majority of cases, MVA removes the amniotic fluid, placenta, and early fetus intact (see figure 4.1), thus making it easier to confirm that the procedure is complete.[6]

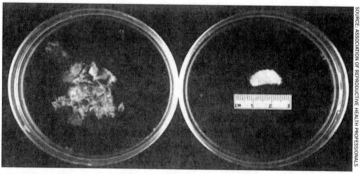

SOURCE: ASSOCIATION OF REPRODUCTIVE HEALTH PROFESSIONALS

FIGURE 4.1. The intact products of conception, which include the placenta and early fetus, roughly 2 cm in length, following MVA are shown in the right-hand dish, and the nonintact products of conception following EPA are in the left-hand dish.

Medically induced abortions are also now possible up to nine weeks of pregnancy, using RU486.[7] RU486 is a combination of two drugs: mifepristone and misoprostol. The mifepristone is taken orally in the physician's office, and the misoprostol is taken a few days later by the woman at home. Mifepristone decreases the hormones that maintain a pregnancy and causes the embryo to detach from the uterus. Once detached the embryo dies. A few days later, a dose of misoprostol is taken to make the uterus contract and expel the embryo.

In the early part of the second trimester, 13 to 15 weeks of pregnancy, dilation and evacuation (D&E) is the most common procedure. The procedure is similar to EPA, except surgical instruments are used to remove larger pieces of fetal tissue. From 16 weeks of pregnancy on, the mid-second and third trimesters, several procedures can be used for terminating the pregnancy. At this stage, these procedures include D&E (discussed above), intact dilation and extraction (D&X), induction of labor and delivery, and cesarean section (C-section). Intact D&X, a particularly controversial procedure, involves using instruments to turn the baby to the breech position so that its feet are facing out. Once in the breech position, the entire body of the fetus, except its head, is extracted from the woman. The fetus's skull is then collapsed, and the dead but otherwise intact fetus is removed.

Induction of labor and delivery involves administering synthetic hormones or inducing agents to the woman to cause contractions, that is, to cause her to go into labor, and deliver the fetus. This can be done following 16 weeks of pregnancy, once the woman's body has developed the biological receptors to respond to the synthetic hormones. Nothing is done to the fetus directly, except it is expelled from the uterus along with the placenta and amniotic fluid. Most often the fetus survives the delivery, but dies shortly after being born, depending on how far along the pregnancy is at the time labor is induced, how far the baby has developed, and whether it has any life-threatening conditions. A few babies have been known to survive after being born at only 23 weeks of pregnancy (14 to 17 weeks early).[8] In these cases, the baby almost always requires aggressive neonatal intensive care (which is discussed later) for the first few months of its life and has significant disabilities and developmental problems. With every week that the pregnancy can be extended beyond 23 weeks, the baby is more likely to survive and have fewer disabilities and developmental problems. A C-section is similar to the induction of labor and delivery, except that contractions are not started. Rather, the baby is delivered through an incision in the woman's abdomen.

All of the above procedures are clinically accepted ways to terminate a pregnancy. Which method is chosen depends in part on the stage of pregnancy at the time the decision is made to abort and whether that decision is elective or medically indicated. A significant similarity between the procedures of EPA, D&C, D&E, and intact D&X is that they all result in the death of the fetus before its being removed from the womb. Indeed, all of these procedures require destroying the fetus as part of the process of removing it. In the case of MVA, the fetus is not necessarily destroyed as a direct result of the procedure used to evacuate the uterus but nonetheless dies as a result of being detached from it. In the cases of induction of labor and delivery and C-section, the fetus is not destroyed in the process of removing it from the womb, but the fetus often dies as a result of being born prematurely. When the fetus dies as a "side effect" of the induction of labor and delivery or a C-section performed primarily for the purpose of saving the mother's life, this is sometimes referred to in the moral context as an "indirect abortion." Generally speaking, an indirect abortion occurs when the primary purpose of the procedure is to save the life of the mother and the fetus dies as a side effect of the lifesaving treatment. In a "direct abortion," the primary purpose is ending the life of the fetus for some other ultimate goal besides eliminating a threat to the woman's life.

As the case of Laura (4B) illustrates, often the reason for an abortion is not a matter of choice, but the pregnancy is being terminated for medical reasons, that is, to save the life of the woman. Some conditions in which pregnancy termination might be clinically indicated for the purpose of saving the life of the mother include cardiomyopathy (as in Case 4A), pulmonary hypertension (a similar condition to that of cardiomyopathy but involving the lungs), renal failure, chorioamnionitis (as in Case 4B), preeclampsia (pregnancy-related high blood pressure), extreme cases of hyperemesis gravidarum (excessive pregnancy-induced vomiting), and placental abruption, previa, or accrete (conditions involving an abnormal placental attachment that carries a risk of hemorrhaging). In other cases, abortion might be pursued not because of the physical health of the mother but because of a medical condition affecting the unborn child, as in the case of Tanya (4A).

In these types of cases, the decision to abort a pregnancy might be driven by the potential that the fetus will have an abnormality perceived to negatively affect the child's future quality of life or add a significant burden on the parents raising such a child. Today, many tests are available that can reveal the presence of such conditions well before birth. In particular, advances in prenatal diagnosis have increased the ability to identify a fetus with a genetic anomaly or other birth defect, such as anencephaly or Down syndrome (as in Case 4A), earlier in the course of pregnancy. For example, in 2007, the American College of Obstetrics and Gynecology (AGOC) issued a new set of clinical guidelines that recommend screening for chromosome aneuploidy, an abnormal number of chromosomes, for all women in the first trimester of pregnancy "regardless of maternal age."[9] If a woman is found to be at risk of having a baby with a chromosomal abnormality, such as Trisomy 21 (Down syndrome), Trisomy 18, or Trisomy 13, she would then undergo amniocentesis, in which medical personnel draw out a sample of amniotic fluid, or chorionic villus sampling (CVS), similar to amniocentesis but involving the small projections from the chorionic membrane that help ensure sufficient maternal blood flow to the fetus, to test for more conclusive indicators that the baby does actually have the chromosomal abnormality. As alluded to in Case 4A, however, these tests cannot indicate the severity (or lack thereof) of the condition, and there are no curative interventions.

The practice of prenatal screening or diagnosis for genetic conditions that cannot be cured raises several significant ethical issues. First is the issue of ensuring adequate informed consent. This particularly applies when the woman is being provided with the information about false-positive rates, exactly what information the tests will and will not yield, and what options are available for responding to a positive test. If this information is not provided until after the first round of screening has been done, as in Case 4A, then we would view this as an ethically problematic practice. Also of ethical concern is the fact that the pregnancy termination rate following a prenatal diagnosis of Trisomy 21 is between 85 and 95 percent.[10] In these circumstances, what are the implications of such a high rate of abortion? Does this mean that pro-life individuals should never consider prenatal diagnoses? Should pro-life organizations, such as Catholic health care, always and everywhere refrain from providing these services? How ought we to ensure that such information is provided as part of counseling in a way that does not bias the decision-making process? Another ethical concern raised by the prevalence of first-trimester screening relates to the distribution of resources, the common good, and stewardship. Is there a high enough risk of chromosome aneuploidy for all women, regardless of maternal age, to justify the expense of such screening? Are we as a society dedicating enough resources so that families who have children with chromosome abnormalities are supported and have access to services needed to care for such children? Although prenatal diagnosis is clearly related to maternal decisions to pursue abortion as an individual reproductive choice in the clinical context, it also raises less obvious questions regarding the social factors that contribute to abortion. We discuss different types of prenatal diagnosis in more detail in chapter 6, but for now we turn to the social factors that contribute to decisions to terminate a pregnancy.

The Social and Legal Status of Abortion in the United States

Often, the reason for an abortion is related not to a medical condition but to social pressures. A review of nineteen studies from eight countries identifying reasons women give for having an abortion found that the most common were a sense of being too young to be a mother, not wanting a disabled child, the absence of a partner to help raise the child, being in an abusive relationship, pressure from the genetic father, the pregnancy resulted from sexual assault, and a lack of financial resources.[11] It has not always been the case, however, that abortion was as socially or legally accepted as it is today.

Throughout most of U.S. history, abortion has been illegal. In fact, as recently as 1965, abortion at all stages of pregnancy was prohibited by law, though forty-six states and the District of Columbia allowed abortions to save the life of the mother. The legal landscape changed with the landmark case *Roe v. Wade* (1973).[12] In this case, the Supreme Court struck down as unconstitutional almost all state laws that restricted abortion. The court ruled that laws prohibiting abortion violated a woman's right to privacy, which is not explicit in the U.S. Constitution but has its basis in the Bill of Rights and in the concept of liberty as guaranteed by the Fourteenth Amendment. The Fourteenth Amendment provides protection for each person regarding due process and equal protection under the Constitution. However, as part of its decision in *Roe v. Wade*, the court ruled that the unborn fetus is not a person in the "whole sense" and, therefore, not deserving of protection under the Fourteenth Amendment.

Rather than entitling the fetus to protection under the Fourteenth Amendment, the ruling in *Roe v. Wade* sets limits on the laws states can enact to prohibit abortion, based on which trimester of pregnancy has been reached. Specifically, the ruling declares that during the first trimester, the decision to abort is a medical judgment belonging to the woman's physician and cannot be prohibited by law. During the second trimester, states may regulate abortion, as long as they allow for exceptions to protect the woman's health, as defined by the state. In the third trimester, states are permitted to regulate and even prohibit abortions, as long as they permit exceptions for protecting the woman's health and preserving her life. *Roe v. Wade* is not the only case in which the U.S. Supreme Court has ruled on the question of abortion.

In the case of *Planned Parenthood v. Casey*,[13] the *Roe v. Wade* ruling was affirmed and even expanded. In this case the Court stated that only a pregnant woman—not the state—has the authority to determine whether the unborn fetus should be counted as a member of the community, deserving of protection. The court's rationale in *Casey* for giving the woman this authority was twofold. First, the "mother who carries a child to full term is subject to the anxieties, to physical constraints, to pain that only she must bear." Second, the court ruled that the state cannot impose an undue burden on a woman's right to have an abortion by placing a "substantial obstacle in the path of the woman seeking an abortion before the fetus attains viability." Again the stage of pregnancy is given legal weight in the context of abortion insofar as the fetus is provided additional protections once it has attained "viability" (the point at which it would be capable of surviving outside of the uterus).

In legal contexts unrelated to abortion, however, more than half of the states consider human life as beginning with conception, that is, with the completion of fertilization. Indeed, many states give the embryo legal protection outside the context of abortion either by statute, resolution, or court decisions. For example, Missouri law states that "the life of a human being begins at conception," and legally defines the term *unborn child* as including embryos and fetuses "from the moment of conception until birth at every stage of biological development."[14] If someone murders a pregnant woman in Missouri, that person could be found guilty of two homicides. Thus the legal status of early human life in this country represents a somewhat schizophrenic outlook. On the one hand, pregnant women have, as stated in the ruling in *Planned Parenthood v. Casey*, the "right to define one's own concept of existence, of meaning, of the universe, and the mystery of life," within the context of deciding whether to have an abortion. On the other hand, outside the context of abortion, states can and do offer the embryo and fetus the same legal protections afforded to other human beings. Somewhat ironically, some states give legal protection to the embryo even earlier than most doctors would recognize a woman as being pregnant: the common medical definition recognizes pregnancy as beginning with implantation of the embryo.

The Intersection of Law, Public Policy, Ethics, and Abortion

The U.S. Supreme Court used the stages of fetal development in pregnancy as criteria for certain restrictions on what individual states could and could not prohibit. The Supreme Court later tightened restrictions on what individual states could prohibit, using the point of viability as the key consideration. The question of when viability begins and who gets to define it is truly significant from both a legal and ethical standpoint. If, for example, a fetus could survive on its own outside the womb, that is, if it were truly viable, the induction of labor and delivery or a C-section, or indeed any method of terminating pregnancy that did not entail the destruction of the fetus, would not be considered an abortion from either an ethical or a legal perspective (by implication of the ruling in *Planned Parenthood v. Casey*). These considerations illustrate how the legal and ethical questions regarding abortion intersect.

The question of when viability begins, however, is not the only significant question in the legal and ethical contexts of abortion. As is clear from the preceding discussion of the Supreme Court's rationale, the question of whether and when human life ought to be deserving of our respect and protection has been central to the legal debate regarding abortion. For example, the decision in *Planned Parenthood v. Casey* explicitly turned on the consideration of whether the fetus should be considered a person deserving of the same respect and protection as other members of the community.

Debate in the public sphere was reignited in 2009, when President Barack Obama introduced health care reform legislation known as the Patient Protection and Affordable Care Act (PPACA). This legislation, which eventually passed, included government-funded multistate insurance exchanges. With regard to abortion, the legislation required that at least one insurance plan in the exchange not cover elective abortions. Many pro-life organizations, including the U.S. Conference of Catholic Bishops (USCCB), saw this as possibly forcing families with complex medical circumstances to contribute to and fund insurance plans that include abortion in the event that the one plan that does not cover abortion may not cover all the complex medical needs of all families. Another point of contention held by pro-life individuals and groups was that the PPACA could create a loophole—an area not covered under the Hyde Amendment, which prohibits the use of federal tax money for funding abortions—that might enable the appropriation of millions of tax dollars for funding abortions.

Although the practical implications of the legislation in these respects remains open for debate, few have recognized or acknowledged that the legislation contains provisions intended to address social factors leading to abortion. For example, the PPACA includes a permanent tax credit for parents who adopt a child. Moreover, the PPACA allocates $250 million ($25 million per year for 10 years) for the express purpose of supporting women who are pregnant or parenting and considered vulnerable members of society. The social services named for funding include counseling and community services, job training, housing assistance, and individual and group counseling aimed at preventing domestic violence, sexual violence, sexual assault, or stalking, as well as services improving care for female victims of sexual assault.[15] In this way, the PPACA actually contains positive provisions intended to address many of the social factors that are often the primary reason a woman may see no other option but to abort.

Discussion: Ethical Issues and Analysis

Respect for Autonomy and the Moral Status of Early Human Life

As in the legal context, the ethical debate on abortion has centered less on the contributing social factors and more on the question of personhood and who counts as a person. When should the product of conception (an embryo, a fetus, or an infant) be considered a person deserving of moral respect and protection? Three primary characteristics of contemporary Western ethical culture have influenced the public debate on the moral status of unborn life: (1) ethical relativism, (2) mind–body dualism, and (3) the supreme value of autonomy.

Ethical Relativism. Ethical relativism (the view that what is right or wrong is relative to a particular group of people or an individual) has given rise to the view that there are no moral truths that hold for everyone everywhere. As in the *Planned Parenthood v. Casey* ruling, ethics and values are defined by each individual or, at best, by social consensus. Within this framework are few shared normative limits, and ethics is viewed as legalistic. Accordingly, public morality is seen as primarily a matter of law. This implies that social ethics is understood as the minimum constraint on freedom necessary for individuals to be able to live together, and consent is the only ethical principle that can bind individuals who do not share the same moral values.[16] As such, the role of ethics in prescribing what one ought to do to promote human flourishing is limited to the individual or private sphere of life.

Mind–Body Dualism. The primary underlying view of human nature in the West is fundamentally dualistic. The idea that a human being is essentially a body inhabited by a mind dates back at least to Plato. Numerous thinkers throughout history—including some within the Christian tradition, such as Augustine—have embraced this perspective. The popularity of this dualistic view in the modern period can be traced to the philosopher René Descartes, who offered the famous adage *"cogito ergo sum"* ("I think, therefore I am"). The dualistic view holds that the body and the mind are two distinct, independent realities. The body is most closely associated with being human, while the mind and one's mental capacities are more closely associated with what makes someone a person.

Supreme value of autonomy. Autonomy (understood as the capacity for rational thought and the ability to determine for oneself what is right and wrong, good and bad) is seen as the supreme value within contemporary Western secular culture. In light of the supreme value of autonomy, human life is often seen as having value only when an individual has the capacity to act autonomously. However, in some religious traditions, such as Christianity and Judaism, human life is seen as having a basic intrinsic value because people are made in the image and likeness of God. Moreover, we have autonomy precisely *because* we are made in the image and likeness of God. Viewed theologically, life—the most basic of values, enabling all other values to be pursued—places constraints on autonomous action. In secular ethical thought, however, autonomy has been given such significance that the ability to exercise one's autonomous capacities has become synonymous with what it means to be a human person.[17] Thus the question of when personhood begins has long been the center of the abortion debate. Regarding the moral status of the fetus, two of the more predominant views can be described as the nonpersonal position and the personal position.

1. **Nonpersonal Position.** The nonpersonal view of the fetus is influenced by, and consistent with, the moral relativism and dualism described above and has been reinforced in the legal context by *Roe v. Wade* and *Planned Parenthood v. Casey*. According to this position, a fetus does not deserve the same respect and protection as other members of the moral community because it is not capable of functioning in ways characteristically associated with being a person. That is, it cannot make free choices, communicate, plan for the future, participate in social life, or do anything else commonly associated with fully conscious, autonomous, rational individuals. Consequently, a fetus is not a person but only a "potential person." This view is based on a strong distinction between and separation of being "human" and being a "person." As the philosopher Peter Singer writes,

> These two senses of "human being" overlap but do not coincide. The embryo, the later fetus, the profoundly

intellectually disabled child, even the newborn infant—
all are indisputably members of the species Homo sapi-
ens, but none are self-aware, have a sense of the future,
or the capacity to relate to others.[18]

The philosopher H. Tristam Engelhardt Jr. writes,

> Not every person need be human, and not every human
> is a person. In order to understand the geography of
> obligations in health care regarding fetuses, infants,
> the profoundly mentally retarded and the severely
> brain damaged, one will need to determine the moral
> status of a "person" and of mere human biological life,
> and then develop criteria to distinguish between these
> classes of entities.[19]

From a theological perspective, the nonpersonal position is
inadequate for two main reasons. First, according to the view of
the human person as made in the image and likeness of God,
there is much more to being a human person than being fully
conscious, autonomous, and rational. Rather, humans are insepa-
rably physical and material, creative and spiritual, relational and
social, as well as morally free and responsible.[20] Simply because
a human being may not have the capacity to actualize or realize
fully one of these innate capacities does not necessarily make
that human being less than a person.

Second, the nonpersonal position fails to recognize the
developmental dimension of human life. That is, the fact that
we grow through different developmental stages at which we
have different capabilities does not imply that we are not the
same human being that existed as a six-cell embryo when we are
80 years old. We are, in fact, one and the same individual, just
at different stages in our natural course of development. That
we exhibit different capacities at different life stages does not
mean our underlying nature (what kind of being we are, and
what form our ultimate fulfillment takes) also changes. To claim
otherwise is to ignore not only the developmental dimension of
human life but also its inherent and necessary continuity. As the
philosopher Stephen Schwarz argues,

The fact that my capabilities to function as a person have changed and grown does not alter the absolute continuity of my essential being, that of a person. In fact, this variation in capabilities presupposes the continuity of my being as a person. It is as a person that I develop my capabilities to function as a person.[21]

From a theological perspective, the nonpersonal position is arbitrary. Moreover, a social consensus regarding what criteria ought to be included in the definition of a *person* has never been reached. The debate regarding what should be included in this definition goes nowhere in the face of moral pluralism (competing and irreducible views of morality). Furthermore, the nonpersonal position lacks any inherent reason for why only a *person* is deserving of moral respect and protection.

From the perspective of our normative basis, the question of personhood is not the only, or even the main, question regarding abortion. Rather, four other interrelated questions are of primary importance: What value does early human life have? What respect does it deserve? What is the nature of our relationship as individuals and as communities with early human life? Who are we called to be in that relationship?

2. **Personal Position:** The personal position represents the strongest claims regarding the moral status of unborn life. According to this position, the product of conception deserves absolute respect and protection from the time the process of fertilization is complete. Moreover, the product of fertilization (the zygote) deserves moral respect and protection regardless of whether it ever actually becomes capable of conscious, autonomous, and rational thought. To call this the personal position is perhaps somewhat ironic, because this position does not rest on the assumption that the product of fertilization is in fact a person. According to this view, moral respect and protection are deserved not because we attribute "personhood" to a living being, but because that being is a human life. Still it is appropriate to refer to this position as the personal position precisely because it grants the moral respect and protection that

we would give to a person to all human life, at every stage of development from conception to death.

The strongest supporter of the personal position has been the Catholic Church. According to Church teaching,

> In reality, respect of human life is called for from the time that the process of generation begins. From the time that the ovum is fertilized, a life is begun which is neither that of the father nor of the mother; it is rather the life of a new human being with its own growth. It would never be made human if it were not human already.[22]

This position has been reaffirmed in subsequent Church teachings:

> The fruit of human generation from the first moment of its existence, that is to say, from the moment the zygote has formed, demands the unconditional respect that is morally due to the human being in his bodily and spiritual totality. The human being is to be respected and treated as a person from the moment of conception and therefore from the same moment his [or her] rights as a person must be recognized, among which in the first place is the individual right of every innocent human being to life.[23]

The personal position on the moral status of unborn life is based on three key claims.[24] First, a genetically unique human life comes into being at the moment the process of fertilization is complete. Second, science alone cannot answer the philosophical question of when personhood begins but can only confirm the biological point at which human life begins. Third, regardless of whether the embryo is a person, it is a grave sin to disrupt the biological process of human development once started. Ultimately, the foundation for this position is the inherent value of all human life, considered as a gift of divine love freely given by a beneficent creator, God. For those who recognize all human life as having some inherent moral worth, the question of abortion in the clinical context does not concern when personhood begins so much as what the sanctity of human life requires of us morally, particularly in the presence of a complex maternal-fetal care situation.

Abortion and the Sanctity and Dignity of Life

Within our normative basis, the sanctity of life is founded on the intrinsic moral worth of all human life, that is, human dignity, considered as the basis of our rights and moral responsibilities. Within the Christian and Judaic religious traditions, the sanctity of life and its inherent dignity is rooted in the concept of *imago Dei* (Latin for "image of God"). This concept denotes the theological view that human beings are made in the image and likeness of God and destined for eternal union with God. Biblically, this means that we are all God's children. Philosophically, this is usually understood as referring to the physical and material, spiritual and intellectual, social and relational, and moral dimensions of human life. It also refers to our responsibility as "created cocreators" to use our autonomy and other rational capabilities to care for our human brothers and sisters and all of God's creation. Insofar as we are created cocreators, that is, made in the image and likeness of God, we are not restricted to obeying God blindly but are able to obey God intelligently and freely. Obeying God intelligently and freely means that we use our intelligence and experience to carry out God's purpose creatively and discern for ourselves what is right and wrong as understood in light of human flourishing, virtue, and right relationships.

A direct implication of this understanding of the sanctity of human life is that every human being should be acknowledged as an inherently valuable member of the human community and as a unique expression of life. In this way, the sanctity of life and its inherent dignity provide the foundation for a Christian understanding of the right to life. According to this understanding, the right to life establishes an absolute obligation never to intend the destruction of innocent human life. Understood in this context, the right to life does not necessarily imply a positive obligation always to do everything that can be done to save human life. Nor does the right to life so understood imply an obligation never to do something that might indirectly result in the death of a human being.

This understanding of the human person as created in the image and likeness of God taken together with the fact that human flourishing is only possible in and through community implies that we all have a responsibility to foster right relationships and help others to achieve human well-being and to live a flourishing life to the greatest extent possible. In this sense, we also have positive responsibilities to form right relationships and to help others, not just negative obligations to avoid harming others. Together these implications of the sanctity and dignity of human life give rise to the first principle of ethics: do good and avoid evil. In the clinical context, the ethical questions related to the termination of pregnancy are especially difficult when we acknowledge the reality of the sanctity and dignity of human life and the fact that we are already in a community (i.e., in a relationship) with early human life. How do we do good when evil cannot be avoided, as in cases of maternal-fetal vital conflict? Whose life should we save? Which course of action best promotes human flourishing in a community? What should we do when we have information regarding a fetal anomaly, but there is no therapeutic or curative intervention? To whom do we have the greater obligation, the mother or the unborn baby, when conflicting values are at stake?

Addressing the Tension

Consider again the case of Laura (4B), the 29-year-old woman who is 20 weeks pregnant and is developing a life-threatening infection (chorioamnionitis). If the pregnancy is terminated at this stage, the fetus will probably not survive more than a few hours. After trying to control the infection with antibiotics, Laura's physician recommends induction of labor and delivery, even though he foresees that the fetus will die as a result. The moral tension in this case arises from the fact that the physician wants to save Laura's life, but the only way to do so involves terminating the pregnancy before the fetus can survive outside the womb. Within our normative framework, resolving this tension depends largely on whether the primary purpose for terminating the pregnancy can be considered consistent with the sanctity and dignity of human life, the requirements of virtue, and our responsibilities as created cocreators to help others achieve human well-being.

In this case, the primary purpose, or intention, of inducing labor and delivery is to rid Laura's body of the amniotic fluid and chorion containing the source of the infection, thereby eliminating the threat to her life. We have a pretty good idea that this is the primary purpose because the physician first tried to cure or at least control the infection by using antibiotics. Thus the physician only recommended induction of labor and delivery once the only other way of eliminating the threat to Laura's life, which did not involve terminating the pregnancy, had failed. We also know that the primary purpose is to cure Laura, because the physician did not recommend the induction until the infection became severe enough to present a real threat to Laura's life. We can sum up the physician's recommendation to terminate the pregnancy through induction of labor and delivery as a "last resort" for saving Laura's life.

Insofar as the physician's primary purpose is to save Laura's life, we can see that the choice to induce labor and delivery in this case is not out of any disrespect for the sanctity and dignity of the fetus's life, despite the fact that the physician foresees that it will die as a result of the lifesaving procedure. In the moral context, labor and delivery in this case is what we would call an "indirect" abortion. It is "indirect" insofar as the death of the fetus is a foreseen side effect that is tolerated for only a proportionately serious reason, namely, saving the life of the mother.

While we would have preferred that both Laura's life and the life of the fetus could have been saved, that is not a possible outcome, and the physician should not be blamed or held morally responsible for the death of the fetus. In fact, not only should the physician not be held morally responsible for the fetus's death in this case, but one could make a strong case from our normative basis that his actions are virtuous. If labor and delivery are not induced, both Laura and her baby will die. Thus by not inducing labor and delivery, we would allow the loss of two lives. If, on the other hand, Laura consents to the induction and is saved, she and Keith can continue caring for one another and possibly try to have another baby, if they desire. Thus in this case, inducing labor and delivery is the course of action that best promotes right relationships and human well-being.

Although this scenario provides a relatively clear example of how we might morally reason our way through a dilemma involving a maternal-fetal conflict entailing a threat to the mother's life in light of our normative basis, different circumstances can give rise to a contrary conclusion. Contrast the case of Laura and Keith with that of Tanya and Bill (4A). In the latter case, there is no threat to Tanya's life, but prenatal testing indicates the baby may itself be affected by a genetic anomaly that might be more of a social and economic strain on their family and may negatively influence the *perceived* quality of life of their child. In this case, if Bill and Tanya were to choose to terminate the pregnancy, there would be no therapeutic or curative effect of that action on Tanya, precisely because the baby's condition is not a pathological condition of Tanya and poses no threat to her life. In this case, then, the primary purpose of the act in question is to end the life of the baby for the purpose of not bearing a child with such a condition.

Within our normative framework, terminating the pregnancy in this case would not be considered consistent with respect for human dignity and the sanctity of life. The death of the fetus in this case would not be a foreseen but unintended side effect of a curative treatment for Tanya but rather the primary means by which certain negative consequences of having a child with this condition are avoided. Thus the intentional destruction of the fetus, for whatever perceived benefit might result, would constitute a disregard for the fetus's right to life as understood in its Christian fullness. In this regard, we should take care to remember that an individual's inability to fully actualize the spiritual and moral capacities of human life and the perceived diminished quality of life that some might assign to that individual do not justify the destruction of that life. To the contrary, in such cases, virtue calls us to respond to the individual's inherent moral worth, to recognize that person as a vulnerable member of our community, and to take steps to help that individual actualize his or her human capacities to the greatest extent to which he or she may be able. By responding to the call of virtue, we as individuals and as a community can become more accepting of our own human finitude, as well as the limits of others and, ultimately, more disposed to respond with solidarity to those whose health status makes them vulnerable.

The high rate of termination following a positive prenatal diagnosis for a genetic anomaly, even though such a diagnosis does not yield any information regarding the severity of the condition, would seem to indicate that this is an area of opportunity for our society to grow in compassion and virtue. Moreover, within our framework, prenatal testing should not be undertaken with the intention of aborting a fetus found to have a genetic anomaly. However, we must be careful not to place more responsibility on particular individuals than is appropriate. Although individual virtue is a necessary element for improving our practice within this area, society must also be pro-active in creating the circumstances in which families who choose to raise a child with a genetic condition can flourish.

Of course, this case raises more questions than whether Tanya should or shouldn't terminate her pregnancy. For example, given that within our normative framework no one should ever undergo prenatal testing with the intent of aborting a fetus with a genetic anomaly, are there other reasons that would be morally valid for undertaking prenatal testing? What are these reasons? How does society need to change to better support families that choose to bear and bring up a child known to have a genetic anomaly? What resources does society need to provide for these families? How can we affect a shift in societal attitudes to be more accepting of persons with genetic conditions? These are all important questions within our framework that need to be addressed at the micro, middle, and macro levels of ethics.

While the case of Laura (4B) provides us with a relatively clear example of when terminating a pregnancy would be considered morally just within our normative framework, and the case of Tanya (4A) offers a counterexample of when it would not be so, the case of Jane (4C) provides an example of how different circumstances can give rise to greater complexity and the need for further discernment. Although it may initially appear that Jane's case is more similar to that of Laura (in which the death of the fetus is a side effect of a lifesaving intervention) than to that of Tanya (in which there is no threat to Tanya's life), the complexity and need for further discernment in Jane's case centers on the question of whether the death of the fetus would be a side effect of a lifesaving intervention or is itself the means by which Jane's life would be saved. Some might argue, for example, that because the way to eliminate the increased blood volume, which is a normal, expected, and usually healthy response to pregnancy, is to terminate the pregnancy, doing so constitutes a direct attack against the fetus. Thus, though with the aim of securing the noble end of saving Jane's life, terminating the pregnancy in this case would not be consistent with respect for the sanctity of life and the corresponding right to life.[25] Others might argue, in contrast, that because the danger or threat to Jane's life would not exist but for the pregnancy, the pregnancy is itself a pathological condition. Thus in this case, the procedure of terminating the pregnancy and that of saving Jane's life are one, indivisible human act that is justified for the purpose of saving Jane's life even though it is foreseen that the fetus will die.[26] Moreover, given that if Jane dies, the baby will also die, one might argue that it is better to act to save one life than to do nothing and lose two. How would you analyze this case?

Regardless of how one analyzes Jane's case, it raises a noteworthy consideration to which we have not yet given adequate attention. Namely, in the vast majority of cases, and certainly in those like Jane's and, perhaps to a lesser extent like Tanya's, those who decide to terminate a pregnancy do so not out of any freely made choice but precisely because they do not see that they have any choice. In such cases, one can be said to be acting out of "duress" in circumstances that, for fear of grave harm, restrict one's ability to exercise free will. Although such duress cannot make a morally bad act good, it does mitigate, if not eliminate in some cases, the moral culpability or guilt that an individual assumes for the morally bad act committed. As Pope John Paul II described it in his encyclical *The Gospel of Life*, "Decisions that go against life sometimes arise from difficult or even tragic situations of profound suffering, loneliness, a total lack of economic prospects, depression and anxiety about the future. Such circumstances can mitigate even to a notable degree subjective responsibility and the consequent culpability of those who make these choices."[27]

Conclusion

The question that has dominated the legal and ethical debates regarding abortion in this country is whether the fetus can be considered a person and, therefore, a member of the moral community. From the perspective of our normative basis, however, all human life, including fetal life, whether healthy or sick, has an inherent dignity and the right to life. If we recognize and accept this, the question becomes, under what conditions and through what procedures can terminating a pregnancy be consistent with our commitment to human life and hence morally acceptable? In rare situations, given the brokenness of human life, we will have to make fateful decisions. Nevertheless, we must always do so with an eye on what it means to live in right relationships and ultimately flourish as human beings in the context of community.

In the tragic circumstances of maternal-fetal conflict in which the life of the mother, fetus, or both is threatened, principles alone will carry us only so far. At some point, virtue, prudence, and discernment must illuminate the path to human flourishing, that is, to becoming who God is calling us to be, as individuals and as a community. In these cases, we must turn to the entire network of our human capacities to help us decide what the most loving and virtuous response is in the present circumstances. Moreover, we must realize that the development of virtue is a gradual process that occurs over time. As our own wise mentors once wrote, "Helping people to fulfill the norms of morality is not accomplished through condemnation but through patience and compassion. . . . In all things, moral behavior included, we make progress only by invoking and practicing 'patience, sympathy and time.'"[28]

Additional Case Studies

Case 4D

Stacey M., who is 41 years old and 15 weeks pregnant, has just been told her fetus has a condition known as anencephaly, in which the "higher" brain fails to develop. The baby will never be conscious and never be able to think or talk. It has a brain stem, though, which controls bodily functions, such as breathing, heartbeat, and sucking reflexes. The doctor says that if the baby is carried to term it will die within a week of being born, if not sooner. The condition poses no serious threat to Stacey's health, but the physician suggests to Stacey that it might be better to terminate the pregnancy instead of carrying it to term

cont.

Case 4D cont.

and having to deal with the psychological burden of knowing that her baby will die shortly after it is born. Some of the nurses object, arguing that the fetus should be given the chance to live as long as possible, while others think the decision ought to be Stacey's alone insofar as the baby is going to die anyway.

Discussion Questions. Do you take the side of the nurses who argue the fetus should be given the chance to live as long as possible, even if only for the remaining months of pregnancy, or the nurses who argue that the pregnancy should be terminated, because the baby will die anyway? What would you do if you were this woman or her husband? Why?

Case 4E

An 18-year-old female is admitted to the ER with preterm labor. Ultrasound reveals that she is 32 weeks pregnant. The emergency physician immediately initiates drugs to stop the contractions and stall labor for a time. The physician also administers corticosteroids to strengthen the baby's lungs in the event that the baby is delivered early. The ob-gyn on call is consulted and requests that the woman be brought to the labor and delivery unit. After reviewing the girl's ultrasound, the ob-gyn notes that the baby is in a breech position, which means that a Cesarean section will most likely be required. The girl's labor continues to progress, and fetal monitoring shows that the baby is experiencing significant fetal distress. The ob-gyn informs the girl that an emergency C-section will have to be done to save the baby. The girl, however, states that she "does not want to be cut into" and refuses to give her consent for the procedure. The ob-gyn explains that time is of the essence if the baby is to have the best outcome, but the girl is adamant that no C-section be performed. The ob-gyn insists that it must be done and the girl's grandmother, who has been with her since entering the ER, intervenes and says, "My granddaughter has made her wishes known." Furious, the ob-gyn points out that "the baby will die or be severely impaired if a C-section is not done immediately."

cont.

Case 4E *cont.*

The grandmother does not give in, however, and says that "God will do with the baby what he wills" and that if anything is done against her granddaughter's wishes, she will bring suit against the ob-gyn and the hospital. A staff nurse concerned about the situation calls for an ethics consult.

Questions. Do you think the pregnant girl in this case should be allowed to refuse the C-section even though doing so will most likely harm, maybe even kill, the baby? Does the girl's right to refuse specific medical interventions and her autonomy outweigh the potential benefit to the unborn baby, or should her refusal be overridden?

Case 4F

Christi is 22 weeks pregnant and has been diagnosed with severe preeclampsia (very high blood pressure induced by pregnancy), which has not improved with antihypertensive medications and in-hospital bed rest. The ob-gyn overseeing Christi's care is very concerned about her condition and thinks the best option is to induce delivery immediately, despite the lethal consequences for the baby. She knows, though, that despite the considerable risks to Christi (stroke, impaired kidney and liver function, blood clotting problems, pulmonary edema, seizures, and, rarely in the United States, death), they could take the chance and forestall delivery a little longer to give the baby an opportunity to live. After discussing all this with Christi, they both agree that the risks to Christi are too great and the outcome for the baby is too uncertain to wait any longer; thus, Christi is scheduled for an immediate induction.

Questions. Do you think induction is justified in this case? If so, why? If not, why not? Do you think a pathological condition of a pregnant woman must be life threatening to justify inducing when it is foreseen the baby will die? How immediate a threat to the mother's life does there need to be before induction can be justified?

SUGGESTED READINGS

Cahill, Lisa Sowle. "Abortion, Sex, and Gender: The Church's Public Voice." *America* 168 (May 22, 1993): 6–11.

Gustafson, James M. "Abortion: A Protestant Ethical Approach." In *On Moral Medicine: Theological Perspectives in Medical Ethics.* 2nd ed. Edited by S. Lammers and A. Verhey, 600–611. Grand Rapids, MI: Eerdmans, 1998.

John Paul II. "*Evangelium Vitae* [The Gospel of Life]." *Origins* 24 (April 6, 1995): 689, 691–730.

Kaveny, Cathleen. "Toward a Thomistic Perspective on Abortion and the Law in Contemporary America." *Thomist* 55 (1991): 343–96.

Marquis, Donald B. "Four Versions of Double Effect." *Journal of Medicine and Philosophy* 16 (1991): 515–44.

Walter, James J. "Theological Parameters: Catholic Doctrine on Abortion in a Pluralistic Society." In *Abortion and Public Policy: An Interdisciplinary Investigation within the Catholic Tradition*, ed. R. Rainey and G. Magill, 91–130. Omaha, NE: Creighton University Press, 1996.

MULTIMEDIA AIDS FOR TEACHERS

"The Last Abortion Clinic." *Frontline*. Public Broadcasting System. November 9, 2005. This 60-minute program reviews the history of the abortion debate in the United States, provides many facts and statistics, and examines the volatile political climate regarding *Roe v. Wade* at a time of significant change in the U.S. Supreme Court. For more information or to order copies, see *http://www.pbs.org/wgbh/pages/frontline/clinic/*.

If These Walls Could Talk. Directed by Cher. Starring Demi Moore. Rated R. 1996. This made-for-HBO movie chronicles the moral struggles of three women (one in the 1950s, one in the 1970s, and one in the 1990s) wrestling with the decision of whether to have an abortion. It is available on DVD through Amazon.com and other retailers.

Life's Greatest Miracle. Directed by Mark Davis. Starring Stacy Keach. Not Rated. 2002. This updated version of *Nova*'s original, "The Miracle of Life," narrated by John Lithgow, illustrates the complex processes that result in the birth of a baby. It is available on DVD through Amazon.com and other similar retailers.

ENDNOTES

1. F. Gary Cunningham, Kenneth J. Leveno, Steven L. Bloom, et al., *Williams Obstetrics*, 22nd ed. (New York: McGraw-Hill, 2005), 241.

2. Gilda Sedh, Stanley Henshaw, Susheela Singh, et al., "Induced Abortion: Estimated Rates and Trends Worldwide," *Lancet* 370 (2007): 1338–45.

3. Rachel K. Jones, M. R. S. Zolna, Stanley K. Henshaw, and L. B. Finer, "Abortion in the United States: Incidence and Access to Services, 2005," *Perspectives on Sexual and Reproductive Health* 40 (2008): 6–16. See also, Rachel K. Jones et al., "Trends in Abortion in the United States," *Clinical Obstetrics & Gynecology* 52 (2009): 119–29.

4. Cunningham, *Williams Obstetrics*, 241.

5. For more regarding procedures for terminating pregnancy, see Cunningham, *Williams Obstetrics*.

6. Emily Godfrey and Michelle Forcier, "Management of Early Pregnancy Failures in the Outpatient Setting," presented at ARHP 2006 National Conference, available at *https://www.arhp.org/uploadDocs/RH06_MVAPre-Con*. ppt on 9/28/2010.

7. Regarding the use of RU486, see F. Cadepond, A. Ulmann, and E. E. Baulieu, "RU486 (Mifepristone): Mechanisms of Action and Clinical Uses," *Annual Review of Medicine* 48 (1997): 129–56.

8. Regarding the survival statistics of premature neonates, see Maureen Hack, Jeffrey D. Horbar, Michael H. Malloy, Jon E. Tyson, Elizabeth Wright, and Linda Wright, "Very Low Birth Weight Outcomes of the National Institute of Child Health and Human Development Neonatal Network," *Pediatrics* 87 (May 1991): 587–97. We address the ethical issues related to the care of critically ill newborns in chapter 5.

9. Regarding the ACOG guidelines and an ethical analysis of them, see J. Tuohe and M. Repenshek, "Ethical Considerations Concerning Screening for Chromosome Aneuploidy: A Response to a 2007 American College of Obstetricians and Gynecologists Practice Bulletin," *Linacre Quarterly* 75, no. 2 (2008): 96–111.

10. M. J. Korenromp, C. M. L. Docelieve, J. van den Bout, et al., "Maternal Decision to Terminate Pregnancy after a Diagnosis of Down Syndrome," *American Journal of Obstetrics & Gynecology* 196 (2007): 149.e1–149.e11.

11. Maggie Kirkman, Heather Rowe, Annarella Hardiman, et al., "Reasons Women Give for Abortion: A Review of the Literature," *Archives of Women's Mental Health* 12 (2009): 365–78.

12. *Roe v. Wade,* 410 U.S. 959 (1973). See also B. Furrow, T. Greaney, S. Johnson, et al., *Health Law: Cases, Materials, and Problems,* 3rd ed. (Saint Paul, MN: West Group, 1997), 904–9.

13. *Planned Parenthood of Southeastern Pennsylvania et al. v. Robert P. Casey et al.,* 112 S.Ct. 2791 (1992). See also, Furrow et al., *Health Law,* 909–20.

14. Regarding the states and the different contexts in which the fetus is given legal protection, see Thomas W. Strahan, "Legal Protection of the Unborn Child Outside the Context of Induced Abortion," *Association for Interdisciplinary Research in Values and Social Change* 11 (1997).

15. See H.R. 3590, Patient Protection and Affordable Care Act, Part II, "Support for Pregnant and Parenting Teens and Women," 813–7.

16. For this account of secular ethics in the public sphere, see H. Tristram Engelhardt Jr., *The Foundations of Bioethics,* 2nd ed. (New York: Oxford University Press, 1996), 11–4.

17. See Peter Singer, *Practical Ethics,* 2nd ed. (Oxford: Cambridge University Press, 1993), 86–7. Singer argues that to be a full member of a moral community, one must be rational, self-conscious, and autonomous. For this specific list of characteristics, see Peter Singer, *Rethinking Life and Death: The Collapse of Our Traditional Ethics* (New York: St. Martin's Press, 1995), 191. This conception of the "person" is also espoused by H. Tristram Engelhardt Jr., in *The Foundations of Bioethics,* 135–40.

18. Singer, *Practical Ethics,* 86.

19. Engelhardt, *The Foundations of Bioethics,* 108.

20. This account of the nonpersonal and personal position is adapted in part from Michael R. Panicola, "Three Views on the Preimplantation Embryo," *National Catholic Bioethics Quarterly* 2 (Spring 2002): 69–97.

21. Steven D. Schwarz, *The Moral Question of Abortion* (Chicago: Loyola University Press, 1990), 93.

22. Congregation for the Doctrine of the Faith, "Declaration on Procured Abortion," *Vatican Council II* (1982), 2:441–43.

23. Congregation for the Doctrine of the Faith, "Instruction on Respect for Human Life in Its Origin and on the Dignity of Procreation," *Origins* 16, no. 40 (1987): 701–2.

24. Regarding these bases of the personal position, see Panicola, "Three Views," 69–97.

25. For an explanation of this position see, U.S. Conference of Catholic Bishops, Committee on Doctrine, "The Distinction between Direct Abortion and Legitimate Medical Procedures," at *http://usccb.org/doctrine/direct-abortion-statement2010-06-23.pdf,* accessed on December 16, 2010.

26. Regarding an argument of this nature on the permissibility of terminating pregnancy in these types of cases, see Germain Grisez, *The Way of the Lord Jesus: On Living a Christian Life,* vol. 2 (Chicago: Franciscan Herald Press, 1983), 501–3.

27. Pope John Paul II, *The Gospel of Life, Origins* 24, no. 18 (April 6, 1995).

28. Benedict Ashley, OP, Jean deBlois, CSJ, and Kevin O'Rourke, OP, *Health Care Ethics: A Catholic Theological Analysis,* 5th ed. (Washington, DC: Georgetown University Press, 2006), 89.

CHAPTER 5

Care of Critically Ill Newborns

Michael Panicola

Fateful Decisions in the Neonatal Context

Treatment decisions for critically ill newborns (i.e., newborns with congenital malformations, extremely small and premature newborns, and newborns suffering from brain-damaging conditions) are perhaps the most difficult to make in all of medicine. Several reasons account for this.

First, medically there is more uncertainty surrounding outcomes for critically ill newborns than there is for, say, adult patients with multiple conditions progressing rapidly and inevitably to death. In many instances caregivers may not know precisely the extent of damage a newborn has sustained from a brain-damaging condition or how the newborn will respond to intensive care following a very premature birth.

Second, emotionally such decisions are extremely distressing because the life on the line is that of a newborn, a voiceless and defenseless person whose life has barely begun and whose future should be open to great possibilities. Caregivers often experience a heavy emotional toll when faced with the prospects of losing a newborn to illness. However, this is nothing compared to the parents who wait excitedly and anxiously for the birth of their baby, only to have their hopes and dreams shattered as their baby is severely impaired, beset with a medical condition or constellation of conditions that endanger their newborn's life.

Finally, ethically such decisions present many challenges. For one thing, unlike adult patients, newborns' wishes and values with regard to life, death, and treatment are unknown, because these simply have not yet been formed. We don't know what conditions they would accept or what burdens they might be willing to bear for a chance at life. Consequently, treatment decisions must be made by others who must proceed without this vital information and often must contend with varying degrees of medical uncertainty, as well.

For these and other reasons, the care of critically ill newborns is high on the list of issues considered in health care ethics. In what follows we describe the evolution of neonatal medicine, highlighting how medical advances have forced us to make these seemingly impossible decisions. Then we explore the main ethical issues in the care of critically ill newborns and apply our skills of discernment using our normative basis to outline possible ways of looking at these issues. Before we begin, however, the following case serves as a helpful backdrop for the discussion.

Case 5A

Baby Suzy was delivered at 24 weeks' gestation (16 weeks premature) with a birth weight of 674 grams (1 pound, 7.77 ounces, lighter than a large fountain soda). Immediately after delivery, the neonatologist did a quick test to see how Suzy was doing. The test, called an Apgar, rates the baby's activity, pulse, grimace, appearance, and respiration with a number between 0 and 2 given for each, with 10 being a perfect score. Suzy's Apgar score at 1 minute was only 1. At birth there was a faint heartbeat but no apparent respirations. Resuscitative efforts were initiated quickly. After a considerable amount of time trying to resuscitate Suzy, her caregivers were finally able to stabilize her. Suzy survived the initial onslaught of prematurity. However, she had almost every complication an extremely premature baby could have, as indicated by the following:

cont.

Case 5A *cont.*

- hyperbilirubinemia (yellowish skin color caused by abnormally high amounts of bilirubin in the blood, which can result in brain damage depending on the severity)
- bacterial sepsis (an infection caused by bacteria in the bloodstream, which can be fatal)
- patent ductus arteriosus, or PDA (a heart defect caused by the failure of a vessel to close after birth, which is correctable with surgery)
- intraventricular hemorrhage (excessive bleeding inside the ventricles of the brain, which can harm the brain's nerve cells and lead to brain damage)
- feeding problems
- respiratory distress syndrome (difficulty breathing due to incomplete lung development, which can be fatal)
- seizures

Suzy was connected to a variety of machines and monitors: a breathing machine (mechanical ventilator), heart monitors, intravenous infusion pumps for feeding and administering medications, intra-arterial pressure gauges, and temperature sensors. She was receiving numerous medications. Her physicians informed Suzy's parents that she would need surgery for a shunt to relieve the pressure caused by the bleeding in her brain, possibly another surgery to correct the PDA, and various other treatments would also be necessary to offset the complications that were sure to arise. Moreover, Suzy would be in the hospital for many months—if she survived, which was still questionable. While Suzy's parents wanted nothing more than for their baby to get better, they entertained thoughts of just letting her go so she would not have to suffer any longer and they would not have to incur the huge expenses that were sure to follow. However, they kept these thoughts to themselves because they did not want Suzy's caregivers to think that they were "bad parents."

Setting the Context: The Evolution
of Neonatal Medicine

Baby Suzy's case is filled with many difficulties of a medical and ethical nature. Ironically, just a short time ago we would not have had to contend with such issues, because neonatal medicine was relatively powerless to intervene to save the lives of critically ill infants like Suzy. Pediatrician Clement Smith describes this well:

> So when respiration was delayed or difficult, or the infant particularly tiny and immature, or structural or neurological abnormality was apparent, we troubled ourselves far less about the quality of the infant's future life than about whether he could be given any future at all. . . . If a two-pound baby of 30 weeks gestation could not survive when drained of mucus and placed in a warm isolated environment of extra oxygen, no procedure then known to us seemed very likely to increase his chances. And if he died (as he often did) we presumed he was, in simple terms, unable to live.[1]

All this has changed dramatically as neonatal medicine has developed the means to save many critically ill newborns who previously would have died. One reason for this is that neonatal medicine has become more of a science and less guesswork. Clinical and laboratory research have helped caregivers better understand diseases in newborns, how such diseases manifest themselves and progress, how they might respond to treatment, and what the outcomes might be.[2]

A second reason is that neonatal medicine has become more skilled at diagnosing and treating newborn diseases. Blood gas analysis, electronic monitoring devices, and other diagnostic tools such as computerized tomography (CT) scans, echocardiography, and ultrasonography have permitted caregivers to diagnose most newborn conditions; developments in ventilation, improved resuscitation and surgical techniques, and other therapies such as total parenteral nutrition for feeding, phototherapy for hyperbilirubinemia, and surfactant replacement therapy for respiratory distress have enabled caregivers to treat many newborns who were once beyond treatment.[3] Besides these diagnostic and therapeutic advances, caregivers can now track the development and condition of fetuses through fetal monitoring and prenatal diagnosis, and treat certain diseases or malformations (e.g., bladder outlet obstruction or congenital diaphragmatic hernia) while the fetus is still in the womb.

A third reason is that neonatal medicine has become more specialized and organized. Neonatal care has shifted from general pediatric and obstetric practitioners to specially trained nurses and physicians in neonatology and perinatology.[4] These specialists work within a team setting with various consultants and support staff including obstetric ultrasonographers, obstetric endocrinologists, pediatric neurologists, pediatric cardiologists, pediatric hematologists, pediatric geneticists, respiratory therapists, physical therapists, pharmacologists, lab technicians, chaplains, and social workers.[5] Neonatal teams provide comprehensive care to critically ill newborns in organized hospital units known most commonly as neonatal intensive care units (NICUs). The first NICU in the United States was phased in at Vanderbilt Medical Center, Nashville, Tennessee, in 1962–1963;[6] today literally hundreds of NICUs exist throughout the states.

The diagnostic and therapeutic innovations of the last fifty years in neonatal medicine, coupled with improved prenatal and obstetric care, have contributed substantially to the declining mortality rates of infants (under 1 year) and neonates (less than 28 days). In the United States, the number of deaths per 1,000 live births has fallen from 26.04 in 1960 to 6.68 in 2006 among infants, and from 18.73 in 1960 to 4.46 in 2006 among neonates (see figure 5A).[7] Reductions in

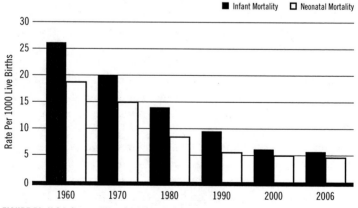

FIGURE 5A U.S Infant and Neonatal Mortality Rates

mortality have been most striking for extremely small and premature newborns, who, along with newborns with congenital malformations and those who die of sudden infant death syndrome (SIDS), account for 46 percent of all infant deaths. Not long ago, few newborns weighing less than 750 grams (1 pound, 10.45 ounces) were actively treated, because treatment was considered futile or useless. Today, however, newborns weighing as little as 400 grams (14.10 ounces) and newborns delivered as early as 22 weeks' gestation receive treatment in the United States, and these limits continue to be challenged.[8]

This change in treatment philosophy is supported by neonatal outcome studies over the last several decades that show improved survival rates for extremely small and premature newborns over time. For instance, Hack and associates[9] evaluated the outcomes of infants weighing less than 1500 grams (3 pounds, 4.91 ounces) and reported survival-to-discharge rates of 34 percent for infants weighing 750 grams or less, 66 percent for infants weighing 751 to 1000 grams, 87 percent for infants weighing 1001 to 1250 grams, and 93 percent for infants weighing 1251 to 1500 grams. These results, particularly those for the extremely low birth weight infants (less than 1000 grams), are staggering, especially when compared with older studies like that reported in the 1950s by the renowned obstetrician and early pioneer of modern neonatal care, Julius Hess (see figure 5B).[10]

Interestingly, this study by Hack and associates does not adequately capture the full extent of improvements in neonatal

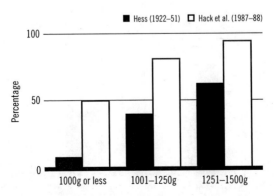

FIGURE 5B Comparative Analysis of Neonatal Survival Rates over Time Based on Birth Weight

survivability, because it involved infants delivered from November 1987 to October 1988, which was before surfactant replacement therapy became widely used as part of Treatment Investigational New Drug protocols in 1989 and eventually licensed for use in the United States in mid-1990.[11] Surfactant is a material normally produced by the lungs that acts by way of coating the tiny air sacs of the lungs (alveoli), allowing them to stay open, which is essential for oxygen to enter the blood and for carbon dioxide to be released from the blood. Infants who are born very prematurely have incomplete lung development and often lack this important substance. Surfactant can be inserted directly into immature lungs to lower surface tension and thus improve a newborn's ability to absorb oxygen. Since its introduction, surfactant replacement therapy has been effective in combating respiratory distress syndrome, a major complication experienced by premature newborns.

Studies analyzing survival rates of extremely small and premature infants presurfactant and postsurfactant have shown significant improvements since surfactant has been used. For instance, Muraskas and colleagues[12] reported neonatal survival rates of 59 percent for infants weighing 500 to 1000 grams and 61 percent for infants born at 22 to 29 weeks' gestation during the presurfactant period 1985 through 1989; in contrast, survival rates were 76 percent for infants weighing 500 to 1000 grams and 78 percent for infants born at 22 to 29 weeks' gestation during the postsurfactant period 1990 through 1994 (see figure 5C).

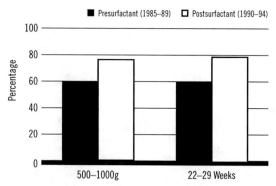

FIGURE 5C Neonatal Survival Rates over a 10-Year Period Based on Birth Weight and Gestational Age

Further improvements in neonatal survivability occurred throughout the 1990s. However, the most recent data suggest that a plateau has been reached, at least in the United States, where survival rates for extremely small and premature infants have remained relatively static since the early 2000s. As an indication of where we stand currently in the United States, we can look to neonatal outcomes of extremely preterm infants from the Eunice Kennedy Shriver National Institute of Child Health and Human Development Neonatal Research Network (NRN), which has monitored trends in mortality and morbidity (diseases and complications) among infants weighing less than 1500 grams born at university centers across the United States for more than two decades. In an NRN neonatal outcome study published in late 2010,[13] Stoll and colleagues reported survival-to-discharge rates of 6 percent for infants born at 22 weeks' gestation, 26 percent for infants born at 23 weeks, 55 percent for infants born at 24 weeks, 72 percent for infants born at 25 weeks, 84 percent for infants born at 26 weeks, 88 percent for infants born at 27 weeks, and 92 percent for infants born at 28 weeks (see figure 5D).

Although improved neonatal care has resulted in better survival rates for critically ill newborns overall, it has not necessarily reduced the incidence of morbidity and disability among extremely small and premature newborn survivors.[14] An alarming number of these

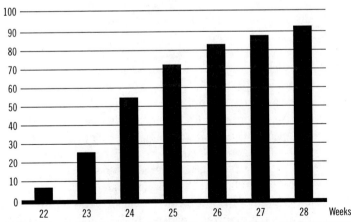

FIGURE 5D Survival Rates According to Gestational Age for Infants Weighing 401–1500g between 2003–2007

infants saved by neonatal medicine experience significant medical complications (such as with Baby Suzy in Case 5A) that include but are not limited to respiratory distress syndrome, apnea of prematurity (periodic episodes where breathing is suspended), hypoglycemia (abnormally low blood-sugar levels), bacterial sepsis, patent ductus arteriosus, intraventricular hemorrhage, necrotizing enterocolitis (a gastrointestinal disease that involves infection and inflammation that causes destruction of part of the bowel or intestine), and hyperbilirubinemia.[15] As such, these infants must often contend with multiple surgeries, chronic pain and suffering, lengthy dependence on breathing machines and other technological interventions, prolonged hospitalization, extensive rehabilitation, and special education.

Numerous outcome studies over the last two decades show this. For instance, Allen, Donohue, and Dusman[16] investigated mortality and morbidity in premature infants and reported that survivors born before 25 weeks had a higher incidence of serious medical conditions such as bronchopulmonary dysplasia (chronic lung disease), retinopathy of prematurity (an eye disorder that can result in blindness), intraventricular hemorrhage, and periventricular leukomalacia (death of white matter of the brain that results in brain damage); in addition, these infants had lengthier stays in the hospital and required oxygen administration for more days. In total, only 2 percent of the infants born at 23 weeks' gestation survived without severe abnormalities on cranial ultrasonography as compared with 21 percent of those born at 24 weeks' gestation and 69 percent of those born at 25 weeks' gestation. Likewise, in the NRN neonatal outcome study mentioned above, Stoll and colleagues reported rates of survival *with morbidity* (including respiratory distress syndrome, bronchopulmonary dysplasia, intraventricular hemorrhage, periventricular leukomalacia, patent ductus arteriosus, necrotizing enterocolitis, and retinopathy of prematurity) of 100 percent for infants born at 22 weeks' gestation, 92 percent for infants born at 23 weeks, 91 percent for infants born at 24 weeks, 80 percent for infants born at 25 weeks, 66 percent for infants born at 26 weeks, 56 percent for infants born at 27 weeks, and 43 percent for infants born at 28 weeks (see figure 5E).

Studies also show that the medical problems extremely small and premature newborn survivors experience in the immediate aftermath of being born can have effects beyond the hospital and even cause

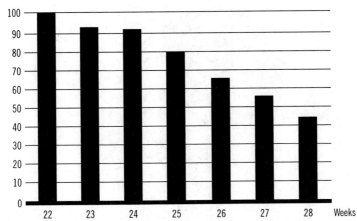

FIGURE 5E Morbidity Rates According to Gestational Age for Infants Weighing 401–1500g between 2003–2007

problems later in life in the form of mental and physical impairments and behavioral problems. For instance, Wood and associates[17] evaluated children who were born at 25 or fewer weeks' gestation when they reached a *median age of 30 months* and reported that 49 percent had no disability but 23 percent had severe disability (defined as one that was likely to put the child in need of physical assistance to perform daily activities, such as inability to walk without assistance, no head control, blind or perceives light only, and so on) and another 25 percent had other disability (defined as disabilities that did not meet the criteria for severe disability, such as abnormal gait with reduced mobility, some difficulty feeding with both hands, delay in speech, and so on) (see figure 5F).

Looking further out, Hack and collaborators[18] compared *school-age outcomes* of surviving children with birth weights of less than 750 grams to children weighing 750 to 1499 grams at birth and children born at term; they reported that survivors in the less than 750 gram group were inferior to both comparison groups in cognitive ability, psychomotor skills, and academic achievement. Children born weighing less than 750 grams also had poorer social skills and adaptive behavior and more behavioral and attention problems; in addition these children had a higher incidence of mental retardation (IQ less than 70), cerebral palsy, severe visual disability, and mild hearing loss.

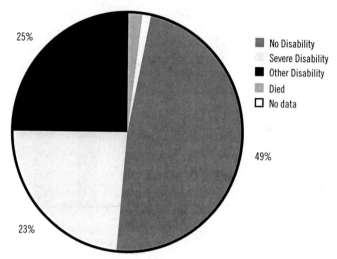

FIGURE 5F Disability at 30 Months for Children Born at 22–25 Weeks' Gestation

In another study, Hack and colleagues[19] compared *outcomes in young adulthood* for very low birth weight infants (less than 1500 grams) against a cohort of normal birth weight infants. They found, among other things, that low birth weight young adults graduated from high school less frequently than normal birth weight adults (74 percent versus 83 percent), had a lower mean IQ score (87 versus 92), and had significantly higher rates of chronic conditions (33 percent versus 21 percent).

These studies are even more distressing when one considers the enormous financial costs associated with neonatal intensive care. Though it is difficult to find an accurate estimate on the overall costs of neonatal care in the United States, the number is conceivably in the tens of billions of dollars, most of which is spent on caring for the more than 500,000 premature infants born annually in this country. Approximately 75 percent of the infants cared for in American NICUs today are premature, and according to the Institute of Medicine's 2006 report *Preterm Birth: Causes, Consequences, and Prevention*, the annual cost of caring for these infants alone is $26 billion.[20] To put this into perspective, consider the story of Heather Ablondi, who delivered her baby, Abigail, at just 27½ weeks' gestation. As one might guess given the studies highlighted above, Abigail experienced serious medical complications, including respiratory distress syndrome and bacterial sepsis, and ended up staying in the NICU for the first three months of her life. By the time of discharge, Abigail's medical bills totaled $750,000.[21]

This tells only part of the story, however. Left out are the additional medical, educational, and social services costs associated with prematurity-related morbidities and disabilities that accrue to families and society in the years following neonatal intensive care. A recent study by Korvenranta and peers[22] captured costs during the first four years of life for infants with a gestational age of less than 32 weeks or a birth weight of less than 1501 grams. They reported, among other things, that the average costs per quality-adjusted life-year ranged from $79,856 for infants born at 23 weeks' gestation to $18,875 for infants born at 30–31 weeks' gestation. Although the bulk of the costs that factor into these averages relates to hospital charges for neonatal intensive care, other costs and financial burdens arise, such as physician or clinic visits, rehabilitation care, emergency outpatient visits, hospital admissions, medical equipment, special education, speech therapy, and so on. Moreover, parents often incur additional costs through lost wages, expenses related to medical travel and lodging during hospitalizations, and child care costs for siblings.

This is the historical context out of which treatment decisions for critically ill newborns have emerged. Before neonatal medicine had the means to prolong the lives of critically ill newborns, we did not have to concern ourselves with such decisions. All we could do was rely on the limited means available and hope for the best. Today, however, this is not the case. Neonatal medicine has progressed to the point that critically ill newborns are surviving with greater frequency through the application of new therapeutic and technologic innovations. Unfortunately, some critically ill newborns saved by the wonders of neonatal medicine survive only a short time despite aggressive attempts to keep them alive, while others survive only to experience severe impairments resulting from their underlying medical conditions or even from the interventions themselves. Progress has a dark side and treatment is not benign. Consequently, intensive care and burdensome, expensive treatments cannot simply be presumed appropriate for every critically ill newborn. We must accept responsibility for the power we have obtained over illness and even, to a certain extent, death, and ask the frightening question of whether what *can* be done *ought* to be done.[23]

This question assumes that survival alone is not sufficient to justify aggressive intervention, that there are goods or values at least as important as the preservation of life itself. If this is true, as experience suggests it is, then we need to determine which critically ill newborns will meaningfully benefit from neonatal medicine's efforts to save them and which will not. How do we make such determinations for these tiny ones? Who decides? What ethical standards or criteria should we use to make such judgments? What role should costs and burdens to families and society play in the overall determination? These questions will be addressed in the next section.

Discussion: Ethical Issues and Analysis

Who Decides?

The first ethical issue has to do with who should have the authority to make treatment decisions for critically ill newborns. The main options are parents (or legal guardians), caregivers, ethics committees, and courts. Arguments could be made for or against each group.

Parents. Parents are generally motivated out of profound love and a deep desire to promote the well-being of their newborn and protect her or him from harm. Moreover, parents have the most at stake because any decision will affect them and their family more than any of the other potential decision makers in multiple ways (emotionally, spiritually, relationally, socially, and financially). However, parents may not understand the medical aspects well enough to make truly informed decisions and could be too involved emotionally to make reasonable decisions. Additionally, not all parents seek to promote the best interests of their newborn and could be motivated by concerns that jeopardize their ability to make sound moral decisions (e.g., costs of care, burdens related to the care of their child, and social stigma of having a disabled child).

Caregivers. Caregivers have the technical knowledge and experience necessary to understand the medical complexities of the situation, the possible treatment options, their effects, and the potential outcomes. Moreover, they tend not to be as emotionally involved as parents and as such may be able to make more objective decisions than parents. However, caregivers could just as easily be driven by technological capacity as by a concern to promote the overall well-being of the newborn, which could lead them to seek overly aggressive treatment when perhaps more limited measures are appropriate. Additionally, treatment decisions have as much to do with personal values (moral, religious, social, and cultural) as they do with medical capacity and possibility. Such decisions are broad human judgments that encompass views about the meaning of life and death, the values that give life its meaning and substance, the obligations we have to others, and our relationship with God. In some instances the values of caregivers may not coincide with those of the parents or with the reality of the situation. What is more, caregivers' objectivity can be compromised just as much as that of parents if they become emotionally attached to the newborn.

Ethics Committees. Ethics committees exist in most hospitals. They consist of health care professionals from diverse fields and usually some community representatives. Ethics committees have a broader perspective than either the parents or the caregivers and are less emotionally involved than either. However, ethics committees may be too distant from the situation to make good judgments that take into consideration the unique elements of the case, as well as the value-laden aspects we mentioned above. What is more, ethics committees may not be able to mobilize quickly enough to provide a timely response to an urgent matter.

Courts. Courts can apply current laws, as well as legal precedent to the situation, and their judgment would be, for the most part, objective and not rushed. However, like ethics committees, courts may be too distant from the situation and may not be able to respond as quickly as is required for the well-being of the newborn and others.

As can be seen, each group has advantages and disadvantages. So who should have the authority to decide the fate of critically ill newborns? Based on the fact that treatment decisions involve personal value factors, as well as medical factors, we believe the best option is a shared decision-making model in which the parents decide in conjunction with the team of caregivers. The authority for most decisions in this model would reside ultimately with the parents, who need always to be enlightened and guided by caring, competent, and compassionate health care professionals. The priority given to parents and the generally responsible action of parents will not guarantee that treatment decisions will always be morally reasonable. Therefore, caregivers and society, through ethics committees and the courts, may intervene so as to protect the well-being of newborns in certain situations. One such situation involves a parental decision opposing a treatment that would clearly benefit the newborn. Another situation involves a parental decision pursuing treatment when treatment would clearly harm or impose an excessive burden on the newborn. A third situation involves a parental decision pursuing treatment for an irreversibly ill and dying newborn, when the newborn clearly would not benefit from treatment and the use of limited health care resources would be disproportionate to any effect the treatment might have.[24] These limits to the authority of parents are simply guidelines and would need to be interpreted and applied in particular situations, but they serve as adequate checks and balances to potential parental abuses of decisional authority.

What Criteria?

The second ethical issue has to do with what ethical standards or criteria we should use when making treatment decisions for critically ill newborns. Over the years, as neonatal medicine increased its capacity to save newborns with devastating diseases, several standards have been proposed. The three most prominent ones are medical indications, best interests, and relational quality of life. Below we briefly describe these standards and point out some of their strengths and weaknesses.[25]

Medical Indications Standard. This ethical standard bases treatment decisions on medical indications and maintains that all newborns, regardless of disability or developmental potential, possess equal dignity and intrinsic worth. Consequently, treatment decisions for such patients should not be made on the basis of disability or projected quality of life, because these considerations open the door to serious abuse by those deciding. Rather, treatment decisions should be made on the more objective grounds of what is medically indicated, such as physiological or clinical data. The medical indications standard asserts that medical treatment should be provided to all critically ill newborns unless it is determined that such newborns are irreversibly or imminently dying or the medical treatment itself is judged to be medically contraindicated. For those impaired newborns who are not in the process of dying, any treatment judged to be medically beneficial, understood as the improvement of biological functioning and physical capabilities, must be provided. The leading proponent of this standard is the late Christian ethicist Paul Ramsey.[26]

The primary strength of the medical indications standard is that it seeks to obtain the greatest objectivity possible by using only medical and clinical data, as opposed to subjective assessments about the newborn's projected quality of life. This reduces the possibility that parents or other decision makers will decide solely on the basis of the newborn's disability or developmental potential. This is a concern because healthy, high-functioning people often cannot imagine living with physical or mental impairments and consequently set a high bar for treatment.[27]

However, the standard also has several weaknesses. First, the standard is too restrictive. Quality of life considerations need to be made or else critically ill newborns could be held hostage by technology. As we have seen, neonatal medicine has the capacity to save many newborns who would have died previously, but sometimes the newborns saved must endure terrible burdens that we would not expect an adult patient to bear. Second, just because something is medically possible or a treatment might be effective does not mean it is beneficial and thus morally required. We can treat most complications that arise for newborns and keep many alive indefinitely, but this is not the point, at least from a moral perspective. The key question is not what we can do but rather whether treatment would provide a meaningful benefit to the newborn. Third, the standard itself would cut parents out of the decision-making process: only medical information is allowed for consideration. This seems unfair and cruel. It would also eliminate values and personal/familial contexts from shaping decisions, including burdens faced by families, which can be considerable. Finally, the standard is too optimistic in regard to neonatal medicine. To say that we should treat based on clinical data assumes that medicine has all the answers about diagnosis, prognosis, treatment, and outcomes. As mentioned above, medical uncertainty frequently shrouds the care and treatment of critically ill newborns.

Best Interests Standard. This ethical standard bases treatment decisions on the newborn's best interests and maintains that potential burdens to the family and society should not be considered. Rather, treatment decisions should be based on the interests of the infants in question and these interests alone. The best interests standard asserts that medical treatment must be provided to impaired newborns unless (1) death is imminent, (2) treatment is medically contraindicated, or (3) continued existence would represent a fate worse than death. This last exception is a quality of life judgment that distinguishes this standard from the medical indications standard. The leading proponent of this standard is the ethicist Robert Weir.[28]

The primary strength of the best interests standard is that by focusing on the overall well-being of the newborn, it allows medical, as well as quality of life and value, factors to shape the decision-making process. In this way the standard recognizes that there are limits to what neonatal medicine can and should do and that other goods are just as important as life itself.

However, the standard has at least one critical weakness: "best interests" is a vague concept, and the standard itself offers little help in defining it. The standard does list exceptions to treatment, which shed some light, but what is "a fate worse than death"? How do we assess this without projecting our own views of quality of life, which can be inflated, onto the decision? How do we evaluate our decisions to ensure that they are morally acceptable? Is this left to the parents to decide? On what grounds would they make such a determination? What limits to their judgments might apply so we can protect critically ill newborns from rash, ill-motivated judgments? Another potential weakness of the best interests standard is that it leaves costs and burdens to families and society out of the decision-making process altogether by focusing exclusively on the newborn's interests. Granted, including such factors as costs and burdens to others can result in utilitarian calculations that undermine principles of justice and exacerbate racial and economic disparities; thus, there is need to be cautious. However, should costs and burdens to others, especially families, be completely left out of the equation, in every case? This is an extremely complex question that we discuss below.

Relational Quality of Life Standard. This ethical standard bases treatment decisions on the relationship between the newborn's overall medical condition and the newborn's ability to pursue the goals of life, understood as material, emotional, moral, intellectual, social, and spiritual values that transcend physical life itself. The rationale underlying this standard is that human life is a basic good, but it is a good that needs to be protected and preserved insofar as it offers a person some hope in striving for other goods or values. The relational quality of life standard holds that when treatment can improve the critically ill newborn's overall condition such that she or he can pursue life's goals, then it is morally obligatory, because it provides a meaningful benefit to the newborn and is in her or his best interests. However, when treatment cannot improve the newborn's overall condition at all or merely maintains a physical condition in which the newborn's pursuit of life's goals will be profoundly frustrated, then it is not morally obligatory, because it contradicts the newborn's best interests. In assessing the quality of this relationship, the standard maintains that the focus should be on the best interests of the newborn and these alone. The roots of this standard are found in the work of the late Catholic theologian Richard McCormick, SJ.[29] It has been developed further by fellow theologians the late Rev. Dennis Brodeur and James Walter.[30]

The relational quality of life standard has the same strengths as those of the best interests standard, and the additional strength of providing some insight into just what "best interests" are. The standard does this by viewing the newborn's overall condition against the backdrop of the newborn's ability to pursue life's goals. These goals help us to understand when treatment is truly beneficial and in a person's best interests.

However, the standard shares one potential weakness with the best interests standard, which is the exclusion of costs and burdens to families and society. The standard also has a critical weakness of its own: assessing the relationship between the newborn's overall condition and her or his ability to pursue life's goals is a broad guideline that is difficult to apply in practice due to the medical uncertainty often surrounding these tiny patients and the lack of any sense of the newborn's as-yet-unformed values or perspective on life's goals.

The relational quality of life standard can be useful in end-of-life settings involving adult patients insofar as illness is often leading inexorably to death; thus there is less medical uncertainty, and adult patients can help us discern (or we can know implicitly) what goals of life are important to them in considering whether to pursue treatment. However, just what "life's goals" means for critically ill newborns is an enigma of sorts. McCormick attempts to address this by noting the newborn's potential to engage in human relationships, which is one of the most important human goods along with life itself. Although helpful to a point, relational potentiality has little significance as an ethical standard for neonatal treatment decisions, aside from situations involving newborns with devastating congenital malformations or brain-damaging conditions that preclude them from taking part in human relationships. For many critically ill newborns, particularly those born extremely small and premature, it is virtually impossible to know whether they will survive and have the capacity to engage in human relationships, without at least starting intensive care. Furthermore, to what degree would a newborn need to be able to one day pursue life's goals, including human relationships, for treatment to become morally obligatory under the relational quality of life standard? In other words, how high or low is the bar set? Does a newborn need to have complete cognitive and physical ability or is bare minimal ability sufficient to justify aggressive intervention? These questions remain unanswered within the standard itself, at least to date.

Given the strengths and weaknesses of these standards, it may be clear but nonetheless bears mentioning that no single standard is sufficient in itself. Rather, elements within all three should be taken into consideration when making treatment decisions for critically ill newborns. As the medical indications standard notes, we need to look at objective clinical data, including those provided by neonatal outcome studies, and consider medical indications for and against treatment. As the best interests standard notes, we need to go beyond mere medical indications and consider the effect of treatment on the newborn holistically, recognizing the limits of neonatal medicine and realizing that there are goods at least as important as mere survival. As the relational quality of life standard notes, we need to consider treatment against, and understand best interests in light of, the newborn's ability to pursue life's goals, while making sure we do not set the bar so high that quality of life factors become a way of systematically weeding out those who will grow up to live with disabilities. As a corrective to this potentially dangerous and discriminatory application of the relational quality of life standard, we would instead like to propose, using language tied to our normative basis, the following treatment guideline, which sets the bar appropriately low: If treatment can enable the newborn to pursue goods bound up with human flourishing, especially human relationships, *at least at a minimal level without experiencing excessive burdens*, then treatment generally should be considered proportionate and hence morally obligatory.[31] If it cannot, then treatment generally should be considered disproportionate and hence morally optional because in such situations, treatment typically ceases to provide a meaningful benefit and as such, the goals of care might best shift to comfort and palliation. The latter, of course, is never an easy determination to make but nevertheless is a determination that must be made at times if neonatal medicine is going to serve the best interests and overall well-being of critically ill newborns.

At What Cost and Whose Burdens?

The final and perhaps most challenging ethical issue is that of the role costs and burdens to families and society should play in treatment decisions for critically ill newborns. As noted above, costs related to neonatal care, as well as subsequent medical, educational, and social services for surviving newborns, are incredibly high when taken collectively. This fact has caused some to ask whether the money and resources spent to save critically ill newborns, especially those born at the edges of viability and at the lowest birth weights where survival is so low and morbidity so high, could be used in more cost-effective ways, such as for universal prenatal care and multidisciplinary research aimed at reducing the incidence of prematurity. This is a crucial question when one considers the following factors:

- Health care is a basic good bound up with our pursuit of human flourishing and as such, all people should have access to a certain level of health care services, namely, preventive, primary, and emergency care.
- Health care resources are limited, and there are further limits to how much we can spend on health care without negatively

affecting other areas closely aligned with personal and societal well-being.

- In many nations people lack even the most basic health care services, while in others, like the United States, overall health care costs are increasing faster annually than employee wages and economic growth and are approaching or already have approached unsustainable levels.

The easy thing to do would be to set aside cost considerations in health care altogether. However, for all the reasons listed above, we simply cannot do this, at least not ethically. Costs have a role to play at the health policy and organizational levels, as well as in clinical decision making, including decisions made in the neonatal context. Interestingly, despite the high costs associated with neonatal care, studies suggest and many people argue that neonatal care is cost-effective, especially when compared against resource use in other health care settings (such as adult intensive care units), because most of the money spent is allocated to survivors. Lantos and Meadow describe this well in their book *Neonatal Bioethics*:

> We calculated the efficiency of neonatal care by looking at the overall number of bed days that were used by babies who ultimately went on to die, compared with the bed days used by babies who went on to survive. We found that most of the bed days, and thus most of the dollars, spent in the NICU go to survivors. . . . Even for the tiniest babies, more than 80 percent of the bed days were used by babies who ultimately survived. We then compared the smallest babies in the NICU with the oldest adults in the medical intensive care unit (MICU). We found a sharp contrast. More than 80 percent of the bed days used for the sickest adults—those over 75 years of age and on a ventilator—were used by patients who went on to die.[32]

This does not necessarily settle the issue, but it does indicate that the money being spent on neonatal care is directed mostly to infants who will go home to their families. It also may suggest that before we begin weighing the costs of and setting limits around neonatal care, we need to make better use of our health care resources at the end of life. Still, on a health policy level, it bears asking whether some limits could or should be set around birth weight, gestational age, or both. This may seem callous at first glance, but viewed another way it could prevent some newborns from suffering unnecessarily when their chances of survival are slim. Consider the NRN neonatal outcome study described above. Of note, only 6 percent of the infants born at 22 weeks' gestation survived, and 100 percent of the survivors had serious morbidities; likewise, at 23 weeks' gestation only 26 percent of the infants survived, and 92 percent of the survivors had serious morbidities. Are these acceptable numbers? Are our limited health care resources best used trying to save these extremely small and premature newborns? Are we doing these newborns a service or a disservice? These are difficult questions that no one really wants to address because it could mean that policy is set in such a way that some newborns, who might live, with or without serious impairments, are denied treatment. Furthermore, some argue that the money potentially saved from setting a birth weight or gestational age cutoff would be so small in comparison to overall health care costs that it would not make much difference. This may be true. Nonetheless, if we are ever going to come close to creating a just health care system in which benefits and burdens are shared equitably among all, we might just have to start considering setting limits that produce small-scale cost savings, which, when taken together, could indeed make a significant difference.

All this says nothing about the burdens to families. Without question, families of critically ill newborns suffer in many ways and must overcome terrible hardships emotionally, spiritually, relationally, socially, and financially. Burdens to families tend to be excluded as factors when it comes to making treatment decisions in the neonatal context. This is understandable to a point, given that we want to ensure that every critically ill newborn who can meaningfully benefit from neonatal intensive care receives it. Familial burdens, though real and often significant, could easily be applied to treatment decisions in an unjust and discriminatory way. Still, is there no place for familial burdens and can we not do better addressing and responding to these burdens? At the least, we need to attend to these burdens, acknowledge them, discuss them with families, and, most of all, provide more social support than we do currently. We need better financial aid programs, technical assistance, respite care for families, and counseling services. And perhaps, *in some cases*, we need to allow familial burdens to be weighed when making treatment decisions in the neonatal context, which we could see limited particularly to cases involving newborns with very poor prognoses and who will have to endure terrible burdens of their own in the mere struggle to survive (e.g., newborns born at 22–23 weeks' gestation and those suffering from severe congenital malformations that may be incompatible with life). In the end, though, if treatment provides a meaningful benefit to a critically ill newborn, then it should be provided regardless of its costs and the burdens to families and society.

Conclusion

Treatment decisions for critically ill newborns are never easy. We have provided some insight and guidance into the ethical issues surrounding these decisions. By way of summary, we now apply these insights and guidelines to the case of Baby Suzy. As you recall, Suzy was very sick and was looking at multiple treatments and surgeries with a lengthy hospitalization and prolonged rehabilitation—if she survived. Given what we said about who should have the authority to make these decisions, Suzy's parents and caregivers will need to work together to decide whether Suzy can benefit meaningfully from continued intensive care and other treatments necessary to her survival. To make this determination, Suzy's caregivers will need to assess the extent of brain damage Suzy has sustained, the effect that her other conditions will have on her overall health, and what mental and physical disabilities she will endure if she survives. Suzy's caregivers will then need to make this information available to her parents and work with them in assessing the benefits and burdens of the various treatment options. Suzy's caregivers should also help her parents navigate the many complexities of the NICU and work with the parents in understanding and responding to the various burdens they face and will continue to face as a family.

As for treatment decisions, if Suzy's parents are given reasonable assurances that continued intensive care and other treatments will improve Suzy's condition such that she will be able to pursue goods bound up with human flourishing, especially human relationships, at least at a minimal level without experiencing excessive burdens, then treatment could be considered proportionate and hence morally obligatory. If, on the other hand, Suzy's parents are told that all treatment will do is (1) prolong Suzy's life for a short time, (2) maintain her in a condition that will not allow her to pursue goods bound up with human flourishing, even at a minimal level, or (3) severely frustrate her in her pursuit of these goods in the mere struggle to survive, then treatment could be considered disproportionate and hence morally optional, and costs and familial burdens could become a tilting factor in deciding whether to pursue treatment or allow Suzy to die free of invasive medical interventions, while under the watchful eye of a palliative care specialist. It needs to be clear that a decision against treatment would not imply that Suzy's life is less valuable than others or that her life is not worth living. Rather, it would quite simply be an acceptance of the fact that this valued person, Suzy, has come to "the end of . . . her pilgrimage and should not be impeded from taking the final step."[33] Because a great deal of uncertainty often surrounds treatment decisions for critically ill newborns, one last caution is in order. Even the best of ethical guidelines are not fail-safe and thus, as McCormick long ago noted, parents and caregivers should proceed with "great humility, caution, and tentativeness" when making these decisions, erring on the side of life when in doubt.[34]

Case Studies

Case 5B

Baby John was delivered at 36 weeks and 5 days' gestational age with a birth weight of 2637 grams (5 pounds, 13 ounces). Delivery was relatively uncomplicated, though at birth Baby John was cyanotic (bluish in color due to lack of oxygen) and had severe tachycardia (increased heart rate) and tachypnea (increased respiratory rate). Baby John was immediately intubated and ventilated with 100-percent oxygen through bag and

cont.

Case 5B *cont.*

endotracheal tube. All of this was expected, however, as ultrasonography at 17 weeks revealed that Baby John suffered from hypoplastic left heart syndrome (HLHS). HLHS is the most common cardiac defect causing death during the first year of life in the United States. The condition is fatal, but with reconstructive surgery many babies survive long-term. In fact, some institutions achieve up to 85 percent long-term survival rates with no significant disability. Still, definite risks are associated with the reconstructive surgery, and medical costs can be very high.

Prior to delivery, Baby John's parents told their ob-gyn that they would seek surgery for their baby. Shortly after delivery, the surgeon scheduled to perform the procedure stops by Baby John's room and discusses things with the parents. Much to her surprise, the parents are now refusing to give their consent for the surgery. Even though the surgeon explains that they often have great outcomes for babies with John's condition, the parents do not relent, even stating that if the surgeon continues to badger them, they will get a lawyer. Dumbfounded and unsure what to do, the surgeon seeks an ethics consult to see if the parents' decision is acceptable ethically and if not, what she should do. Is the parents' decision against surgery in this case justified morally? Would it be supported by the relational quality of life standard? Why or why not? If you disagree with the parents' decision, how would you handle the situation and how would you advise the surgeon?

Case 5C[35]

Carol, a 26-year-old pregnant woman, went with her husband for a routine visit to the ob-gyn. Much to their dismay, the ultrasound showed that the twin girls Carol was carrying were conjoined. As devout Roman Catholics, the couple refused to even consider the option of terminating the pregnancy, and several months later Laura and Jeanne were born. Lying on their backs, the girls' heads and upper bodies emerged at opposite ends of

cont.

Case 5C *cont.*

a torso that was joined from the base of the pelvis to the lower abdomen. The spines were fused at the base, and their legs extended to the sides at right angles. Each twin had her own brain, heart, lungs, liver, and kidneys, and they shared a bladder that lay mostly in Laura's abdomen.

Laura was described as bright and alert; she moved her limbs, squirmed, and appeared to have developmentally normal responses for her age. Her brain appeared to be anatomically and functionally normal, and the same was true of her liver, lungs, kidneys, and heart, with one exception: Laura's aorta fed into Jeanne's, circulating blood through Jeanne's body and back into Laura through a united inferior vena cava. Jeanne's condition was less hopeful from the start. Her brain was described as "primitive" and she was unable to cry because her lungs were severely underdeveloped and virtually devoid of functioning tissue. As a result, she was incapable of breathing on her own. Her heart was abnormally large and had difficulty functioning properly. It was estimated to contribute less than 10 percent of Jeanne's circulatory requirements. Because of these circulatory incapacities, Jeanne relied entirely on Laura's heart and lungs to stay alive.

In the days after birth, physicians at the hospital were grim about the prognosis of the twins. They predicted that Laura's heart would fail under the excess strain in as little as six weeks. They also predicted that Jeanne would develop hydrocephalus (fluid in the brain), which would be very difficult to treat in light of her abnormal abdominal cavity and cardiac defect. The prospect of persistent hypoxia (lack of oxygen) in Jeanne increased the likelihood of further damaging her brain, and doctors also thought it could promote similar destruction in Laura. Surgeons were very optimistic, however, that Laura could survive the surgical separation, giving her at least an 85-percent chance. They believed that if she survived the surgery, she would be able to live out a normal life span with the most serious foreseeable complications limited to possible difficulties walking with support and controlling her bowels. They were certain, though, that

cont.

Case 5C *cont.*

Jeanne would not survive independently of her sister, and that separation would therefore lead to her demise.

Given the urgency of the situation, the surgeons wasted no time in discussing the option of surgical separation with Carol and her husband. They carefully explained the benefits and risks, including the certain death of Jeanne. At first, the couple refuses to give their consent but several days later mention to one of the surgeons that they may be open to the option if they are reassured surgical separation is acceptable morally and not equivalent to murder of one to save another. The surgeon calls the ethics committee to review the case. Given that baby Jeanne will most likely die following surgical separation, is it morally justified to perform the surgery? If so, on what grounds and who should ultimately decide?

SUGGESTED READINGS

Anspach, Renée R. *Deciding Who Lives: Fateful Choices in the Intensive-Care Nursery.* Berkeley: University of California Press, 1993.

Camosy, Charles C. *Too Expensive to Treat? Finitude, Tragedy, and the Neonatal ICU.* Grand Rapids, MI: Eerdmans, 2010.

Fanaroff, Avery A., Am Weindling, and Tom Lissauer. *Neonatology at a Glance.* Malden, MA: Blackwell, 2006.

Guyer, Ruth Levy. *Baby at Risk: The Uncertain Legacies of Medical Miracles for Babies, Families, and Society.* Sterling, VA: Capital Books, 2006.

Hauerwas, Stanley. *Naming the Silences: God, Medicine, and the Problem of Suffering.* Grand Rapids, MI: Eerdmans, 1990.

Lantos, John D. *The Lazarus Case: Life-and-Death Issues in Neonatal Intensive Care.* Baltimore, MD: Johns Hopkins University Press, 2001.

Lantos, John D., and William L. Meadow. *Neonatal Bioethics: The Moral Challenges of Medical Innovation.* Baltimore, MD: Johns Hopkins University Press, 2006.

McCormick, Richard A. "To Save or Let Die: The Dilemma of Modern Medicine." *Journal of the American Medical Association* 229 (July 8, 1974): 172–6.

Miller, Geoffrey. *Extreme Prematurity: Practices, Bioethics, and the Law.* New York: Cambridge University Press, 2006.

Rogoff, Marianne. *Sylvie's Life.* Berkeley, CA: Zenobia Press, 1995.

Sparks, Richard C. *To Treat or Not to Treat? Bioethics and the Handicapped Newborn.* New York: Paulist Press, 1988.

Weir, Robert F. *Selective Nontreatment of Handicapped Newborns: Moral Dilemmas in Neonatal Medicine.* New York: Oxford University Press, 1984.

MULTIMEDIA AIDS FOR TEACHERS

Born Too Soon: Life and Death in the NICU. DIA Learning. 2006. For information see *http://fac.ethicsprograms.com/.* This 30-minute video can be purchased separately or as part of a group of videos on select issues in health care ethics.

Little Man. Reel Indies. Not Rated. 2007. This heart-wrenching film, which has won several "best documentary" awards, tells the story of Nicholas Conn and his family, providing an intimate, behind-the-scenes glimpse into the decisions and struggles that surround the birth of an extremely preterm infant. It is available through Amazon and PreemieWorld Store at *http://www.neoflix.com/store/PRE08/.*

Nurses: Battling for Babies. A Discovery Channel Production. 2000. This 51-minute video shows nurses in the fields of obstetrics and neonatal intensive care using their highly specialized skills to save babies at Johns Hopkins Maternity Center. It is available through *www.films.com.*

ENDNOTES

1. Clement Smith, "Neonatal Medicine and Quality of Life: An Historical Perspective," in *Ethics of Newborn Intensive Care,* ed. Albert R. Jonsen and Michael J. Garland (Berkeley: University of California, Institute of Governmental Studies, 1976), 32–3.

2. Marie C. McCormick, "Survival of Very Tiny Babies—Good News and Bad News," *New England Journal of Medicine* 331 (September 22, 1994): 802–3, at 802; and E. Shelp, *Born to Die? Deciding the Fate of Critically Ill Newborns* (New York: Free Press, 1986), 82.

3. V. L. Cassani III, "We've Come a Long Way Baby! Mechanical Ventilation of the Newborn," *Neonatal Network* 13 (September 1994): 63–8, at 66; Hastings Center Research Project on the Care of Imperiled Newborns, "Imperiled

Newborns: A Report," *Hastings Center Report* 17 (December 1987): 5–32, at 8; Mark Hilberman, "The Evolution of Intensive Care Units," *Critical Care Medicine* 3 (July–August 1975): 159–65, at 163; and Barbara Krollmann, Dona Ayers Brock, Patricia Murray Nader, Patricia Walsh Neiheisel, and Christel Schade Wissmann, "Neonatal Transformation: Thirty Years," *Neonatal Network* 13 (September 1994):17–20, at 20.

4. Peter P. Budetti and Peggy McManus, "Assessing the Effectiveness of Neonatal Intensive Care," *Medical Care* 20 (October 1982): 1027–39, at 1028.

5. Michael LeFevre, Louis Sanner, Sharon Anderson, and Robert Tsutakawa, "The Relationship Between Neonatal Mortality and Hospital Level," *Journal of Family Practice* 35 (September 1992): 259–64, at 260; and Robert Weir, *Selective Nontreatment of Handicapped Newborns: Moral Dilemmas in Neonatal Medicine* (New York: Oxford University Press, 1984), 37–8.

6. Jeff Lyon, *Playing God in the Nursery* (New York: Norton, 1985), 97.

7. T. J. Mathews and Marian F. MacDorman, "Infant Mortality Statistics from the 2006 Period Linked Birth/Infant Death Data Set," *National Vital Statistics Report* 58 (April 30, 2010): 1–32.

8. Marilyn R. Sanders, Pamela K. Donohue, Mary Ann Oberdorf, Ted S. Rosenkrantz, and Marille C. Allen, "Impact of Perception of Viability on Resource Allocation in the Neonatal Intensive Care Unit," *Journal of Perinatology* 18 (September–October 1998): 347–51.

9. Maureen Hack et al., "Very Low Birth Weight Outcomes of the National Institute of Child Health and Human Development Neonatal Network," *Pediatrics* 87 (May 1991): 587–97.

10. Julius H. Hess, "Experiences Gained in a Thirty Year Study of Prematurely Born Infants," *Pediatrics* 11 (May 1953): 425–34.

11. Karen C. Schoendorf and John L. Kiely, "Birth Weight and Age-Specific Analysis of the 1990 U.S. Infant Mortality Drop: Was It Surfactant?" *Archives of Pediatric and Adolescent Medicine* 151 (February 1997): 129–34, at 129.

12. Jonathan Muraskas et al., "Neonatal Viability in the 1990s: Held Hostage by Technology," *Cambridge Quarterly of Healthcare Ethics* 8 (Spring 1999): 160–70.

13. Barbara J. Stoll, Nellie I. Hansen, Edward F. Bell, et al., "Neonatal Outcomes of Extremely Preterm Infants from the NICHD Neonatal Research Network," *Pediatrics* 126 (September 2010): 443-56.

14. Marilee C. Allen, "Preterm Outcomes Research: A Critical Component of Neonatal Intensive Care," *Mental Retardation and Developmental*

Disabilities Research Reviews 8 (2002): 221–33; Maureen Hack and Avroy A. Fanaroff, "Outcomes of Children of Extremely Low Birthweight and Gestational Age in the 1990s," *Early Human Development* 53 (December 1999): 193–218; and N. Marlow, "Neurocognitive Outcome after Very Preterm Birth," *Archives of Disease in Childhood: Fetal and Neonatal Edition* 89 (2004): F224–28.

15. See, for instance, James A. Blackman, "Neonatal Intensive Care: Is It Worth It?" *Pediatric Clinics of North America* 38 (December 1991): 1497–511; Maureen Hack et al., "Very Low Birth Weight Outcomes of the National Institute of Child Health and Human Development Neonatal Network," *Pediatrics* 87 (May 1991): 587–97. Mary Lou Hulseman and Lee A. Norman, "The Neonatal ICU Graduate, Part I: Common Problems," *American Family Physician* 45 (March 1992): 1301–5; and Lyon, *Playing God in the Nursery*, 85–6.

16. Marilee C. Allen, Pamela K. Donohue, and Amy E. Dusman, "The Limit of Viability: Neonatal Outcome of Infants Born at 22 to 25 Weeks' Gestation," *New England Journal of Medicine* 329 (November 25, 1993): 1597–601.

17. Nicholas S. Wood et al., "Neurologic and Developmental Disability after Extremely Preterm Birth," *New England Journal of Medicine* 343 (10 August 2000): 378–84.

18. Maureen Hack et al., "School-Age Outcomes in Children with Birth Weights Under 750g," *New England Journal of Medicine* 331 (September 22, 1994): 753–9.

19. Maureen Hack et al., "Outcomes in Young Adulthood for Very-Low-Birth-Weight Infants," *New England Journal of Medicine* 346 (January 17, 2002): 149–57.

20. Institute of Medicine, *Preterm Birth: Causes, Consequences, and Prevention*, National Academy of Sciences (July 13, 2006).

21. Michelle Andrews, "Insurers Sometimes Reject Neonatal Intensive Care Costs," *Kaiser Health News*, January 4, 2011.

22. Emmi Korvenranta, Miika Linna, Liisi Rautava, et al., "Hospital Costs and Quality of Life during Four Years after Very Preterm Birth," *Archives of Pediatric and Adolescent Medicine* 164 (July 2010): 657–63.

23. Renée R. Anspach, *Deciding Who Lives: Fateful Choices in the Intensive-Care Nursery* (Berkeley: University of California Press, 1993), 4.

24. These situations have been adapted from Paul R. Johnson, "Selective Nontreatment of Defective Newborns: An Ethical Analysis," *Linacre Quarterly* 47 (February 1980): 39–53, at 49–50.

25. For an excellent discussion of these and other ethical standards for making neonatal treatment decisions, see Richard C. Sparks, *To Treat or Not to Treat: Bioethics and the Handicapped Newborn* (New York: Paulist Press, 1988).

26. Ramsey developed this standard in several of his works, namely, "The Sanctity of Life," *Dublin Review* 511 (Spring 1967): 3–23; *The Patient as Person: Explorations of Medical Ethics* (New Haven: Yale University Press, 1970); *Ethics at the Edges of Life: Medical and Legal Interventions* (New Haven: Yale University Press, 1978); and "The Saikewicz Precedent: What's Good for an Incompetent Patient," *Hastings Center Report* 8 (December 1978): 36–42.

27. See, for instance, Saroj Saigal et al., "Differences in Preferences for Neonatal Outcomes among Health Care Professionals, Parents, and Adolescents," *Journal of the American Medical Association* 281 (June 2, 1999): 1991–7.

28. Weir promoted this standard in his landmark book, *Selective Nontreatment of Handicapped Newborns*.

29. See, for instance, Richard A. McCormick, "To Save or Let Die: The Dilemma of Modern Medicine," *Journal of the American Medical Association* 229 (July 8, 1974): 172–6.

30. For Dennis Brodeur's work in this area, see his "Feeding Policy Protects Patients' Rights, Decisions," *Health Progress* 66 (June 1985): 38–43; and "Neonatal Ethical Dilemmas Examined," *Issues: A Critical Examination of Contemporary Ethical Issues in Health Care* 9 (November–December 1994): 1–5, 8. For James J. Walter's work in this area, see his "Food and Water: An Ethical Burden," *Commonweal* 113 (November 21, 1986): 616–9; "Termination of Medical Treatment: The Setting of Moral Limits from Infancy to Old Age," *Religious Studies Review* 16 (October 1990): 302–7; "The Meaning and Validity of Quality of Life Judgments in Contemporary Roman Catholic Medical Ethics," in *Quality of Life: The New Medical Dilemma*, ed. James J. Walter and Thomas A. Shannon (New York: Paulist Press, 1990), 78–88; and "Life, Quality of: Quality of Life in Clinical Decisions," in *Encyclopedia of Bioethics*, ed. Warren T. Reich, rev. ed. (New York: Simon and Schuster, 1995), 1352–8.

31. Walter, "The Meaning and Validity of Quality of Life Judgments," 85.

32. John D. Lantos and William L. Meadow, *Neonatal Bioethics: The Moral Challenges of Medical Innovation* (Baltimore, MD: Johns Hopkins University Press, 2006), 127.

33. Texas Catholic Bishops and the Texas Conference of Catholic Health Facilities, "Interim Pastoral Statement on Artificial Nutrition and Hydration," *Origins* 20 (June 7, 1990): 53–5, at 54.

34. McCormick, "To Save or Let Die," 176.

35. This is an adaptation of the real-life case of the conjoined twins known as Jodie and Mary, who were born on August 8, 2000, in Manchester, United Kingdom. Despite protests from the parents, whose homeland is Gozo, a small Maltese island, the British High Court decided that the twins be separated, which occurred shortly after the ruling on November 7, 2000. Jodie survived the procedure; Mary died during it.

CHAPTER 6

Reproductive Technology and the Quest for Offspring

Mark Repenshek

Ethics at the Intersection of Technology and Procreation

Technology has clearly increased medicine's capacity to diagnose and treat human disease, often extending the lives of patients who previously would have died. One area in which technology has greatly affected medicine is human reproduction. In the recent past, humans were subject to the whims of nature when it came to getting pregnant. Today, we have many means to enhance and even substitute for natural processes in an effort to have children. Many of us have encountered these technological breakthroughs, either directly or indirectly. You may have been born through the wonders of this technology or know of a friend or family member who has used it in one form or another. If not, you have probably heard of fertility treatments and reproductive clinics, read ads in magazines or newspapers seeking sperm and egg donors, or seen stories on television about couples or individuals having one or more children—as many as eight in one highly publicized case—after undergoing reproductive intervention.

Today's technology has expanded our ability to detect the risk of passing along genetic conditions to our offspring even before conception occurs through carrier testing (CT) and carrier screening (CS). Diagnosing fetal anomalies inside the womb through prenatal diagnosis (PD) has also become a part of routine obstetrical medical practice today. It is now possible to detect genetic mutations that will result in an inherited genetic condition before implantation in the womb for embryos created through in vitro fertilization (IVF), a technique known as preimplantation genetic diagnosis (PGD). PGD enables parents to choose which embryos, depending on certain desired or undesired characteristics, they want to have implanted.

While reproductive technologies (RTs) are fascinating and make for compelling news, they also give rise to important ethical issues that are not resolved simply by declaring them matters of personal choice or by reciting absolute prohibitions against any technological intrusion into human reproduction. To avoid such oversimplification, we consider RTs in view of human flourishing and right relationships. Only by considering reproductive interventions in this broader context can we move beyond slogans and adequately reflect on the ethical questions they raise. Because we focus solely on the ethics of RTs, we do not address the issues of contraception or sterilization, which are often included in discussions of human reproduction. Although these are indeed key subjects in health care ethics, much has been written about them and there is little we could add to the discussion.[1] We begin by setting the clinical context, offering a brief description of select reproductive technologies, and highlighting some of the ethical questions involved. Then we discuss the ethics of RTs in detail against the backdrop of our normative basis.

Setting the Context: The Science of Reproductive Technologies

The most frequently used RTs are artificial insemination (AI) and in vitro fertilization.[2] Although there are variations in both of these methods, all separate human reproduction from the act of sexual intercourse.

Artificial Insemination

The least technological of all RTs, AI was the first major intervention in reproduction. Developed more than 200 years ago, AI has become a popular means for achieving pregnancy outside of normal reproduction, particularly in the last fifty years or so. In its simplest form, AI involves collecting sperm from a male (usually by means of masturbation) and injecting the sperm directly into the woman's uterus. Techniques have been developed over the years to increase the likelihood of AI's success (e.g., detecting the timing of ovulation, giving the woman fertility drugs, and "washing" the sperm), and AI has been given a new name: intrauterine insemination (IUI). AI is perhaps the most accessible RT because it is relatively simple and inexpensive, about $300–$500.[3]

Originally, AI was used to overcome infertility in married couples when the couple could not have sexual intercourse or when the husband had a low sperm count or poor sperm motility (an inability of sperm to make the long journey to the egg). This "simple" intervention offered such couples hope for having a baby of their own genetic lineage. This seemed enough to most people, but since 1975 in the United States, third parties in the form of sperm donors, often anonymous, were thrown into the equation. This allowed married couples to use another man's sperm to get pregnant when the husband's sperm was deficient. It allowed persons to use AI outside the context of marriage, even if infertility was not an issue. Heterosexual women without male partners and lesbian women, for instance, have used AI successfully to achieve pregnancy.

While AI has helped married couples and others overcome infertility troubles and have children, the technique itself raises ethical issues, and its expanded use further complicates matters, especially when a donor is involved. What happens to married couples when they have recourse to a donor's sperm? How does this affect their relationship and the way they view resultant offspring? How does it affect the offspring, who may later learn that their genetic (or biological) father is not the person who has raised them all these years? Is it acceptable for men to sell their sperm anonymously and to have no responsibility for their genetic offspring? What are we to make of the use of AI outside the context of marriage? Is this an acceptable application of the technology, or should it be limited to married couples? Are some relational settings more appropriate than others for raising children? How are offspring affected when they are born to unmarried mothers or people in nontraditional relationships? On a more basic level, is infertility a disease that medicine and its technologies are meant to fix? Should we use AI on women who do not have infertility problems?

In Vitro Fertilization

With the birth of the first "test-tube baby," Louise Brown, in 1978, IVF became a popular reproductive intervention, particularly when infertility issues are more complicated than low sperm count or poor function in the male. IVF entails (1) harvesting eggs from a woman's ovaries (this could be either the woman seeking to have a baby or a donor); (2) collecting sperm from a male (husband, partner, or donor), usually obtained through masturbation, though other procedures offer options for such collection; (3) bringing the eggs and sperm together in a small laboratory dish (i.e., in vitro); (4) facilitating fertilization of the eggs outside the body; and (5) transferring one or more of the resulting embryos, after they have incubated for three to five days in a culture medium, into a woman's uterus (this could be either the woman seeking to have a baby or a surrogate who carries the baby and then gives it up at birth).[4]

Unlike AI, IVF is anything but simple. Egg harvesting is a complex process that can be burdensome for the woman. First, the woman must receive fertility drugs so that her ovaries produce an abnormally large number of eggs; side effects may include serious mood swings, as well as physical complications, including abdominal cramping and nausea. Then the woman must have her blood tested every other day to measure hormone levels, and she must have periodic ultrasounds. Before egg retrieval, the woman must receive a hormone shot of human chorionic gonadotropin (HCG) to prepare the eggs for release. The actual retrieval is done under anesthesia, using a long needle to obtain from ten to twenty eggs. There are also potential risks to the woman. In rare situations the fertility drugs can hyperstimulate the woman's ovaries, requiring hospitalization until the ovaries return to normal. In extremely rare cases, the woman's ovaries can rupture, resulting in permanent infertility or even death.[5]

Also unlike AI, IVF can be expensive. Although wide variation exists, each fertilization cycle costs roughly $4,000–$10,000; most women go through two or three cycles before pregnancy occurs. As mentioned above, to provide the best chance of success at minimal cost, eggs are often fertilized ten to twenty. Fertilized eggs are then implanted in the woman's uterus—usually one or two eggs, depending on the age of the recipient. From a simple economics basis, this seems the most beneficial and cost-effective route. However, there are limits to this cost-benefit analysis. If more than three fertilized eggs are transferred at once, the likelihood of multiple pregnancies dramatically increases, which proportionately increases the likelihood of fetal loss and premature birth, with all its attendant costs (see chapter 6).[6] Moreover, multiple pregnancies can lead to selective termination, in which one or more fetuses are destroyed to improve the odds of successful development for the remaining fetuses or to reduce the risks to the woman, who cannot safely carry all of the fetuses.

To eliminate the need to harvest eggs multiple times and thus reduce the burdens and risks to the woman supplying the eggs, the remaining fertilized eggs not transferred in an IVF cycle are often saved through a technique known as cryopreservation.[7] This involves freezing the "excess" or "spare" embryos at appropriate temperatures so they can be used later if needed. Consequently, when an early treatment cycle succeeds, there may be leftover embryos in cryopreservation. What can or should be done with them? Should they remain in a state of suspended animation? Should they be donated to another person or couple? Should they be donated and used for research purposes? Should we simply discard them? Interestingly though, it is not the complexity of these questions that has led to freezing only the egg (oocyte cryopreservation), but rather implantation success rates.

With live birth success rates of 45–57 percent per egg retrieval for women under 35, IVF has helped thousands of women achieve pregnancy and have children. The technique itself and some of its uses raise significant ethical concerns, however. Some of these concerns are similar to those related to AI, while many go further. Is IVF an acceptable means of achieving pregnancy in the first place, because (unlike AI) it goes beyond assisting natural processes and actually replaces them with a technology in which fertilization occurs outside a woman's body? Does IVF impose disproportionate burdens on women who, among other things, have to endure the difficult egg harvesting process and potentially carry multiple embryos to term, thus increasing the risks associated with pregnancy? What are we to make of sperm and egg donation and the use of surrogates? Is it acceptable to pay these third parties for their services? Does third-party involvement cheapen and degrade human reproduction and result in the commercialization of baby-making and the exploitation of potential donors? Is it wise to separate the components of parenting—genetic, gestational, and social? What is the effect on children born through IVF? What effect does this have on our views of marriage, childbearing, childrearing, and parenting? Is it acceptable to fertilize more embryos than can be safely transferred into a woman and then freeze those that are not used? Does this undermine the value of early human life and further weaken our view of it? What about the use of genetic screening techniques that are often employed before transferring embryos into the woman's uterus? Can we discard those embryos with genetic anomalies or even those who may not be the "right" sex? Finally, what about issues of access and equitable distribution? Is it acceptable that IVF, given its expense, is available to only select members of our society, namely, those who have significant financial means or generous health care coverage? Ought we to be spending our money on IVF when the basic needs of so many go unmet?

Methods of Prenatal Testing

RTs are not limited to those techniques that enable otherwise infertile couples to achieve pregnancy; they also include technologies that can not only help ensure that offspring are healthy but even that they have certain desired characteristics. In particular, the following are some specific types of prenatal testing: carrier testing and carrier screening, prenatal diagnosis, and preimplantation diagnosis.

CT is done to assess whether an individual carries one copy of an altered gene for an autosomal or X-linked recessive disorder. CT is usually performed on people who have a family history of an inherited condition to determine if they carry the associated recessive mutated gene. CT can be used in planning pregnancies so individuals can avoid passing on the mutated gene to their offspring. CS refers to genetic testing applied to a whole population or to a defined group that has a greater than average chance of carrying a particular mutated gene, due, for example, to their ancestry or ethnic background. Examples of genetic diseases that are linked to ethnic background and for which CS may be used are cystic fibrosis (in Caucasians), sickle cell disease (in individuals of African and Mediterranean descent), thalassemia (in Asians and individuals of Mediterranean descent), and Tay-Sachs and canavan disease (in Ashkenazi Jews).

PD refers broadly to a number of different techniques and procedures that can be performed during pregnancy to provide information about the health of the fetus. Initial screening tests may indicate whether the fetus has an average, above-average, or below-average risk of being affected by a particular genetic condition or birth defect. When screening results show increased risk, pregnant women may be offered other diagnostic tests to confirm if the fetus is affected. PD may also be offered directly to women whose pregnancies are considered high risk because of age, family history, or other factors.[8]

Several different prenatal diagnostic tests can be offered at various stages in pregnancy:

- *Ultrasound:* a noninvasive procedure that can be done at any time in a pregnancy. High-frequency sound waves are used to produce an image of the fetus inside the uterus. Ultrasound is often used to determine the age of a fetus based on fetal measurements, to monitor fetal growth, to determine why bleeding is occurring, to check the baby's position in the uterus, to detect multiple births, or to evaluate the general development of the fetus. Most recently, however, first trimester ultrasound has become a method for detecting Down syndrome. A significant ethical concern is raised by the use of ultrasound as a screening tool: what if the mother wishes to terminate her pregnancy because the fetus is positive for Down's?[9]

- *Nuchal fold translucency:* an ultrasound performed by a specially trained physician-sonographer at 10½–13½ weeks that measures the thickness of the skin in the back of the baby's neck. If the skin folds are thickened, there is an increased risk of Trisomy 21 or 18 and further testing and counseling are recommended.

- *Chorionic villi sampling (CVS):* a test performed at 11–12 weeks to detect specific genetic abnormalities by obtaining cells from the developing placenta (villi) and examining the chromosomes or DNA in the lab. CVS is performed by inserting either a catheter through the vagina and cervix or a needle through the abdomen into the villi. The risk of miscarriage is about 1 percent, but the procedure can be done earlier than amniocentesis.

- *Maternal serum marker screening (MMS):* a simple blood test that is offered to pregnant women at 15–18 weeks to screen for neural tube defects (such as spina bifida and anencephaly) and two chromosome disorders (Trisomy 21 and 18). The MMS for the Trisomies have a detection rate of 85 percent and 60 percent respectively. MMS measures the concentration of proteins (alpha-fetoprotein, unconjugated estriol, human chorionic gonadotropin, and inhibin A) that are made by the fetus during pregnancy and that circulate in the blood of a pregnant woman.

- *Amniocentesis:* a diagnostic test performed at 15–20 weeks in which a fine needle is inserted through the abdomen to withdraw a small amount of amniotic fluid from the sac holding the developing fetus. The fetal cells found in the amniotic fluid are then grown in a cell culture and studied to detect chromosome abnormalities. Specific enzyme or DNA analyses, which may be indicated based on family or medical history, can also be performed on the fetal cells derived from amniotic fluid. The risk of miscarriage is less than 1 percent.[10]

Preimplantation genetic diagnosis involves removing and testing a polar body (a small cell that is the by-product of meiosis) from an egg cell or, more commonly, a single cell from an early embryo before implantation for identification of genetic mutations associated with disorders. Two procedures are testing polar body and testing embryonic cells.

- *Testing polar body:* IVF techniques are used to obtain eggs from the mother, and the genetic makeup of the egg is inferred from the genetic makeup of the polar body cells; eggs determined to be free of the particular disease under scrutiny are then fertilized in the lab with the sperm of the father or donor, and the embryo is implanted.

- *Testing embryonic cells:* one or two cells are removed from the developing embryo two to four days after fertilization, and the DNA from these cells is examined; results can be obtained within 12 to 24 hours, and the embryos without the genetic abnormality or with the desired genetic traits are then transferred into the uterine cavity.

Almost all genetically inherited conditions that can be diagnosed in the prenatal period can also be detected during the preimplantation period.

Discussion: Ethical Issues and Analysis

Having briefly reviewed the clinical aspects of reproductive technology, we now move to an ethical analysis of the issues related to RTs. We have already raised these issues in the form of numerous questions. Because there are so many, we cannot do justice to them all here. Instead, we examine some of the more pressing questions, starting with whether it is morally acceptable to intervene in reproduction.

Intervening in Reproduction

This may not seem like an important issue, because we are accustomed to babies being born as a result of reproductive interventions. However, when AI and, especially, IVF first became widely available, the main ethical question was whether these budding technologies ought to be used. The concern was that we could be overstepping natural limits by creating life apart from sexual intercourse within marriage, and that by doing so, the "humanness" of reproduction could be lost as technology replaces the generative, life-giving act of the spouses. To put it more simply, the concern was that creating babies through technological as opposed to natural means could cheapen the reproductive process and undermine the good of marriage, as well as the dignity of those born through the use of such technology.

This discussion unfolded mostly within Christian religious circles but rapidly spilled over into the public debate. Interestingly, apart from the Roman Catholic Church, most Christian religious traditions ultimately decided that interventions into reproduction, such as AI and IVF, could be morally acceptable despite the so-called unnatural means of achieving pregnancy. Although there were some reservations as to how the interventions might be used, there was general agreement that their use within marriage could be justified morally. The thinking behind these various Christian viewpoints is that procreation is a great good of marriage. As such, remedies to correct infertility, within the context of marriage, are encouraged and welcomed. Just as we use technological means to overcome biological limitations caused by illness, so too can such means be used to treat infertility, especially because it enables couples to bring their love to fruition and to grow in relationship with one another. There is nothing that says procreation has to be achieved solely by "natural means" of conceiving and "life-giving." We can get an assist from technology as we do in many other areas of our lives.[11]

A steadfast opponent of this viewpoint is the Roman Catholic Church, which holds that reproductive interventions, such as AI and IVF, are not morally permissible when they go beyond assisting natural processes and instead substitute for them to help married couples achieve pregnancy. Although procreation within the context of marriage is indeed a good, the integrity of the marriage and the dignity of the child demand that pregnancy be achieved through natural means as the marriage partners express their love for one another in the intimate act of sexual intercourse ("marriage act") and cooperate with God in the creation of a new human being. This viewpoint is summarized well in the introduction to part 4 of the *Ethical and Religious Directives for Catholic Health Care Services:*

> With the advance of the biological and medical sciences, society has at its disposal new technologies for responding to the problem of infertility. While we rejoice in the potential for good inherent in many of these technologies, we cannot assume that what is technically possible is always morally right. Reproductive technologies that substitute for the marriage act are not consistent with human dignity. Just as the marriage act is joined naturally to procreation, so procreation is joined naturally to the marriage act.[12]

The Catholic tradition presents its unique Christian perspective in its moral evaluation of reproductive interventions, which is concerned primarily with the intervention or individual act, and only secondarily with the couple's intentions or any potential good consequences (i.e., having a baby). We see this in the following statement of the Second Vatican Council:

> When there is question of harmonizing conjugal love with the responsible transmission of life, the moral aspect of any procedure *does not depend solely* on sincere *intentions* or on an evaluation of motives. It must be determined by objective standards. These, based on the nature of the human person and *his acts,* preserve the full sense of mutual self-giving and human procreation in the context of true love.[13]

According to Catholic teaching, then, any intervention into reproduction that substitutes for the natural act of sexual intercourse within marriage is absolutely prohibited, no matter what good may come from it. IVF, in particular, moves procreation from the purview of the married partners into a clinic, where fertilization occurs outside the woman's body. In this way, procreation is deprived of its essential "mutual self-giving" of the partners as manifest through the natural act of sexual intercourse. Catholic teaching does hold, however, that "certain artificial means designed only to facilitate the natural act or to enable that act, performed in a normal manner, to attain its end" are not necessarily off limits or forbidden.[14]

So what are we to make of RTs? Are they a morally acceptable means of achieving pregnancy, or do they represent an unwarranted technological intrusion into reproduction? Considering this question against the backdrop of our normative basis, it seems to us the objection raised by the Catholic Church focuses too heavily on the intervention itself and whether pregnancy is achieved through natural or technological means.[15] This is certainly a concern, because we are dealing with the delicate area of human reproduction, and there is always the potential for abuse of the technology. Yet our normative basis, which is grounded in human flourishing and right relationship, would consider RTs in a much broader context by reflecting on whether reproductive interventions can help married people grow in their relationship with one another and progress on the path of human flourishing through the life-giving role of becoming parents.

In saying this, we do not mean that people have an absolute right to have children regardless of the means used or that having children of one's own is necessary for human flourishing. We agree with Maura Ryan that "as a dimension of human flourishing, the opportunity to conceive or bear a child of one's own can be called basic without being necessary, central without being essential."[16] Rather, we are saying that any moral evaluation of RTs must go deeper than merely looking at the intervention itself and include an assessment of how the intervention contributes to the overall development and flourishing of the married couple. When viewed in this way, we may come to the conclusion that *in certain circumstances*, reproductive technologies are a morally acceptable means of enhancing the relationship of married people who are committed to one another and to expressing their love in the creation of a new human being.

All this assumes that marriage is the normative or ideal context for having children. With no disrespect to single parents or parents in nontraditional relationships, experience suggests that, all things considered, marriage offers a certain level of stability for raising children that other relationships may not. This, of course, is not always the case.

Additionally, the use of RTs outside of marriage often involves donors or surrogates and this, to us, is unacceptable for three reasons: First, it degrades human reproduction, as the baby that results is not the fruit of love between two committed individuals but the choice of individuals who contract with third parties and pay for their "services" (whether it be eggs, sperm, or uterus). Second, it distorts our collective view of human reproduction and responsible parenting. Although AI using donor sperm raises concerns, IVF adds further concern in that one can have a sperm donor, an egg donor, and a surrogate mother, all with the possibility that the person or couple who eventually raises the baby had no part in any of this. In effect, a baby produced through IVF could have five "parents": the genetic parents (those who donate the eggs and sperm), the gestational parent (the woman who carries and delivers the baby), and the social parents (those who rear the baby). Third, IVF could negatively affect offspring who must, if truth be told, deal with the fact they were conceived through the use of a donor or donors and carried by a surrogate whom they most likely will never know. Empirical evidence is mixed on this. You might try an experiment: ask yourself how you would feel if you found out you were born through the use of eggs bought over the Internet after a careful screening process that involved selecting just the "right" woman with just the "right" traits.

Disproportionate Burdens to Women

An often overlooked issue with RTs is that women tend to bear most of the burdens, whether these are the burdens associated with egg harvesting, with the actual intervention, with carrying and delivering the embryo, or with raising any resulting children. Is it fair that the woman must undergo this grueling process, especially if it is not the woman's infertility issue but the male's? To some extent nothing can be done about this. The burdens are what they are, and unfortunately they fall disproportionately to women. And women always have a choice to participate or not—or do they? Society has a way of telling women they must have children, that they can be complete only through this experience. Psychologically and spiritually this can have devastating effects on women. Is there not subtle coercion, then, for women to use reproductive technologies in an effort to get pregnant when infertility gets in the way?

What about egg donors and surrogates, who do not even get a baby in the end? Is it fair to them that they have to participate in this process and endure the burdens, which can be significant with egg harvesting and with surrogacy, especially if multiple embryos are transferred? Of course, they do not have to participate. They, too, have a choice—or do they? Surrogacy arrangements can be lucrative, as can payment for eggs (on average about $3,000–$5,000, but sometimes higher for the "right" eggs). How enticing might it be to women who may be struggling financially to offer themselves up so that another person or couple can achieve their dream of having a baby? What do they have to go through when they are being screened for their eggs or picked for surrogacy, having to answer sensitive questions, submit health records, and be looked over physically? Is this how we want to treat women? Does it not objectify them and exploit them for the personal gain of others?

These are all difficult questions. Outside the context of a particular case, it is hard to say whether the burdens of reproductive interventions that women are made to endure undermine their dignity and threaten their integral well-being. Nevertheless, as we consider the ethics of RTs against the backdrop of our normative basis, we must keep these questions in mind, as they can have a significant effect on our overall moral evaluation. In the end it may come down to a matter of consent on the part of the woman. Still, we must be mindful of this overarching issue, too often cast aside in ethical discussions of reproductive interventions.

Access and Equitable Distribution

Two closely connected issues that get too little attention when considering the ethics of RTs are the access to and the equitable distribution of health care resources. As noted above, IVF is expensive, prohibitively so for many people in the United States and for people in many other parts of the world where access to even basic health care services is lacking. Is it fair that IVF is available to some but not others? We could fix this problem perhaps, at least in developed nations, by requiring all health insurance plans to provide coverage for it. Currently some do, but most do not. Adding this coverage, however, would significantly increase overall health care spending, which is already high ($1.023 billion in 2010) and continues to rise at a furious pace. Is IVF important enough that we are willing to make it more fairly accessible? Probably not, because there are more basic areas of health to which we need to attend (e.g., immunization, clean water, and preventative health programs for chronic illness), and the option of adoption is always available.

Even if we did add IVF coverage to health plans, however, it would not completely solve the problem, given that more than 50.7 million Americans (16.7 percent of the U.S. population) are presently uninsured. This brings us to the question of whether we should be doing IVF at all when so many of our fellow Americans lack even minimal health care coverage. Even though the costs of all RTs are high (about $2 billion a year in the United States alone), they are assumed mostly by individuals, not by health plans or the federal government. Thus, a dollar saved on IVF or some other reproductive technology does not necessarily mean an extra dollar for basic health care for the uninsured. Still, we do dedicate health care resources to technological reproduction in the form of time, money, equipment, research, and personnel. Wouldn't such resources be better used in other ways that improved more significant health problems? What is more, is it ethical for a society to pursue expensive, elective interventions when so many people, mostly women, children, and the working poor, have to rely on emergency rooms or overcrowded free clinics for their care or go without?

Unfortunately, in our society the market tends to dictate access to health care services and distribution of health care resources. In effect, if you have the money, you can get the services. This is largely how the reproductive technology industry works. Put simply, those with the means can have the babies. Although this may satisfy economists, it is clearly not the best system from an ethical perspective. Health care should be more coordinated, and if we were prioritizing in terms of basic health requirements, reproductive technologies might fall far down the list. Given these concerns, particularly when they are viewed in light of human flourishing and right relationships, it seems inconceivable that we could look on RTs favorably. But given that interventions are available and will continue to be so in the future, we have to make more prudent and discerning choices regarding their use. Rather than letting the market make our decisions for us and assuming that we have unlimited procreative liberty, we need to recognize our responsibility to the common good. Although the leap from the individual to society may not seem natural, our normative basis demands it insofar as we are social beings connected to others in our pursuit of human flourishing.

Value of Early Human Life

Another important issue involves the treatment of embryos in reproductive interventions in which fertilization occurs outside the woman's body, such as IVF. Though it is clear from the abortion and stem cell debates that many people do not consider the four- to five-day-old embryo a person, no one can reasonably deny that it is human life at an early stage of development. Everyone reading this book passed through this stage of human development. However we may view the embryo individually or collectively, the least we can say is that it is valuable and deserves respect as a beginning form of human life. If this statement is true, then we have to ask whether our current handling of embryos is morally acceptable in our attempts to achieve reproduction technologically.

Wouldn't it be more respectful to human life to develop only the number of embryos that could be safely transferred into the woman without having to submit "extra" embryos to the cryopreservation process, which is not without risks? Admittedly, this would be more expensive, because a failed intervention would mean starting over again and instead of using excess embryos. Yet how much more respectful is this of human life than creating excess embryos that not only need to be stored in freezers but also are often discarded because they are no longer needed or are donated for research where they are manipulated and dissected for the "good" of science? By instituting this change, wouldn't we be saying that human life matters, and wouldn't this translate into a deeper respect for all life that spills over into all our relationships and to our views of creation? At least it would be better than what we are currently doing.

There are also concerns about genetic screening techniques before embryo transfer (e.g., preimplantation genetic diagnosis) to weed out undesirable embryos that might have a genetic mutation or, even worse, might be the "wrong" gender. What does this say about who we are as individuals and as a society? Does this practice undermine the gift of life by turning embryos into products for which we can select traits, or gender—as already clearly occurs in other parts of the world? If we are serious about pursuing human flourishing and fostering right relationships, then we have to be more respectful of early human life in all its dynamism. We ought to find this type of treatment of embryos in reproductive interventions simply unacceptable when viewed against this larger backdrop.

Case Studies in Assisted Reproduction

We have described the science of AR and discussed some of the ethical questions they raise. By way of summary, let us now consider case studies that allow us to apply some of our reflections.

Case 6A

Sam and Camory, happily married for more than eight years, have been trying to have children for some time without success. Examination by a physician reveals that Camory has blocked fallopian tubes, and surgery would not rectify the condition—quite simply, they are unable to have children through conventional means. They strongly desire to have a child that is their own genetic offspring, and although their insurance does not cover reproductive interventions other than fertility drugs, they are willing to make the financial sacrifice. Sam and Camory's deep longing for children leaves no reason to doubt they will be loving parents. To a certain extent they also feel their marriage is lacking because they are unable to have children. Faced with this situation, IVF seems like the best solution. Camory is a prime candidate for the intervention because her uterus and ovaries are healthy. Also Sam has an adequate sperm count and the sperm function properly. Thus neither a donor nor surrogate will be necessary. IVF seems to offer them a good chance at having genetic offspring.[17]

This is a common situation in the context of reproductive technology. Like so many other individuals and couples, Sam and Camory's deep longing for children and feelings of emptiness stem from problems related to infertility. IVF offers them hope of overcoming these challenges. The question is whether it is morally acceptable for Sam and Camory to pursue this reproductive intervention in an effort to have a child. The first thing to consider as we think about this case is how having a child through technological means will affect their relationship. Will it bring them closer together in their love for each other? Will it satisfy the deep longing and fill the emptiness they have? What kind of parents will they be? Will their love for each other be reflected in how they care for the child should the procedure succeed? Given what we know, it seems that Sam and Camory's relationship could be enhanced by having a child. Though happily married for eight years, they long to have a child, which they would very much welcome into their lives and for which they would take full parental responsibility. Yet is this adequate? This would suggest that any committed, married couple experiencing infertility could pursue reproductive technologies if they are willing and able. Our normative basis requires a deeper look.

The use of a donor or surrogate is not an issue here. If they were to have recourse to a donor or surrogate, we would have to object given the potential negative effect on the marriage, offspring, and society at large.

We also must consider whether the burdens on Camory are acceptable. Is Camory aware of what IVF entails in terms of fertility drugs, egg harvesting, the transfer of multiple embryos, and the possibility of multiple pregnancies and associated risks? If her physician explained all this to her and she is willing to accept the burdens, it is hard to argue that these burdens are too heavy, especially because she will not be asking another to carry these burdens for her (through egg donation or surrogacy).

How will Sam and Camory's decision affect their financial well-being and the common good? Because their health insurance does not cover IVF, they are going to have to assume all the costs. We don't know what effect this will have on them, but if they can reasonably afford it without undermining their overall well-being, then it would be hard to deny them this opportunity on these grounds. If they were receiving help or coverage from their health plan, one could argue that their use of IVF could drive up the overall costs of the plan and result in increased premiums for all members, but that is not the case here.

Will Sam and Camory elect to create multiple embryos and choose to freeze any that are not transferred in the first cycle of treatment? Respect for early human life demands that they create only the number of embryos that could be safely transferred for implantation without having recourse to cryopreservation. If they insist on this point, we would have no objections on these grounds.

Finally, we must consider whether there are any viable alternatives for Sam and Camory, such as becoming foster parents or adopting. Would one of these options satisfy their deep longing to have a child? Either of these options would allow Sam and Camory the opportunity to be parents while at the same time providing a safe, loving home for a child in need. For many people with problems of infertility, though, these are options of last resort because of their strong desire to have children of their own genetic lineage. Though ideal, these options seem to demand more from Sam and Camory than we can reasonably expect.

The case of Camory and Sam again reveals that one must not isolate individual decisions about reproductive interventions from the broader context of human flourishing and right relationships. We may not have satisfied a desire for definitive answers to the ethical questions raised by RTs, but hopefully through the discussion of the ethical issues and the analysis of this case we have shown what needs to be considered. Perhaps the most we can say about reproductive interventions outside of concrete situations is that there are certain circumstances in which their use may be morally permissible. Like many of the Christian religious traditions noted above, the circumstances we would find acceptable would be within the context of a loving, committed marriage, where there is no recourse to donors or surrogates, where the health and safety of the woman is protected, where embryos are not destroyed, where financial burdens are borne by the couple, and where the common good is not negatively affected. The use of RTs in such a context and under these circumstances would be conducive to fostering right relationships and ultimately contributing to the well-being of the married couple and their children without undermining that of others.

Now consider another case:

Case 6B

A 35-year-old female contacts you regarding a letter she received from an infertility clinic where she contracted services for in vitro fertilization some fifteen years ago. The letter states that she has five embryos frozen in cryopreservation and her agreement is due to expire in six months. The infertility clinic is asking what she would like to have done with the embryos at the expiration of the contract. The contract

cont.

Case 6B *cont.*

stipulated that she could continue the cryopreservation process on a year-to-year basis at $300 annually. The woman was unaware that she had any embryos still in cryopreservation and is stunned to find out that she is now responsible for determining their fate. She is currently divorced from the man whose sperm was used in the in vitro fertilization process and she has sole custody of their children.

At the same time, the former husband received the same letter due to legal stipulations in the informed consent process at the time of the in vitro process. The letter states the mother has the right to determine what to do with the embryos (which includes offering the embryos for adoption or donating them for research purposes), unless she chooses to have the embryos destroyed. In the latter case, the partner's consent would be necessary, regardless of marital status. Further complicating the matter is that the ex-husband's visitation rights had been taken away due to allegations surrounding child neglect and abuse, and the woman does not want to reopen a custody battle in the courts for fear her ex-husband might gain visitation rights. Also she had recently lost her job and, although she has found new employment, it pays substantially less. She says she is barely getting by and is not financially prepared to handle the $300 fee to keep the embryos in cryopreservation. The woman tells you she is a Roman Catholic. She has not gone to church in quite some time but is aware of the Catholic Church's position on abortion and does not feel it is right to simply dispose of the embryos. Furthermore, destruction of the embryos would require the husband's consent, and she does not want to reestablish contact if avoidable.

Despite financial hardship, does the divorced couple (or at least the woman) have an obligation to maintain the embryos in cryopreservation? Or should the woman simply offer the embryos for adoption to avoid reestablishing contact with her former husband and the corresponding risks to her children should contact occur? Is there another ethically permissible option?

Beyond Assisted Reproduction: Ethics and Prenatal Testing

The ethical issues and questions brought about by RTs are not limited to those ARs that people may use to try to become pregnant. RTs also enable us to gain knowledge about the child with which one has already become pregnant or may become pregnant. Indeed, many ethical issues arise in the context of what ought one to do in light of this knowledge given a current or desired pregnancy.

Issues in Carrier Testing and Screening. The acquisition of knowledge is not in itself a justification for CT or CS. Yet such technologies can be extremely beneficial to individuals with a genetic predisposition to a particular disease. For example, those with the gene for xerodermapigmentosum are extremely sensitive to ultraviolet radiation, and exposure to such radiation is likely to lead to a form of melanoma that is usually incurable. However, avoiding such exposure usually allows one to avoid developing melanoma; knowledge leads to benefit.

Take, however, the case of Duchenne muscular dystrophy (DMD), an X-linked recessive disease. Because females have two X chromosomes, a female can be a carrier of a DMD gene mutation but will usually not develop the condition, because she has a normal copy of the gene on her second X chromosome. Knowledge of being a carrier for this condition will in no way lead to treatment or cure. In other words, no way of preventing the disease is known, and early diagnosis and intervention makes no difference in the outcome of the disease progression. Some may wish to know whether they are a carrier of the deleterious gene so as to make informed decisions about marriage, childbearing, and lifestyle. Others might prefer blissful ignorance. This raises an ethical question: in cases where treatment or cure cannot change the outcome of the disease progression, should genetic testing be done as a matter of responsibility to future offspring and society? That is, does an individual with a terminal genetic diagnosis have an obligation to undergo testing so as not to reproduce? If so, the deleterious gene would not harm future offspring, and the lineage with the genetic anomaly would cease.[18]

The normative basis offered in this work suggests that the question of what constitutes right relationships between parent and child (or potential child) is relevant in a discussion about CT. Specific to the case of DMD and future children, it is important to recognize that a male child would be at significantly greater risk for having DMD than a female child. Thus the question of whether to reproduce or the obligation not to reproduce begs further ethical questions: should one screen embryos positive for the DMD gene mutation and select only those embryos negative for the mutation, or select only females (who may be carriers but would likely not be otherwise affected)? The question of whether one has an obligation not to reproduce also begs the question of obligations to future generations. Certainly, our commitment to human flourishing would suggest that where known gene-based disorders would be clearly transmitted to a future generation, one has an obligation to avoid reproduction to the extent that such a disease would arguably impair that person's ability to flourish. However, such an assertion cannot suggest the person currently living with DMD somehow lacks human dignity or the ability to flourish as a human person. We will address this line of argumentation in the section on prenatal diagnosis.

What if a gene-based disease is identified as specific to an ethnic background, as in the case of sickle-cell disease, which is an inherited autosomal recessive genetic disorder found mainly in people of West African descent and people of Mediterranean origin? The disease affects the ability of hemoglobin in the blood to carry oxygen. In a sickle-cell crisis, hemoglobin is distorted and trapped in small blood vessels, which results in severe pain, blood clots, and even stroke or heart attack. In 1972, the U.S. government adopted a national screening program. Unfortunately, the program did not include education regarding the disorder. African American schoolchildren, athletes, and military cadets were targeted in many states, and leaders of these communities argued that the mandatory screenings were racially motivated and discriminatory. As a result of these state-sponsored screenings, many individuals, including carriers who were quite healthy, faced discrimination in employment and insurance.[19]

Further ethical questions concern informed consent, that is, whether people are forced to undergo such testing or screening or are fully informed of the implications of such testing or screening. Another concern is whether people are given proper education, support, and counseling related to the test results and the possible applications of such knowledge. Other questions concern whether individuals should disclose genetic knowledge to their offspring, and who should decide when and how much the offspring should know. Finally, what might be the effect of this genetic information on the individual's family?

Ethical Issues in Prenatal Diagnosis. A central tenet of the practice of prenatal diagnosis is the claim that there is no connection between the test, the documentation of fetal abnormalities, and the decision of whether to terminate the pregnancy. The assertion is often made that prenatal diagnosis is for the purpose of providing information to couples about what they can expect. Is this a naïve or overly limited perspective? Does one have a responsibility to early human life irrespective of the child's genetic makeup? Once the information is disclosed to a parent about the genetic makeup of his or her child, can one truly obtain noncoercive, unbiased counseling related to matters like selective termination and alternatives?[20] Some argue that knowledge gained from prenatal diagnoses and screening can significantly prepare parents for what they are to expect. Additionally, in cases where outcomes can be affected, prenatal screening may allow for significant changes in obstetrical care (e.g., children with ventral wall defects or neural tube defects can be delivered in an environment that can immediately address these issues as well as adapt modes of delivery to significantly reduce comorbidities). But can these distinctions be drawn so clearly for parents, who may be in the midst of decisions related to the results of a genetic test or screen?

Given that answers to many of these questions are rooted in specific definitions of what constitutes human life, imperfection, normalcy, and health, it is important that ethical reflection consider what constitutes a genetic disorder.[21] In other words, if one's genetic makeup is increasingly the basis for evaluations of normalcy, should parents have their fetuses tested for obesity, shortness, asthma, migraine headaches, alcoholism, depression, aggressiveness, Alzheimer's disease, and sexual orientation? In an attempt to define these terms, questions arise. If there were a test for determining a predisposition for homosexuality, what if someone wished to use it as a prelude to selective abortion? Should geneticists withhold certain information if they feel it will be used for selective abortion because, for instance, the baby is considered the "wrong sex"? Ought society or the medical profession set limits on individual autonomy in the age of genomics? Is nondirective counseling for parents at odds with public health considerations? In other words, what if, from a societal perspective, genetic testing is confirming that the gene pool continues to be weakened? Do we have social eugenic responsibilities to correct this negative effect?[22]

Genetic information is deeply personal and yet has profound social implications. If individuals in their reproductive years have deleterious genes that may lead to genetic disorders, the possibility of passing those genes along or the potential harm caused to future generations sets up a unique set of circumstances in an age of genomics. Rosamond Rhodes has proposed an interesting argument suggesting "there is no right to genetic ignorance."[23] She argues there is a duty to inform one's family of one's genomic heritage based on traditional kinship bonds and a duty of fidelity. Genetic knowledge may be viewed like any other sort of knowledge that allows us to make life decisions. Failing to act in accord with genetic knowledge constitutes failure to accept our human condition and treat ourselves with the inherent respect deserving of human beings. Many of these ethical issues are illustrated in the following case:

Case 6C

In 1983 a group of Orthodox Jews in New York and Israel initiated a screening program to eliminate diseases transmitted as recessive genes within their community. The group called itself Dor Yeshorim, "the generation of the righteous." A couple familiar with this program is working with Dr. Cowan and decide they are going to take their chances despite both of them testing as carriers for Tay-Sachs. Unfortunately, amniocentesis reveals the fetus is positive for Tay-Sachs.

The couple knew the odds were stacked against them in terms of their fetus testing positive for Tay-Sachs, but they felt they had a right to try to have genetic offspring. Now they

cont.

Case 6C *cont.*

are wondering whether the unfavorable odds might suggest they had an obligation not to reproduce. They are struggling with feelings that they knowingly put their child in harm's way. They are knowledgeable about Tay-Sachs, but it is still difficult for them to conceptualize that it is their child who has the disease. Finally, they are struggling with their emotional pain, knowing they will be raising a child who will live less than a year and die as a result of this condition.

The couple in the case study is struggling with Rhodes's idea that they may have an obligation not to reproduce. Our normative basis suggests that although there is no right to reproduce, offspring is certainly a significant component of human flourishing as it relates to married couples. Yet in this set of circumstances, the couple is presented with unique knowledge before a decision to attempt to procreate. This knowledge seems to create responsibility based on the human dignity of the future person.[24] This is a difficult discussion to process, however. What are our obligations to future individuals? We commonly refer to these sorts of obligations in such contexts as the reduction in nuclear arms, the removal and treatment of nuclear waste, education regarding the prevention and spread of disease, and concerns about the national debt. However, given that future individuals do not yet exist (and may never exist), the notion of obligation becomes problematic at best.[25] In other words, one must question the extent to which persons who do not exist can place obligations on persons who do. Nonetheless, human dignity suggests the fetus the couple is going to bring into the world does possess inherent dignity and worth as a human being and must be treated as such despite its limited life span and potential for great suffering. The obligations of the couple are now those related to becoming parents as with any other offspring. The question of flourishing as a married couple and the matter of offspring might have been addressed through other means, perhaps, like adoption.[26] Although often considered less satisfactory than having genetic offspring, parenthood through other means could have provided an avenue for human flourishing. Yet now that possibility is beside the point: a fetus has been conceived, that fetus possesses inherent human dignity, and the parents of that fetus have obligations to their child's well-being as any parents do.

Ethical Issues in Preimplantation Genetic Diagnosis. An advantage of PGD allows a person to detect genetic defects that cause inherited disease in human embryos before they are implanted. PGD offers selection of healthy embryos leading to presumptively healthy pregnancies and the ability to discard unhealthy embryos at a stage earlier than conventional methods. However, because of PGD's link to IVF, ethical issues that burden the mother include all those related to both technologies (see chapter 9). Other issues are associated with the moral status of the human embryo. Although this issue was discussed more substantively in previous chapters, specific concerns related to the moral status of the human embryo and PGD also require discussion here.

At the eight-cell stage of embryonic development, the embryo is apparently unharmed by the process of "cellular biopsy"; however, the research is somewhat ambiguous. Hence, polar body PGD or preconception PGD may be ethically more acceptable to those opposed to the manipulation of the human embryo. These forms of PGD have their limits in terms of reliability and, in the case of preconception, PGD has so far failed to establish a pregnancy.

To date, steps have been taken through legislation or public policy to set parameters around the use of PGD. For example, in the United Kingdom alteration of an embryo's genes, even for gene therapy or cloning embryos, is illegal. All IVF clinics must be licensed by a government-appointed authority; this authority can withhold a license if the proposed use of PGD is not ethically acceptable or otherwise justified. This may include the use of PGD for sex selection exclusively.

Several ethical questions call for reflection. If harmful effects could occur to the embryo, can the benefits of genetic knowledge ever outweigh the harm? What is our responsibility to early human life even if it does exhibit deleterious genes? What are the obligations of medical practitioners who offer IVF in conjunction with PGD to the prospective parents, and what are their obligations to any embryos created? What of questions of access and distributive justice? Do all prospective parents have access to the technology? Is knowledge of the technology made available to all people regardless of socioeconomic status, race, ethnicity, education, and other factors that often limit access?[27] Consider the following case:

Case 6D

Mark and Cory are little people. They feel they would not know how to raise a child that is not a little person. They have made numerous changes to their living environment to accommodate their size and wonder what it would be like if their son or daughter soon surpassed their height. Further, Cory comments, "We want a child like us. We understand our culture and wish to emphasize that this life is just as dignified as others." Mark and Cory decide they want to speak with a geneticist to screen embryos before implantation for those that are positive for the genetic mutation that produces dwarfism. Mark and Cory are confident that in speaking with a genetic counselor, they will get unbiased information as to the likelihood of PGD allowing them to achieve their goals. Yet when they meet with the genetic counselor, Mark and Cory are dismayed that the counselor starts her conversation by asking whether Mark and Cory have considered whether such a selection might be in the best interests of their child.

Mark is outraged. He comments, "I thought genetic counselors were supposed to be value neutral. We came to you precisely to avoid this type of discussion." Mark goes on to ask, "Do you begin your discussion with prospective parents in a similar manner when they are blind or deaf and make similar requests? What is so different in our situation?"

May a prospective parent, as in the case of Mark and Cory, use PGD to screen embryos for conditions like dwarfism, deafness, or blindness? Is it appropriate to consider, as Mark implicitly asserts, all such conditions as equal? Our normative basis would definitely affirm that all such people are equally valued as human beings and in their inherent dignity and worth because they are all created in the image of God. Yet the issue is not whether such people maintain such dignity and worth but rather can prospective parents intentionally use technology to try to bring only individuals positive for these conditions into existence? A simplistic view of autonomy might suggest that prospective parents with the means to do so should be allowed to screen their embryos for a variety of conditions to achieve the ends they desire. However, recall that we are framing these ethical issues in the context of human flourishing and right relationships. In that context one must ask whether the parents are selfishly restricting their offspring's abilities in order to feel more comfortable about their ability as parents. Should the parents use technology as a means to legitimize a culture, or should it be more a matter of how actively they pursue such a cause to the exclusion of purposefully screening their embryos for particular characteristics?

Addressing such a question would require our conception of human anthropology and human flourishing to suggest that blindness, deafness, and dwarfism are conditions that prospective parents ought to, at the least, purposefully choose for their offspring. Laura Purdy attempts to deal with this difficult issue in what she calls criteria for a "minimally satisfying life."[28] Admittedly, the term *minimally satisfying* is a shifting concept based on the relative concept of normal health in a given culture. It is difficult to know what to make of this claim, or even what demands it places on us presently.[29] Yet as argued earlier, to ignore such a claim would result in creating unnecessary constraints on human flourishing and, in certain cases, suffering and purposeful disadvantage for some people.[30] Hence, despite its relativity, the claim is somewhat satisfactory, for it implies that "parents ought to try to provide for their children health normal for that culture, even though it may be inadequate if measured by some outside standard."[31]

Additional Case Studies

Case 6E

In January 2007, the American College of Obstetricians and Gynecologists (ACOG) released new recommendations for Down syndrome screening. The recommendations suggest that all

cont.

Case 6E *cont.*

pregnant women, regardless of their age, should be offered screening for Down syndrome. Previously, only women age 35 and older were offered genetic and diagnostic testing for Down syndrome. According to the new guidelines, the goal is to provide screening tests with high detection rates and low false positive rates that "provide patients with diagnostic testing options if the screening test indicates that the patient is at an increased risk for having a child with Down syndrome." Given that there are a variety of approaches to this level of early screening strategies, the recommendations are intended to offer guidelines to meet the best interests of the patient.

You are the director of benefits for a nonprofit, faith-based organization whose health plan is self-funded. You also have a daughter with Down syndrome. You wonder why your organization would fund screening tests for Down syndrome earlier in a woman's pregnancy. You suspect the reason the ACOG recommendations have changed is to allow women to terminate pregnancies positive for Down syndrome early in the pregnancy, although you hope this is not true. Through inquiry you find that some people suggest earlier screening allows parents to prepare early for a child diagnosed with Down syndrome. You approach your vice president of human resources to inquire whether the benefits plan should cover this set of screening tests.

Given the strong correlation between pregnancy termination and a diagnosis of Down Syndrome, might there be an undisclosed motivation behind earlier testing that includes, but is not limited to, detection specificity early enough to allow for first-trimester termination? Given the risks associated with follow-up testing after the first-trimester screening, especially given ACOG's recommendation to open screening to all women (not just those 35 and older), are there plan cost implications without commensurate value added in terms of information for the mother making the decision?

Case 6F

John, a 22-year-old man married just under a year, has just been diagnosed as brain-dead after a severe car accident. His wife, Dana, who has the legal right to make decisions for him, agrees to multiple organ donations to be coordinated by a local organ procurement organization. Dana also makes an unusual request: can sperm be obtained from John so that she can become impregnated through IVF? Dana states, "This is one way that John can live on." John's primary physician is obviously uneasy about this request and probes into the situation further. The physician finds out that John never really discussed having kids with Dana. Nevertheless, Dana insists, "This is what John would have wanted."

Should the sperm be retrieved from John so Dana can have his baby? Why or why not? Does this formulation call into question the nature of family? What role should society have in answering that question?

SUGGESTED READINGS

Congregation for the Doctrine of the Faith. *Donum vitae.http://www. vatican.va/roman_curia/congregations/cfaith/documents/rc_con_cfaith_ doc_19870222_respect-for-human-life_en.html.*

Congregation for the Doctrine of the Faith. *Dignitas Personae. http:// www.vatican.va/roman_curia/congregations/cfaith/documents/rc_con_ cfaith_doc_20081212_sintesi-dignitas-personae_en.html.*

Harwood, Karey A. *The Infertility Treadmill: Feminist Ethics, Personal Choice, and the Use of Reproductive Technologies.* Chapel Hill: University of North Carolina Press, 2007.

Kohl, Beth. *Embryo Culture: Making Babies in the Twenty-First Century.* New York: Farrar, Straus, and Giroux, 2007.

Ryan, Maura. *The Ethics and Economics of Assisted Reproduction: The Cost of Longing.* Washington, DC: Georgetown University Press, 2001

Sontag, Sherry. *One in a Million: The Real Story of IVF and the Fight to Forge a Family.* New York: PublicAffairs, 2007.

Spar, Debora L. *The Baby Business: How Money, Science, and Politics Drive the Commerce of Conception.* Boston: Harvard Business School Press, 2006.

Spencer, John R., and Antje du Bois-Pedain, eds. *Freedom and Responsibility in Reproductive Choice.* Oxford: Hart, 2006.

Winston, Robert. *The IVF Revolution: The Definitive Guide to Assisted Reproductive Techniques.* London: Vermillion, 1999. Excerpts at *http://www. pbs.org/wgbh/pages/frontline/shows/fertility.*

MULTIMEDIA AIDS FOR TEACHERS

"Making Babies: An Examination of the Booming Infertility Business." *Frontline.* PBS. 1999. Excerpts at *http://www.pbs.org/wgbh/pages/ frontline/shows/fertility.*

Nova *Online.* "18 Ways to Make a Baby." PBS Airdate: October 9, 2001. Found at *http://www.pbs.org/wgbh/nova/baby/18ways.html#18ways.*

ENDNOTES

1. For further reading on these topics, see, among others, Charles E. Curran and Richard A. McCormick, eds., *Dialogue about Catholic Sexual Teaching: Readings in Moral Theology,* no. 8 (Mahwah, NJ: Paulist Press, 1993); Michel Foucault, "An Introduction," in *The History of Sexuality,* vol. 1, trans. Robert Hurley (New York: Penguin, 1978); John T. Noonan Jr., *Contraception: A History of Its Treatment by the Catholic Theologians and Canonists* (Cambridge, MA: Harvard University Press, 1986); and Jael Silliman, Marlene Gerber Fried, Loretta Ross, and Elena R. Gutierrez, *Undivided Rights: Women of Color Organize for Reproductive Justice* (Cambridge, MA: South End Press, 2004).

2. There are other reproductive interventions, such as gamete intrafallopian transfer (GIFT), zygote intrafallopian transfer (ZIFT), intravaginal culture (IVC), uterine lavage embryo retrieval (ULER), partial zona dissection (PZD), and intracytoplasmic sperm injection (ICSI). We will not discuss these due to space limitations.

3. The cost of just the IUI and sperm washing is usually $200–$300. However, if there is a need for medication, ultrasounds, blood work, or additional monitoring, then the cost can rise to as much as $6,000.

4. For an excellent source on the process of in vitro fertilization, see Robert Winston, *The IVF Revolution: The Definitive Guide to Assisted Reproductive Techniques* (London: Vermillion, 1999), 1–12.

5. This discussion of egg retrieval is based on the excellent article by Jessica Cohen, "Grade A: The Market for a Yale Woman's Eggs," *Atlantic* 289 (December 2002): 74–8.

6. Evangelos G. Papanikolaou et al., "In Vitro Fertilization with Single Blastocyst-Stage versus Single Cleavage-Stage Embyos," *New England Journal of Medicine* 354 (March 16, 2006): 1139–46; Ann Thurin et al., "Elective Single-Embryo Transfer versus Double-Embryo Transfer," in "In Vitro Fertilization," *New England Journal of Medicine* 351 (December 2, 2004): 2392–402.

7. F. Nawroth et al., "Cryopreservation in Assisted Reproductive Technology: New Trends," *Seminars in Reproductive Medicine* 23 (November 2005): 325–35.

8. C. Slack, K. Lurix, S. Lewis, and L. Lichten, "Prenatal Genetics: The Evolution and Future Directions of Screening and Diagnosis," *Journal of Perinatal and Neonatal Nursing* 20, no. 1 (January–March 2006): 93–7.

9. B. Bromley, E. Lieberman, T. D. Shipp, and B. R. Benacerraf, "The Genetic Sonogram: A Method of Risk Assessment for Down Syndrome in the Second Trimester," *Journal of Ultrasound Medicine* 21 (2002): 1087–96.

10. D. A. Driscoll, "Second Trimester Maternal Serum Screening for Fetal Open Neural Tube Defects and Aneuploidy," *Genetic Medicine* 6 (2004): 540–41; I. R. Merkatz, H. M. Nitowsky, J. N. Macri, and W. E. Johnson, "An Association between Low Maternal Serum Alpha-Fetoprotein and Fetal Chromosomal Abnormalities," *American Journal of Obstetrics and Gynecology* 1 (1984): 926–9.

11. Eric Gregory. "The Ethics of Embryo Adoption and the Catholic Tradition." *Philosophy and Medicine* 95 (2007): 199–218; Board for Social Responsibility [Church of England], "Personal Origins: The Report of a Working Party on Human Fertilization and Embryology of the Board for Social Responsibility," London, 1985.

12. *Ethical and Religious Directives for Catholic Health Care Services*, 4th ed. (U.S. Conference of Catholic Bishops) available at *http://www.usccb.org/bishops/directives.shtml*. See also Congregation for the Doctrine of the Faith, *Donum vitae, On Respect for Human Life in Its Origin, http://www.vatican.va/roman_curia/congregations/cfaith/documents/rc_con_cfaith_doc_19870222_respect-for-human-life_en.html*.

13. Cf. Second Vatican Council, *Gaudium et spes*, 51 (emphasis added).

14. Pius XII, "Address to the 4th International Convention of Catholic Physicians," in *Readings in Moral Theology*, no.8, ed. Charles E. Curran and Richard A. McCormick (New York: Paulist Press, 1993), 224.

15. Congregation for the Doctrine of the Faith, *Donum vitae*.

16. Maura A. Ryan. *The Ethics and Economics of Assisted Reproduction: The Cost of Longing* (Washington, DC: Georgetown University Press, 2001), 172.

17. This case is an adaptation of one found in Craig Paterson, "A Case of Misdirected Love? In Vitro Fertilization and the Quest for Fertility," *Health Care Ethics USA* 8 (2000): 4–5.

18. B. Modell and A. Darr, "Science and Society: Genetic Counseling and Customary Consanguineous Marriage," *Nature Reviews Genetics* 3, no. 3 (March 2002): 225–9; R. M. Nelson, J. R. Botkjin, E. D. Levetown et al., "Ethical Issues with Genetic Testing in Pediatrics," *Pediatrics* 107, no. 6 (June 2001): 1451–5.

19. J. E. Bowman, "To Screen or Not to Screen: When Should Screening Be Offered?" *Community Genetics* 1, no. 3 (1998): 145–7; M. S. Yesley, "Genetic Privacy, Discrimination, and Social Policy: Challenges and Dilemmas," *Microbial and Comparative Genomics* 2, no. 1 (1997): 19–35.

20. M. B. Mahowald, M. S. Verp, and R. R. Anderson, "Genetic Counseling: Clinical and Ethical Challenges," *Annual Review of Genetics* 32 (1998): 547–59.

21. W. French Anderson, "Human Gene Therapy: Why Draw a Line?" in *Bioethics*, ed. Thomas A. Shannon, 4th ed. (Mahwah, NJ: Paulist Press, 1993), 140–51. He states, "Because our knowledge of the human body and mind is so limited, and because we do not know what harm we might inadvertently cause by gene transfer technology, the use of genetic engineering to insert a gene into a human being should first be used only in the treatment of serious disease. . . . The initial 'line' should be those diseases that produce significant suffering and premature death." See also Carol A. Tauer, "Preventing the Transmission of Genetic Diseases," *Chicago Studies* 33, no. 3 (November 1994): 213–39. She writes, "The fact that reasonable people may disagree about the seriousness of particular conditions does not mean that no distinctions can be made."

22. U. Kortner, "The Challenge of Genetic Engineering to Medical Anthropology and Ethics," *Human Reproduction and Genetic Ethics: An International Journal* 7, no. 1 (2001): 21–4.

23. R. Rhodes, "Genetic Links, Family Ties, and Social Bonds: Rights and Responsibilities in the Face of Genetic Knowledge," in *Healthcare Ethics in a Diverse Society*, ed. M. C. Brannigan and J. A. Boss (Mountain View, CA: Mayfield, 2001), 291–303.

24. L. M. Purdy, "Children of Choice: Whose Children? At What Cost?" *Washington and Lee Law Review* 52 (1995): 197–224; L. M. Purdy, "Genetic Diseases: Can Having Children Be Immoral?" in *Genetics Now: Ethical Issues in Genetic Research*, ed. John J. Buckley (Washington, DC: University Press of America, 1978), 25–39.

25. Carol A. Tauer, "Preventing the Transmission of Genetic Diseases," *Chicago Studies* 33, no. 3 (November 1994): 213–39; Jan Christian Heller, *Human Genome Research and the Challenge of Contingent Future Persons* (Omaha, NE: Creighton University Press, 1996).

26. There are other options, such as adoption (in which the parent forgoes genetic offspring to prevent the potential spread of disastrous genetic disease), egg or sperm donation (in which the parent with the deleterious genetic makeup would forego contribution to the genome of the offspring to prevent possible genetic disease), and voluntary sterilization (in which the diseased contributor makes the "genetic sacrifice" to forgo possible reproduction so damaged genes cannot be passed to future generations). Joseph Fletcher made this argument when he considered the possibility of such an act to be virtuous in the context of a technologically advanced society: J. Fletcher, *The Ethics of Genetic Control* (New York: Prometheus Books, 1988).

27. G. Pennings and G. de Wert, "Evolving Ethics in Medically Assisted Reproduction," *Human Reproduction Update* 9, no. 4 (2003): 397–404; G. Pennings, R. Schots, and I. Liebaers, "Ethical Considerations on Preimplantation Genetic Diagnosis for HLA Typing to Match a Future Child as a Donor of Haematopoietic Stem Cells to a Sibling," *Human Reproduction* 17, no. 3 (March 2002): 534–8; R. J. Boyle and J. Savulescu, "Ethics of Using Pre-Implantation Genetic Diagnosis to Select a Stem Cell Donor for an Existing Person," *BMJ* 323 (2001): 1240–43.

28. Laura M. Purdy, "Genetics and Reproductive Risk: Can Having Children Be Immoral?" in *Biomedical Ethics*, ed. Thomas A. Mappes and David DeGrazia (New York: McGraw-Hill, 2001), 520–27.

29. Though some claim that there exists a duty to avoid human suffering for future generations through interventions in the human genome, others feel that such a view is antifeminist and places a huge burden on women to give birth to perfect babies. See Abby Lippman, "Prenatal Genetic Testing and Geneticization: Mother Matters for All," *Fetal Diagnosis and Therapy* 8, Supplement (April 1993): 175–88; Abby Lippman, "Mother Matters: A Fresh Look at Prenatal Genetic Testing," *Issues in Reproductive and Genetic Engineering: Journal of International Feminist Analysis* 5 (1992): 141–54; Abby Lippman, "Prenatal Genetic Testing and Screening: Constructing Needs and Reinforcing Inequities," *American Journal of Law and Medicine* 17 (1991): 15–50. Others argue that a duty to avoid human suffering for future generations may imply genetic interventions in utero without considering the effect of that intervention on the mother; see Purdy, "Children of Choice," 197–224; L. M. Purdy, "Genetic Diseases: Can Having Children Be Immoral?" in *Genetics Now: Ethical Issues in Genetic Research*, ed. John J. Buckley (Washington, DC: University Press of America, 1978), 25–39; L. M. Purdy, "Are Pregnant Women Fetal Containers?" *Bioethics* 4 (1990): 273–91. Still other feminist writers focus on the differing roles related to reproduction and caregiving between the sexes insofar as those roles are affected differently by current advances in genetics: see Mary B. Mahowald, "A Feminist Standpoint for Genetics," *Journal of Clinical Ethics* 7 (1996): 333–40; R. Rapp, "Gender, Body, Biomedicine: How Some Feminist

Concerns Dragged Reproduction to the Center of Social Theory," *Medical Anthropology Quarterly* 15 (December 2001): 466–77; Maura A. Ryan, "Cloning, Genetic Engineering, and the Limits of Procreative Liberty," *Valparaiso University Law Review* 32 (Spring 1998): 753–71; Patricia Spallone and Deborah Lynn Steinberg, eds., *Made to Order: The Myth of Reproductive and Genetic Progress* (New York: Pergamon, 1987); Maura A. Ryan, "The Argument for Unlimited Procreative Liberty: A Feminist Critique," *Hastings Center Report* (July/August 1990): 6–12; S. Squier, "Fetal Subjects and Maternal Objects: Reproductive Technology and the New Fetal/Maternal Relation," *Journal of Medicine and Philosophy* 21 (October 1996): 515–35.

30. John Harris, *Clones, Genes, and Immortality: Ethics and the Genetic Revolution* (Oxford: Oxford University Press, 1998), 211–4; See also Andrew Czeizel, *The Right to Be Born Healthy* (New York: Alan R. Liss, 1988), 65–81.

31. Purdy, "Genetics and Reproductive Risk," 524.

CHAPTER 7

Embryonic Stem Cell Research, Human Cloning, and Regenerative Medicine

John Paul Slosar

What Cost a Cure?

In 1877 Louis Pasteur discovered antibiotics. In 1929, antibiotics were first used as a medical therapy with the discovery of penicillin. By 1946 antibiotics had been credited with saving countless lives and extending the average human life span.[1] In 1998, human embryonic stem cells were isolated (found) and cultured (grown outside the body) for the first time, by scientists working separately at the University of Wisconsin and at Johns Hopkins University.[2] Like antibiotics, stem cell research offers the promise of relieving the suffering and saving the lives of millions of people and possibly extending the human life span even more. Broadly, the potential benefits of stem cell research include generating cells and tissues in the lab for transplantation and creating replacement cells and tissues in the body (regenerative medicine) to cure diseases such as Parkinson's, Alzheimer's, heart disease, cancer, and arthritis. The actual and potential medical uses of stem cells and the types of ethical issues raised by stem cell research and human cloning can be illustrated by the following cases.

Case 7A

In 2001, Erica Nader was injured in an automobile accident that left her paralyzed from the neck down. With her father's

cont.

Case 7A *cont.*

assistance, she spent years searching for possible treatments that might restore at least some of her mobility. She underwent an experimental treatment in Lisbon, Portugal, in 2003, in which her own stem cells were removed from her nasal cavity and injected into her spine at the site of the injury, using a technique called "autograft." Two years later, magnetic resonance imagining (MRI) scans confirmed that the injected cells had successfully promoted the development of spinal cord synapses and blood cells. Through a complementary regimen of rigorous rehabilitation, Erica has been able to regain the use of her arms and walk with braces for brief amounts of time. She now owns a company that specializes in aggressive, exercise-based rehabilitation for persons with spinal cord injury.

Case 7B

You are a member of an executive leadership team for a prominent Catholic health system that is opening a new facility. A key component of this new facility will be a state-of-the-art research program that will attract leading physicians from around the world and ensure the facility remains competitive long into the future. At a recent meeting, the vice president of strategy and business development proposed that in addition to pharmaceutical trials, the research program should contain a focus on stem cell research, including research on human embryonic stem cells. As part of the business plan, he suggests the facility need not be involved in obtaining the cells from the embryos directly but could simply purchase existing cells. Thus, he argues, the organization would not be involved in the prior act of destroying the embryos that is required to obtain the stem cells and would still be acting in a manner consistent with the moral teachings of the Catholic Church, by which the organization is required to abide.

Case 7C

Twenty years from now, you find yourself staring blankly at your mother's physician as she tells you the genetic tests they have

cont.

Case 7C *cont.*

just run confirm that your mom's severe headaches are the first symptoms of Alzheimer's disease. The doctor explains the prognosis is not as bad as it once was. Because they caught the disease early enough, they can take the stem cells of a cloned human embryo and inject them into your mom, and the brain cells being destroyed by the Alzheimer's disease will be replaced. There is, however, a 90 percent chance your mom will have to receive these injections several times a year for the rest of her life, and because they involve destroying a newly cloned embryo every time she receives an injection, the treatment is very expensive. Thankfully, she and your father can afford to pay for a supplemental health insurance plan that will cover the costs of the treatments.

Stem cell research has already begun to save lives, and its potential to find cures for other currently untreatable diseases is strong. Some types of stem cell research, however, are ethically controversial. For example, some people question whether research on human embryonic stem cells, like that suggested in case 7B, should be done at all. Moreover, human cloning is highly controversial, and there are many—including some who are advocates for embryonic stem cell research—who oppose attempts at human cloning. Embryonic stem cell research and the possibility of human cloning raise many ethical questions about the value of human life in its earliest stages, the goals and limits of medicine, and who we, as a society, are becoming through the use of medical technology. In this chapter we consider some of the primary ethical questions raised by embryonic stem cell research and the possibility of human cloning. But first, we must familiarize ourselves with some of the basic science.

Setting the Context: The Science and Politics of Stem Cell Research and Human Cloning

What Are Stem Cells?

Stem cells are "blank slate" cells that have not yet developed a specialized function within the body or have not yet become a specific type of cell.[3] Stem cells are therefore referred to as *undifferentiated*. As stem cells replenish other cells within the body that die due to normal wear and tear or due to disease or injury, they become specific types of body cells or tissues, such as heart cells, skin cells, blood cells, pancreatic cells, or nerve cells, through the process of differentiation. Like the stem of a plant out of which the leaves grow, stem cells give rise to the other cells of the body. Stem cells are also capable of dividing and renewing themselves through a process termed *proliferation*. Stem cells can proliferate many times over to replenish other specialized cells. This ability to divide and renew themselves allows stem cells to be grown continually for an almost indefinite period of time outside the body in the laboratory setting. When a group of stem cells is cultured in this way, the result is known as a stem cell line.

Types of Stem Cells

Until recently, stem cells have been classified into two main categories: embryonic and adult. Embryonic stem cells (ESCs) are obtained from five- to seven-day-old embryos (called *blastocysts*), which at this stage of development consist only of an inner cell mass made up of stem cells and a thin outer membrane called the *trophoblast*, which makes up all the extra-embryonic material such as the placenta. To obtain ESCs, a needle is inserted into the trophoblast and the stem cells are sucked out, thereby destroying the embryo. Today, the most common source of ESCs are "spare"—that is, unwanted—embryos left over from in vitro fertilization. According to current estimates, there are roughly 500,000 such embryos in fertility clinics in the United States, though the utility of all of these embryos for stem cell research may be limited.[4] ESCs are attractive to research scientists because they are pluripotent, which means they can, at least theoretically, become any type of cell or tissue in the body. Because they are pluripotent, it is believed ESCs will be more useful than other types of stem cells for treating more diseases, once scientists figure out how to make them become what they want them to be (such as cardiac muscle cells for heart attack victims or pancreatic islet cells for insulin-dependent diabetics).

Adult stem cells (ASCs) are found in the human body once it has developed beyond the blastocyst stage. The term *adult* stem cell, however, is somewhat misleading, because it suggests they are only found in fully grown adults. Actually, ASCs can be found in the bodies of adults, children, and infants, in umbilical cord blood (which can be retained after the umbilical cord is removed from a newborn baby), in the placenta (or afterbirth), in amniotic fluid, and even in women's menstrual blood. ASCs have been found in the bone marrow (the spongy tissue inside bones that makes blood cells), peripheral blood, the eyes, the brain, skeletal muscle, teeth, liver, skin, the lining of the gastrointestinal tract, the pancreas, and even belly fat. The primary distinction between adult and embryonic stem cells is not who or what they are found in, but that the former are considered to be multipotent rather than pluripotent. Multipotent means ASCs are believed to be limited to becoming only the type of cell of the tissue in which they are found. For example, an ASC taken from bone marrow, though still undifferentiated, will only be capable of becoming a bone marrow cell, at least theoretically. For this reason ASCs were generally thought to offer less therapeutic promise for the treatment of disease than ESCs, though new scientific evidence is raising questions about that. Recent studies suggest some ASCs may be capable of transdifferentiation similar to, but not to the same extent as, pluripotent ESCs.[5] Still, many scientists, and some politicians on their behalf, have argued they should have unfettered access to ESCs and embryos from which to derive those cells, including in some cases the ability to create new embryos through human cloning (a process known as somatic cell nuclear transfer). This, they argue, is necessary to allow sufficient research to harness the full potential of stem cells; limiting research to those benefits that might arise from research on multipotent ASCs alone would be too restrictive, they contend.

The Debate Among Scientists

The potential therapeutic usefulness of ESCs and ASCs has been at the heart of the scientific debate regarding stem cell research. Many scientists argue that, because ESCs are pluripotent, they offer the greatest potential for advances in the treatment of disease. Another advantage of ESC research over ASC research posited by some in the scientific community is that ESCs are more readily available, are more easily found, and can proliferate outside the body much longer than ASCs. Consequently, many scientists want unfettered access to ESCs. However, currently there are no proven uses of ESCs in treating human disease, while it has been reported that ASCs have been used in 73 different therapeutic applications.[6] Before any therapeutic uses of ESCs are realized, scientists still need to better understand how undifferentiated cells become differentiated and how to control or direct this process. There are also safety issues associated with ESCs that ASCs do not have. For example, ESCs in mice have been shown to grow uncontrollably into cell and tissue masses, forming benign tumors known as *teratomas*.[7]

Contrary to previously held beliefs, there is evidence that some ASCs may be able to "cross over" and differentiate into cells found in organs and tissues other than those from which the ASCs were derived.[8] For example, bone marrow stem cells have been found to differentiate into brain cells, skeletal muscle cells, and liver cells. Brain stem cells have also been found to differentiate into blood cells and skeletal muscle cells. This ability to cross over from being a stem cell of one tissue or organ to a differentiated cell of another tissue or organ is termed *plasticity*. The case of Erica Nader (Case 10A) is an example of a successful use of ASCs crossing over from one type of cell (mucosal or nasal cell) to another (spinal cord). Also recent research and human subjects trials show some ASCs can be reprogrammed into various cell types, further calling into question the scientific arguments favoring ESC research, but the debate continues.

One reason for this debate is the concern that, because we have fewer and fewer ASCs in our bodies as we age and stem cell therapies often require the use of literally millions of cells, a person may not have a sufficient supply of ASCs for certain therapies that might be developed in the future for devastating diseases, such as Alzheimer's and Parkinson's. Why not just use someone else's ASCs in that case? As with organ transplantation, there are concerns that if ASCs come from someone else, the recipient's body might attack and reject the cells, mistaking them for the cells of a disease. One possibility for avoiding this scenario, some scientists argue, could be to take ESCs from a cloned embryo, an embryo that shares most of its DNA, with the exception of its mitochondrial DNA, with the person from whom the embryo was cloned. Recall the hypothetical scenario in Case 7C.

By taking a stem cell from a cloned embryo, made from the cell of the patient who would receive the treatment, the body would be more likely to recognize it as one of its own cells, though some concern of rejection remains insofar as the mitochondrial DNA is not the same. Still some scientists argue that ESC research combined with human cloning is the most effective and safest way to develop new treatments for especially devastating and currently incurable diseases.

The Science of Human Cloning

Cloning is the process of replicating genetic material and even whole organisms. Cloning is an asexual method of reproduction in which offspring are created from a single "parent." In 1997, Scottish scientists successfully cloned a sheep.[9] Dolly, as she was called, was genetically identical to her "mother." The scientists obtained the DNA from the "mother" and were able to get it to grow into Dolly, a living, breathing genetic replica of another sheep, through a process known as somatic cell nuclear transfer (SCNT). Though Dolly was born only after 300 unsuccessful attempts, many people now believe that SCNT could be used to clone human beings.[10] In SCNT, a nonreproductive (somatic) cell, such as a skin cell, is taken from an individual. The nucleus (the part of the cell containing the person's entire genetic code) is then extracted from that cell. That nucleus is then inserted into an ovum (egg) that has had its own nucleus and DNA removed. The egg with the nucleus from the somatic cell is then mixed with chemicals and given a small electric shock to start it growing. The result is a living embryo who shares most of the genetic makeup of the individual from whom the somatic or nonreproductive cell was originally obtained, with the exception of the mitochondrial DNA of the ovum with which it was joined. The embryo then could develop for a short time in a petri dish or could be implanted in the womb of a surrogate mother or gestational carrier.

Human cloning (SCNT) can be categorized as either therapeutic or reproductive, depending on its intended purpose. In reproductive cloning, the purpose is to implant the embryo in the uterus of a woman who would later give birth to a child. In therapeutic cloning, the purpose is not to create a child (i.e., the purpose is not reproductive) but to create an embryo that will be allowed to develop only to the blastocyst stage (3–5 days) and then be destroyed for its stem cells. To call cloning for this purpose "therapeutic" is a little misleading for two reasons. First, it is not therapeutic for the embryo, which has to be destroyed for its stem cells to be obtained. Second, as we have noted, ESCs have yet to yield any proven medical therapies. Although it would be more accurate to call it "research cloning," the prevailing trend is to refer to SCNT for the purpose of obtaining ESCs for use in research as "therapeutic" cloning. The emphasis is on the hope that medical therapies might one day be derived from research on ESCs taken from three- to five-day-old cloned human embryos, and that cloning would provide an almost endless supply of ESCs for use in those therapies.

Reproductive cloning has been widely rejected by mainstream society, though some fringe groups do continue to advocate for it, and some have claimed—without substantiation—to have done it successfully. Therapeutic cloning, however, is advocated by many scientists and politicians who support ESC research. Therapeutic cloning is even legal in some countries and has been legally approved in some states in the United States.[11] In addition to the rejection issue related to ESCs, the push for therapeutic cloning is also being driven by the human thirst for knowledge, the desire to remain scientifically and commercially competitive in the global context, and the desire for prestige.

Recent research, however, has demonstrated that it is possible to induce pluripotency in ASCs. This ability to take a multipotent stem cell and reprogram it to revert to a pluripotent state may eventually lead to a resolution of the scientific debate and eliminate the perceived need for therapeutic cloning as a source of ESCs. These induced pluripotent stem cells (IPSC) can be generated without using human embryos, thus bypassing the primary ethical concern associated with ESC research. The process entails taking somatic (nonreproductive) cells, such as skin cells or lymphocytes, and reprogramming their DNA so that they resemble and function like pluripotent ESCs. In addition to avoiding the ethical pitfalls associated with ESCs, IPSCs may be more useful than ESCs for the study and treatment of human diseases because they can be generated from the patient who is to be treated, thus minimizing the risk of immune rejection associated with ESCs.[12] However, safety concerns regarding IPSCs remain, and until those obstacles are overcome, the scientific debate will continue to fuel debate in the public and political spheres.

U.S. Public Policy, Human Cloning, and Stem Cell Research

The science of stem cell research and human cloning gives rise to complex public policy questions. Should ESC research be allowed, regulated, or even encouraged by the government? Should taxpayer money be used to fund ESC research? Should therapeutic cloning be legal? These are not only public policy questions but also ethical questions at the macro or health policy level.

The Politics of Human Cloning. While there is more consensus at the federal and state legislative levels that reproductive cloning should be banned, opinions are mixed regarding therapeutic cloning. Fourteen states have or have had laws pertaining to human cloning. California was the first state to ban reproductive cloning, or cloning to initiate a pregnancy, in 1997. According to the National Conference of State Legislatures, Arkansas, Connecticut, Indiana, Iowa, Maryland, Massachusetts, Michigan, Rhode Island, New Jersey, North Dakota, South Dakota, and Virginia have enacted measures to prohibit reproductive cloning. Arkansas, Indiana, Iowa (whose ban was repealed in 2007), Michigan, North Dakota, and South Dakota laws extend their prohibitions to therapeutic cloning. Rhode Island law does not prohibit cloning for research, and California, Missouri, Arizona, and New Jersey all have laws that specifically permit cloning for the purpose of research. Missouri and Arizona even permit the use of public funds to be used for the specific type of cloning known as SCNT for the purpose of creating stem cells for research.[13]

Although bills to ban human cloning have been proposed at the federal level, none have successfully passed both the House and the Senate, and thus there is currently no federal law banning human cloning for any reason. the U.S. House of Representatives has twice passed a bill banning both reproductive and therapeutic cloning, but neither was successful in passing the Senate. Two other bills have, however, been introduced in the Senate. The Human Cloning Prohibition Act of 2003 (SB 245) would ban both therapeutic and reproductive cloning, while the Human Cloning Ban and Stem Cell Research Protection Act (SB 303) would ban reproductive cloning but permit therapeutic cloning. Though then-president George W. Bush openly stated he would support a total ban on all human cloning, many Republican and traditionally pro-life senators have crossed party lines on the issue of therapeutic cloning. Likewise, the President's Council on Bioethics has publicly supported a prohibition of reproductive cloning but stopped short of supporting a total prohibition of therapeutic cloning, instead supporting a moratorium on the practice until sufficient regulations can be worked out.[14] In 2007 Sen. Orrin Hatch (R-UT) introduced a law that would have banned reproductive cloning but not restricted therapeutic cloning. However, the bill never made it out of committee and thus never went up for a vote, suggesting the wide variation in views among politicians on cloning for stem cell research persists.

Stem Cell Research in the Public Arena. There is even more variation in the views of politicians regarding ESC research. Several senators who traditionally have held pro-life positions also advocated for the unfettered and publicly funded pursuit of ESC research. This shift can be attributed largely to their views regarding the moral status of unwanted embryos in fertility clinic storage units as somehow different from other human life. For example, Senator Hatch, who introduced a bill in 2007 that would have permitted therapeutic cloning, has asserted that a frozen embryo in a refrigerator in a clinic is not the same as a fetus developing in a mother's womb.[15] Likewise, former Sen. Connie Mack (R-FL), another traditionally pro-life politician, supported ESC research arguing as long as an embryo is destined not to be placed in a uterus, it cannot become life.[16]

Although such reasoning can be persuasive, it would seem to reflect an inconsistent ethic of life. It is true that an embryo that remains in a cryopreservation tank in a fertility clinic is not actually progressing through its developmental stages like a fetus in the womb. However, limiting moral standing to the developing fetus in the womb implies the moral worth of life is ultimately attached to achieving a particular developmental stage of growth rather than the inherent value of human life itself. This view either posits the accidental circumstances of individual lives as the basis of moral worth or assumes the right to life is conditioned on the actual or even potential capability to function as a person rather than on life itself. Ultimately, such views undermine the arguments that pro-life politicians have put forth in different contexts. If an embryo, even one in a cryopreservation tank, is not human life, then what is it?

How could it become human life simply by being placed in a uterus, if it is not already a human life to begin with?

At the time that human ESCs were first isolated and grown by private researchers, federal regulations did not allow federal money to be used for funding any research that involved the destruction of human embryos, under what is known as the Dickey-Wicker Amendment (named after its two congressional sponsors, Jay Dickey [R-AR] and Roger Wicker [R-MS]). According to the amendment, no federal funds can be expended by the National Institutes for Health (NIH) for "(1) the creation of a human embryo or embryos for research purposes; or (2) research in which a human embryo or embryos are destroyed, discarded, or knowingly subjected to risks of injury or death."[17] Nonetheless, in 1999, during President Bill Clinton's administration, the NIH published draft guidelines outlining the conditions under which it would allow federal funds to be used for ESC research for the first time.[18] However, the Clinton administration did not approve the guidelines until September 2000, just before the president's final term in office ended. No government funds were dispensed for the purpose of ESC research before President George W. Bush came into office, and the Clinton guidelines therefore were not formally challenged under the rubric of Dickey-Wicker. The guidelines were subsequently put on hold until the Bush administration could review them and make a decision as to whether they should stand or be revised.

In August 2001, in his first address to the nation, President Bush announced the creation of new stem cell research guidelines that would permit federal funding to be used for ESC research. Under these guidelines, only existing ESC lines could be eligible for tax-funded research, and no tax monies could go to research that would contribute to the destruction of existing embryos. To ensure federal funds would not be used for research that entailed the destruction of existing embryos, the Bush administration created a stem cell registry consisting of sixty-four ESC lines worldwide. Many in the scientific community questioned the feasibility of using these ESC lines. Advocates of ESC research questioned whether U.S. researchers would be given access to ESC lines in foreign countries, whether the existing cell lines would be sufficiently genetically diverse, whether they would be reliably capable of differentiation, and whether they would be reliably capable of proliferation. Despite these questions and growing political support for ESC research, President Bush vetoed a bill passed by both the House and Senate in July 2006 that would have allowed funding for ESC research to create new stem cell lines from additional embryos. According to President Bush, such a bill "would support the taking of innocent human life in the hope of finding medical benefit for others. It crosses a moral boundary that our decent society needs to respect."[19] Insofar as no funds were eligible to be used for research that would entail the destruction of embryos, it was seen as consistent with the Dickey-Wicker Amendment. As President Bush himself said, "The life and death decision for these embryos has already been made." President Bush's stem cell decision was not limited to the issue of federal funding for ESC research; he also dedicated $250 million in federal funds to go toward ASC research and created the President's Council on Bioethics to provide guidance on public policy matters related to stem cell research and many other ethical issues in health care and the life sciences.

Though the Bush administration's approach to the question of federal funding for ESC research actually expanded the scope of research for which federal funds could be used, it did not go as far in permitting the use of federal funds for ESC research as the original NIH guidelines proposed under the Clinton administration. Rather, President Bush's approach constituted a compromise position, both on the question of federal funding for research that involves the destruction of human embryos, as well as the primary ethical considerations underlying the competing ethical views. However, on March 9, 2009, shortly after taking office, President Barack Obama issued an executive order overturning the Bush administration guidelines and instructing the NIH to develop new guidelines within 120 days. On April 23, 2009, the NIH published a new set of guidelines for public comment that became final on July 7, 2009. Like the Bush guidelines, these guidelines required that federal funding could go only toward research on stem cell lines developed from embryos created for the purpose of IVF and which were donated with informed consent and without monetary compensation. Also like the Bush guidelines, these new guidelines banned federal funds from being used for research on stem cell lines originating from embryos created specifically for the purpose of research and on embryos created through therapeutic cloning (though it did not ban the practice of cloning). The primary difference between the 2009 guidelines and the 2001 guidelines is that the former did away with any deadline by which the stem cell line had to be created, thus opening up federal funding to be used on new stem cell lines created through the destruction of new embryos. Thus the number of ESC lines eligible for federal funding is unlimited.

Later in 2009, two scientists who specialize in ASC research joined with several pro-life groups in bringing suit against the Obama administration, claiming the new guidelines caused irreparable damage to them by creating greater competition for federal funding that could be allocated to stem cell research. U.S. District Court Judge Royce Lamberth dismissed the case because not all of the plaintiffs, in particular, the pro-life groups, had legal standing to file suit. Later, in 2010, the two research scientists filed suit again, this time without the pro-life groups; Judge Lamberth found in their favor and ordered an injunction prohibiting the NIH from allocating any federal funds for the purpose of ESC research. The NIH has appealed the decision, and a three-judge panel has decided to lift the injunction, so that the NIH can distribute funds for the purpose of ESC research while the appeals process proceeds.

Discussion: Ethical Issues and Analysis

It should be clear by now the ethical issues raised by ASC research are not as controversial as those raised by ESC research. Although there are ethical issues related to ASC research, these issues are much the same as those raised by any other type of research involving human subjects. ESC research is more controversial, because obtaining the ESC entails the destruction of human embryos. As the political debate shows, four main ethical questions are raised by ESC research, in addition to the medical and scientific questions about ease and effectiveness:

1. Is a three- to five-day-old embryo deserving of moral respect and protection?

2. If unwanted embryos in fertility clinics are going to be destroyed anyway, why not harvest their stem cells first and reap the potential benefits?

3. Should pro-life organizations, such as Catholic health care institutions, participate in research on ESC lines if doing so would not entail the destruction of any more embryos?

4. If we don't use these unwanted embryos in fertility clinics for research, how do we respond to those patients, now suffering from diseases, who might have benefited from such research?

The Moral Status of the Preimplantation Embryo

As we saw in more detail in chapter 4 on issues related to maternal-fetal care, there are competing views regarding the moral status of prenatal human life. According to one view, consistent with our normative basis, human life has an inherent human dignity and deserves the moral respect owed to all human beings from the moment it comes into existence. At the other end of the spectrum is what can be termed the nonpersonal view, which holds that the fetus does not deserve the same respect and protection as other members of the moral community. Also recall that this view is based on the fact that early human life is not yet capable of functioning in ways characteristically associated with being a person; it is not capable of making free choices, communicating, planning for the future, or participating in social life, nor does it share other characteristics commonly associated with fully conscious, autonomous, and rational individuals. As the previous discussions in this chapter illustrate, this view also applies to the preimplantation embryo, that is, an embryo that has not yet been implanted in the uterus of a woman. In this context, however, a third view emerges.

In contrast to the personal and nonpersonal positions, there is the prepersonal position.[20] According to this view, the embryo deserves the respect and protection due to other human beings at a stage of development long before it has developed the capability to function in ways commonly associated with fully functional, autonomous individuals. However, according to this view, the embryo is not in fact due such respect and protection from the moment it comes into existence.

Rather, the human embryo deserves respect and protection only once it reaches the biological point of development in which *twinning* (dividing into two distinct but genetically identical embryos) is no longer possible. The morally relevant consideration here is that individual members of the human species have an innate and ordained natural end to which all human life is inherently and developmentally oriented and thus have a right not to be subjected to interference in their biological and personal development toward this end. However, because a certain biological stability oriented toward that fulfillment is not present until the point of development at which twinning is no longer possible, preimplantation embryos would not be included as full members of the moral community. Hence this position can be called "prepersonal" regarding preimplantation embryos, which—though human—cannot be said to be unique individual human lives.

The prepersonal position is much less arbitrary than the nonpersonal position insofar as it grounds moral worth in being a member of the human species rather than being a "person" (however defined). This view is less arbitrary in the sense that being a living member of the human species is a matter of biological fact, whereas "personhood" is an elusive and variable philosophical category. However, the prepersonal position can still be criticized for overemphasizing the moral relevance of individuality. That twinning is still a possibility at an early stage of development does not necessarily mean the preimplantation embryo is not an individual human being. When twinning does occur, it is invariably preceded by the biological development of a single organism. Thus, "the fact that a group of cells is able after separation to develop independently into a second individuated organism in no way refutes the prior existence of an individual organism, but confirms it."[21] The prepersonal position can also be criticized for being arbitrary in a different way than the nonpersonal position. In particular, if human life, rather than personhood, is the basis for membership in the moral community, then what basis is there for granting this moral status only to *individual* human lives? In the end, the key difference between the prepersonal and nonpersonal views is that the prepersonal view associates moral status with "individuality" rather than "personhood." Both views still preclude, however, certain members of the human species, namely, preimplantation embryos, as deserving moral respect and protection.

Responding to the Questions of ESC Research. According to the view of the human person in our normative basis, we, as rational beings created in the image and likeness of God, have both the capability and the responsibility to participate in God's ongoing act of creation. In other words, we have a moral responsibility to use our intelligence and freedom to help create a human community in which the basic human goods of individuals are met and flourishing is made a real possibility. From this perspective, stem cell research in general is not necessarily ruled out or forbidden as "playing God." Indeed, stem cell research can be a valuable tool for helping people to pursue human flourishing if the associated ethical issues can be resolved. Rather than an outright rejection, our normative basis provides a framework for responding to the ethical questions raised by stem cell research, both adult and embryonic, and for placing limits on stem cell research in general.

Clearly, one limit that arises from the personal view of the moral status of the preimplantation human embryo is the moral rejection of ESC research. This limit would apply to all forms of ESC research, whether using embryos left over from infertility treatments or those that are the direct result of "therapeutic" human cloning. The source of the embryo is not the problem. From the perspective of our normative basis the problem is that systematic, socially sanctioned destruction of one category of human life is the basis for medical treatments to save other human lives. This is morally inconsistent with the concepts of the sanctity of life, solidarity, right relationships, and human flourishing in community. These concepts also give rise to other limits on stem cell research related specifically to the goals of medicine.

From our perspective, the value of medicine is achieved when it helps people function better as human beings and more closely achieve human flourishing. Simply stated, medicine should serve the good of human life and of the human person; neither human life nor the human person should be used merely as a means in the service of medicine, that is, for the advancement of medicine. Giving priority to the goals of medicine over the good of a human life suggests society has its priorities backward. Although the advancement of medical technology and the discovery of new cures for devastating diseases are noble goals, they should be supported only to the extent they are truly done in service to the goals of human life. We as a society must not allow medical research and science generally to be driven by other factors—such as political or economic interests—that may lead to the devaluation, commercialization, or instrumentalization of human life.

Finding new ways to cure devastating diseases, though a great good in and of itself, is not the only way medicine can serve right relationships and human flourishing. Other appropriate goals of medicine include preventing illness and finding other ways to alleviate suffering, which is an inevitable result of our being part of the created world. For example, providing pain management, spiritual care, and emotional comfort to those who are suffering are reasonable goals of medicine, which acknowledge the dignity of the spiritual, social, and emotional dimensions of the human person in addition to the physical and material dimension. Indeed, these goals are not only appropriate, they also are ways that medicine can help to make the sick or dying person more whole and thereby foster right relationships and human flourishing even in the face of human frailty. Focusing our energies and resources on overcoming the inevitable reality of death, an impossible task, will likely lead us to overlook other ways to alleviate suffering—ways that promote the value of human life rather than devalue it.

To be sure, this line of thought goes against the grain of the prevailing consequentialist view in our society, that a potential cure for millions of people suffering from devastating diseases justifies the use of early human life for ESC research. The consequentialist justification of ESC research is not only put forth by politicians and medical scientists but is also espoused by some medical ethicists. Art Caplan and Glenn McGee have argued in favor of ESC research:

> It is the moral imperative of compassion that compels stem cell research. The stem cell research consortium Patient's Coalition for Urgent Research estimates that as many as 128 million Americans suffer from diseases that might respond to pluripotent stem cell therapies. . . . More than half of the world's population will suffer at some point in life with one of these three conditions [cancer, heart disease, Parkinson's disease], and more humans die every year from cancer than were killed in both the Kosovo and Vietnam conflicts. Stem cell research is a pursuit of known and

important goods. . . . [There] is no need more obvious or compelling than the suffering of half the world at the hand of miserable disease.[22]

Though our normative basis would not lead us to share in this conclusion, the argument raises an important question that needs to be addressed; namely, how should we reply to the accusation that we are neglecting the needs of those who suffer from diseases that might be cured through ESC research? Gilbert Meilander, a Protestant theologian who also rejects the consequentialist justification of ESC research, provides us with a starting point:

> To permit such research is to suppose, as modernity has taught us, that suffering has no point other than to be overcome by human will and technical mastery—that compassion means not readiness to suffer with others but a determination always to oppose suffering as an affront to our humanity. We could have helped you only by destroying in the present the sort of world in which both we and you want to live—a world in which justice is done now, not permanently mortgaged in service of future good. Only in short, pretending to be something other than the human beings we are.[23]

Meilander has articulated one of the sentiments at the core of our normative basis regarding right relationships, social virtues, and principles of justice, including solidarity, relationality, the common good, and ultimately human flourishing.

Practical Implications

Consider again the cases that opened this chapter. Given the normative foundations we have set, how should we evaluate the case of Erica Nader? As we have alluded, the main ethical issues in this case are the same as those accompanying any experimental therapeutic interventions; for example, appropriate human subjects protections, adequate informed consent, avoiding financial conflicts of interest, and so on. Because the therapy in question used Erica's own ASCs and did not involve ESCs, there is no controversy surrounding the destruction of human embryos and no moral concern about reducing innocent human lives (embryos) to merely a means of benefiting another (Erica). However, what about research that uses existing stem cell lines that do not necessarily entail the destruction of any additional embryos? Should pro-life organizations with the mission of improving the lives of individuals and the health of communities make use of such ESC lines, as is proposed in Case 7B?

Though our normative framework would clearly lead to the rejection of destroying embryos to obtain their stem cells, might using those cells once already obtained, without any participation on the part of those who object to embryo destruction, constitute an attempt to extract some good from the evil that others have already done? Though it may be true that at least some scientists who conduct research with existing ESC lines may not approve of the *past* destruction of embryos, it would seem difficult to argue they would not be contributing to the ongoing destruction of embryos for future medical use. Indeed, such use will likely continue in the future in light of the Obama administration's new guidelines. Moreover, by acquiring these cells from those who destroyed the embryos in the first place, the researchers (who might object to the original destruction) would be contributing to the continued demand for more cells.[24] In the end, we conclude that such research is contrary to the development of such virtues as respect for human life, solidarity, and an appropriate recognition of the limits of medicine, which we argue should be the moral ideal toward which we as a society and moral community should strive.

Consider for example, Case 7C in which a cure for Alzheimer's disease is created, but the therapy entails destroying a cloned human embryo each time it is used. In this scenario, large numbers of human reproductive eggs (ova) would be required to generate the cloned embryos for the therapy. This could lead to a situation in which women could sell their eggs. This has already begun to occur in some contexts.[25] Such commercialization of human ova could involve the exploitation of women who are economically vulnerable and lead to serious physical harms and risks associated with the process of hyperstimulation. Moreover, if treatments should be discovered for some diseases using stem cells from cloned three- to five-day-old embryos, would society be able to resist using the cells, tissues, and even organs from more-developed clones, perhaps at the fetal stage of development, to cure other devastating diseases? Admittedly, "slippery slope" arguments (i.e., if one type of behavior is allowed, then others will likely follow) rely less on logic and more on emotions evoked by hypothetical possibilities, but the use of human embryos in the service of other people's interests or, worse, in the service of political and economic interests could have serious consequences for society's moral attitudes toward human life.

Although these concerns regard what may happen, there are current concerns for anyone who rejects as immoral ESC research and human cloning. For example, faith-based organizations, such as Catholic hospitals, already address concerns regarding ESC research. Clearly, Catholic hospitals should not permit ESC research in their facilities, given the Catholic Church's teaching on the sanctity of human life. But there are other questions, as well. To what extent should an individual who objects to the killing of innocent human life cooperate with organizations that fund or engage in ESC research? Many such organizations exist primarily to eradicate certain forms of cancer or childhood diseases—causes that ethical people should and do promote. Should individuals who reject the moral permissibility of ESC research give money to such organizations? In terms of our normative basis, we would put the question this way: Are relationships that encourage and facilitate the destruction of human life, even in the service of other human life, right relationships?

What if therapeutic treatments requiring ESC stem cells become the standard of care? Would it be morally justifiable to use treatments that use such stem cell lines but do not entail the destruction of more embryos (essentially the position of President Bush)? Within our normative framework, it is clear a preferred alternative would be to seek other means for care that do not entail destruction of early human life because this would uphold the dignity and sanctity of human life and foster right relationships at a societal level.

According to our normative basis, ASC research and the therapies derived from it, as in Case 7A, are a morally acceptable alternative to ESC research and human cloning. However, ASCs should not be blindly encouraged and recklessly funded. Fostering right relationships at the societal level requires attending to all dimensions of the common good. Understood thus, ASC research does raise ethical questions, though these questions are more akin to those attached to any medical research rather than to ESC research. All medical research raises questions regarding how much of society's resources, how much of the common good, should be dedicated to the search for new therapies. As just one example, how much suffering could we relieve by dedicating funds that advocates want put toward ESC stem cell research toward instead providing basic preventive care to some of the 50 million Americans who lack health insurance?

Though relevant to all medical research, this question becomes especially pressing given the huge amounts of money and attention that stem cell research receives.[26] In keeping with the normative basis we have outlined, along with the principle of solidarity, perhaps our first concern should be to meet the needs of millions of people who suffer and die today from fully preventable and treatable diseases rather than how to reply to those who might be helped by a therapy that doesn't yet exist. We must also ask whether right relationships would be better fostered by creating unfettered access and dedicating significant funding toward any form of stem cell research or by dedicating those funds to those whom we know can be served now by such resources.

Conclusion

From our perspective the moral questions surrounding ESC research and human cloning are rooted in a concern not only for embryonic human life but also for what kind of society we would become by providing unfettered access, encouragement, and funding for scientific and medical research that entails the destruction of early human life. From this perspective, the debate over the personhood of preimplantation embryos as the basis for the moral status of ESC research can be considered misplaced. Regardless of whether one is willing to give personal moral status to individual embryos, treating early embryonic human life as merely an instrument to benefit others ultimately leads to commercialization, a further eroding of respect for life, and the narrow edge of that slippery slope. Once society heads down that slope, will we be able to recognize any limits to the goals of medicine, or will we let the pursuit of new medical technology and cures undermine the value of the very lives medicine intends to help?

In the end, we must ask what kind of a society we want to become by and through our collective actions. Are we content to let millions of our fellow community members suffer needlessly from illnesses that are fully preventable, while we search for cures for others? Or do we want to become a society that fosters and exhibits genuine human love for all our neighbors so that we and they can achieve human well-being and human flourishing? Even if we agree on the latter, we still must find a way to balance the need to respect all human life, including those not yet born, with the need to improve the lives of those already in community with us. Our normative basis does not provide easy answers to these questions, but it does appropriately reframe ethical questions about ESC research and human cloning in view of promoting right relationships and social virtues that lead to individual and communal human flourishing.

Additional Case Studies

Case 7D

Having had a sibling with juvenile diabetes, you have long supported the Regional Juvenile Diabetes Fund. Even as a young adult, you donated what you could to the charity in hopes of their one day finding a cure. Now that you have amassed a modest personal fortune through your long career as an innovative CEO of one of the country's largest health systems, you have been giving substantial donations on an annual basis. You have recently learned, however, that the Regional Juvenile Diabetes Fund funds embryonic stem cell research. You discuss this with a friend and colleague who also considers herself to be pro-life. She says she donates anyway because the research is going to continue whether she donates or not, and the embryos they are using for the research are destined to be destroyed regardless.

Discussion questions. Would you continue to donate to the Regional Juvenile Diabetes Fund? Why or why not? Would you donate if you could specify your donation not be used for embryonic stem cell research? Are you persuaded by the argument that embryonic stem cell research is not ethically problematic because the embryos are going to be destroyed anyway?

Case 7 E

Your state has recently added a constitutional amendment to the ballot for the upcoming election. If it passes, this amendment would give scientists a constitutional right to engage in human embryonic stem cell research in your state. Although the proposed amendment also claims to ban "human cloning," it specifically defines human cloning as implanting an embryo resulting from somatic cell nuclear transfer in the uterus of a woman with the intent of bringing about a live birth. In effect, the amendment would also make it a constitutional right to conduct somatic cell nuclear transfer for the purpose of creating stem cells for research. There are further provisions in the proposed amendment that would allow women to be "fairly reimbursed" for any time and burdens involved in the process of donating their eggs to science.

Discussion questions. Would you support this proposed legislative amendment in its current form? Would you support such a bill with some revisions? Why? What revisions would you like to see?

SUGGESTED READINGS

Branick, Vincent, and Therese M. Lysaught. "Stem Cell Research: Licit or Complicit? Is a Medical Breakthrough Based on Embryonic and Fetal Tissue Compatible with Catholic Teaching?" *Health Progress* 80, no. 5 (September–October 1999): 37–42.

Brock, Dan W. "Is a Consensus Possible on Stem Cell Research? Moral and Political Obstacles." *Journal of Medical Ethics* 32 (2006): 36–42.

Fabbro, Ronald. "Stem Cell Research, Cloning, and Catholic Moral Theology." *Linacre Quarterly* 72 (2005): 294–306.

Hall, Stephen S. "Stem Cells: A Status Report." *Hastings Center Report* 36, no. 1 (2006): 16–22.

Kavanaugh, John F. "Cloning, by Whatever Name, Smells Bad." *America* 194, no. 21 (June 19, 2006): 6.

Walter, James J. "A Catholic Reflection on Embryonic Stem Cell Research." *Linacre Quarterly* 73, no. 3 (2006): 255–63.

MULTIMEDIA AIDS FOR TEACHERS

Accidental Advocate. Astrid Media. Not Rated. 2009. This film profiles Dr. Claude Gerstle, a surgeon and athlete who suffered a tragic bicycle accident in 2003 that left him quadriplegic. The film follows his efforts to explore the hope, hype, passions, and fears entailed in the scientific, social, and political debates regarding stem cell research. Available at *http://theaccidentaladvocate.com/screenings-2/buy-the-dvd/.*

American Association of for the Advancement of Science. http://www.aaas.org/spp/cstc/briefs/stemcells/. This Web site provides a comprehensive overview of the scientific and political history of stem sell research.

Miracle Cell. Films for the Humanities and Sciences. Not Rated. 2004. This 60-minute video depicts several patients who are undergoing therapies derived from adult stem cells. It is available in DVD or VHS. For information, see *http://www.films.com/id/6674/Miracle_Cell.htm.*

Stem Cell Research: Frontier of Hope and Concern. DIA Productions. Not Rated. 2004. This 30-minute video can be purchased separately or in a group with other videos on select issues in health care ethics. For information, see *http://fac.ethicsprograms.com/.*

My Sisters' Keeper. Directed by Nick Cassavetes. Rated PG-13. 2009. Based on the novel of the same name by Judy Picoult, this feature-length film follows the story of a girl who was conceived through in vitro fertilization to be a genetic match for her older sister, who is sick with acute promyelocytic leukemia. Available on Warner Home Video.

"Stem Cell Information: The Official National Institutes of Health Resource for Stem Cell Research." National Institutes of Health. *http://stemcells.nih.gov/.* This Web site contains a variety of resources regarding the science and politics of embryonic and adult stem cell research.

ENDNOTES

1. Milton Wainwright, *Miracle Cure: The Story of Penicillin and the Golden Age of Antibiotics* (Oxford: Basil Blackwell, 1990).

2. See James A. Thomson, Joseph Itskovitz-Eldor, Sander S. Shapiro, et al., "Embryonic Stem Cell Lines Derived from Human Blastocysts," *Science* 282 (1998): 1145–7; Michael J. Schamblott, Joyce Axelman, Shunping Wang, et al., "Derivation of Pluripotent Stem Cells from Cultured Human Primordial Germ Cells," *Proceedings of the National Academy of Sciences* 95 (1998): 13726–31.

3. On the science of stem cells, see National Institutes of Health, "Stem Cells: Scientific Progress and Future Research Directions," (2001), *http://stemcells.nih.gov/info/scireport/* (accessed June 11, 2011).

4. Peter A. Clark, SJ, "Frozen Embryos: Application of the Extraordinary/Ordinary Means Distinction from the Catholic Perspective," *The Internet Journal of Gynecology and Obstetrics* 12 , no. 2 (2010).

5. See *http://stemcells.nih.gov/info/basicsbasics4.asp* (accessed February 22, 2007). In *Stem Cell Information* [World Wide Web site]. Bethesda, MD: National Institutes of Health, U.S. Department of Health and Human Services, 2011 [cited Saturday, June 18, 2011].

6. For a list of the different therapeutic uses of ASCs, see *http://www.stemcellresearch.org/facts/treatments.htm* (accessed February 2, 2010).

7. Martin F. Pera and Alan O. Trounson, "Human Embryonic Stem Cells: Prospects for Development," *Development* 131 (2004): 5515–25.

8. See, for example, Malcolm Alison, Richard Poulsom, Rosemary Jeffery, et al., "Cell Differentiation: Hepatocytes from Non-Hepatic Adult Stem Cells," *Nature* 418 (2002): 41–9.

9. Wilmut Ian, A. E. Schnieke, J. McWhir, et al., "Viable Offspring Derived from Fetal and Adult Mammalian Cells," *Nature* 385 (1997): 810–13.

10. However, according to researchers at the Roslin Institute, where Dolly was cloned, the cloning of one human being for reproductive purposes could require, given existing technology, the use of 1,000 oocytes (eggs) and twenty to fifty surrogate mothers. See Arlene Judith Klotzko, "Voices from Roslin: The Creators of Dolly Discuss Science, Ethics, and Social Responsibility," *Cambridge Quarterly of Healthcare Ethics* 7 (1998): 121–40.

11. For a chart of state laws regarding therapeutic and reproductive cloning, see the National Conference of State Legislators Web site at *http://www.ncsl.org/programs/health/Genetics/rt-shcl.htm* (accessed June 11, 2011).

12. Joanna Hanley, Ghasem Rastegarlari, and Amit C. Nathwani, "An Introduction to Induced Pluripotent Stem Cells," *British Journal of Haematology* 1, no. 151 (2010): 16–24.

13. For a summary of these states' laws, see the National Conference of State Legislatures at *http://www.ncsl.org/default.aspx?tabid=14284.*

14. *The President's Council on Bioethics, Human Cloning, and Human Dignity: An Ethical Inquiry,* Washington, DC: GPO, 2002, 205.

15. Transcripts from the *Jim Lehrer News Hour* on PBS, July 10, 2001, *http://www.pbs.org/newshour/bb/health/july-dec01/stem_cells_7-10.html* (accessed June 11, 2011).

16. Anonymous, "Stem Cell Politics," *Religion and Ethics News Weekly*, July 6, 2001, *http://www.pbs.org/wnet/religionandethics/week445/news.html* (accessed June 11, 2011).

17. George J. Annas, JD, MPH, "Resurrection of a Stem Cell Funding Barrier: Dickey-Wicker in Court," *New England Journal of Medicine* 363, no. 18 (2010): 1687–9.

18. David Korn, "The NIH Guidelines on Stem Cell Research," *Science* 289 (2000): 1877.

19. Charles Bagington, "Stem Cell Bill Gets Bush's First Veto," *Washington Post*, July 21, 2006, A4.

20. See, Michael R. Panicola, "Three Views on the Preimplantation Embryo," *National Catholic Bioethics Quarterly* 2 (Spring 2002): 69–97.

21. Benedict M. Ashley and Kevin D. O'Rourke, *Health Care Ethics: A Theological Analysis*, 4th ed. (Washington, DC: Georgetown University Press, 1997), 234.

22. G. McGee and A. Caplan, "The Ethics and Politics of Small Sacrifices in Stem Cell Research," *Kennedy of Ethics Institute Journal* 9 (1999): 151–8.

23. G. Meilander, "The Point of a Ban, or How to Think about Stem Cell Research," *The Hastings Center Report* 31 (2001): 9–16.

24. On the following argument, see John Paul Slosar, "Genomics and Neurology: An Ethical View," *Health Progress* 81, no. 1 (January–February 2006): 68–72.

25. Ethics Committee of the American Society for Reproductive Medicine, "Financial Incentives in Recruitment of Oocyte Donors," *Fertility and Sterility* 82 (2004 Suppl.): S240–4.

26. On adult stem cell research and the common good, see Lisa Sowle Cahill, "Stem Cells: A Bioethical Balancing Act," *America* 184, no. 10 (2001): 14–9.

CHAPTER 8

Current and Future Applications of Genomic Technologies

John Paul Slosar

"Quest for Humanity's Blueprint": Ethical, Legal, and Social Implications

In 1988 Congress appropriated funds for the Department of Energy and the National Institutes of Health to begin planning the Human Genome Project (HGP), which was to begin in earnest in 1990 to detail the complete set of genetic instructions of the human being. The estimated cost was $3 billion with a timetable of fifteen years; the actual cost was $2.7 billion over 12.5 years.[1] The public imagination was captured immediately. The project was dubbed "the search for the holy grail of biology," "a quest for humanity's blueprint," and the uncovering of the "Book of Life."[2] Despite the hype surrounding this event, scientists were united in their goal toward a common good: to understand the genetic contribution to human disease and eventually eradicate those genetic anomalies. This represented possibly the first attempt in the history of medicine to cure people by changing the genetic codes that underlay their diseases.[3]

Amid the fervor for scientific truth about our genetic basis were fears of what might be discovered, the ends to which such discoveries might lead, and the magnitude of the project itself.[4] The HGP was the largest genomics project attempted to date. Critical questions were raised as to whether we could develop the technology required to perform the task, whether the cost of the technology was justified, and what other research would need to be sacrificed as a result of taking on this huge endeavor. Further questions faced society: Would this project settle the nature/nurture debate (i.e., are we predominantly the product of our genes or our environment)? Is one's right to privacy violated if one's genetic code is made public? What about discrimination against those who may have an "inferior" genetic makeup or may be more prone to particular diseases? Questions such as these fed Frankensteinian notions of what might come of the knowledge gleaned from the HGP.[5] In response to these and other questions, the HGP devoted 5 percent of its overall budget for the purpose of studying the ethical, legal, and social implications (ELSI) of the research. This amounted to roughly $1.5 million. Unprecedented at the time, ELSI projects and grants helped shape public policy to deal with ethical and legal issues raised by the research, sometimes in advance of the science.[6]

The scientific publication of the completion of the HGP in April 2003, nearly fifty years to the month after the publication of James Watson and Francis Crick's report of the double helix structure of DNA, marked far more than just the completion of the mapping and sequencing of the human genome. The implication was that medicine would now be able to understand the genetic basis of illness and disease and that the information would revolutionize clinical care. Former president Bill Clinton was so swept up with the accomplishment that at a public speaking engagement announcing the completion of the HGP, he remarked,

> Today we are learning the language in which God created life. We are gaining ever more awe for the complexity, the beauty, and the wonder of God's most divine and sacred gift. With this profound new knowledge, humankind is on the verge of gaining immense new power to heal.

Although the full promise of the HGP has yet to be realized, the information has furthered our knowledge about genetics in general and genetic disease in particular. We now know that humans have approximately 25,000 genes—as opposed to 100,000, as was once thought—which means that we have only twice as many as a roundworm, three times as many as a fruit fly, and six times as many as baker's yeast. We also know that 99.9 percent of all genes in the human genome are the same regardless of ethnicity, sex, and other variables. Information obtained from the HGP has allowed us to identify hundreds of genes located on specific chromosomes responsible for numerous diseases, including colon cancer, amyotrophic lateral sclerosis (ALS, also known as Lou Gehrig's disease), type 2 (adult onset) diabetes, late-onset Alzheimer's disease, and X-linked severe combined immunodeficiency disease (SCID). The list continues to expand as science learns more about disease-causing mutations.[7]

The discovery of a disease-causing mutation often leads to the development of a test for that mutation. Although this research continues at an astounding pace, the concept of a genetic disease is not as straightforward as it may seem. First, it is not the case that a person who carries a certain disease-causing mutation will necessarily develop the disease. This reflects the degree of penetrance of the specific mutation. About 75 percent of women with certain mutations in the BRCA1 gene, for example, develop breast or ovarian cancer. The penetrance of those mutations therefore is 75 percent.[8] Second, someone may be a "carrier" of a genetically based disease but be unaffected by that disease because the gene is "recessive" insofar as the person only has one copy, which does not manifest itself as a dominant trait. Third, it may be that a person is merely rendered more susceptible to a particular disease by the presence of one or more gene mutations, a combination of alleles, or both, not necessarily abnormal, associated with the disease (i.e., genetic predisposition).[9]

Though genetic testing is the most prevalent application of genetic technology today, advances in genomic medicine continue to increase our ability to (1) individualize preventive care based on the predicted risk of a disease as assessed from one's genome, (2) develop gene-based therapies by replacing defective genes with healthy ones, (3) provide drugs that are more compatible with a person's genome, as well as develop new drugs targeted to counteract specific disease-causing mutations, (4) build organs in cell cultures to replace "worn-out" or "diseased" ones, and (5) potentially, at least, practice genetic engineering and enhancement.[10] The following cases may help to illustrate some current and future applications of genetic technologies and the types of ethical issues associated with them.

Case 8A

Jeb, a 62-year-old father of two, had not been feeling well. He figured the fuzzy-headed forgetful state he had been experiencing lately was just the result of his chemotherapy for his stomach cancer. Before that he had been functioning fine with no other symptoms. Finally, after a few months of complaining to his oncologist, she referred him to a neurologist. After learning that his mother, grandmother, and great grandmother had all developed Alzheimer's disease in their 60s, the neurologist recommended that Jeb undergo a predictive test to determine his chances of developing an inheritable form of Alzheimer's. The test was simple; a blood draw followed by a quick genetic assay to determine if he had the APOE e4 allele, which indicates susceptibility to Alzheimer's. If he had the gene, he would have a 75-percent chance of having Alzheimer's at some point in his life. Moreover, if Jeb has the allele, his children have a 50-percent chance of inheriting that allele and a 75-percent chance of developing late-onset Alzheimer's.

Case 8B

Mark was only 3 years old when he was diagnosed with "idiopathic short stature," which basically means he was far below the normal growth curve for height, but his physicians did not know why. After running a battery of genetic tests, they still could not tell his parents why he was so short. What they could tell them was that at his current growth rate, he would most likely grow to be only between 4 foot, 8 inches and 5 foot, 4 inches. The good news, though, was that through the use of human growth hormone (HGH), they could increase and even regulate his height so he would grow to be anywhere from 5 foot, 8 inches to 6 foot, 6 inches. With the use of HGH, his parents were free to choose how tall they wanted him to be, and because he was so far under the bell curve of normal growth, it would even be covered by their insurance.

The year is 2060, and a definitive cure for the genetic mutation that causes cystic fibrosis has recently been discovered, tested, and perfected. This gene therapy takes a properly functioning gene and places it at the site of the mutated gene it replaces. The technique is applied to both the somatic (i.e., nonreproductive) cells and the germ-line (i.e., reproductive) cells of the person who has the gene. Your state, like many others, has just added the test for the cystic fibrosis gene to the list of required newborn screening. Moreover, every newborn found to be a carrier of the mutation or to be affected by the gene is required to undergo both the somatic and germ-line gene therapy. The goal is to ultimately eradicate the genetic mutation.[11]

Setting the Context: The Science of Genes and Genomics

To understand the full potential of genetic technologies and the accompanying ethical issues, we begin by focusing on the relationship between genetics and disease as currently understood. Our bodies consist of about 100 billion cells, all of which, except mature red blood cells, contain a complete copy of our genetic code. This genetic code is packaged in chromosomes in the nucleus (or "control center") of every cell. The chromosomes are made up of strands of the chemical deoxyribonucleic acid, or DNA. Genes are specific clusters of DNA that are located on the chromosomes. A small number of genes are also contained in tiny packages in the cell called mitochondria (the "powerhouse" of the cell). The entire DNA in the cell makes up the human genome.[12]

There are forty-six chromosomes in our body (or somatic) cells—twenty-three from mom and twenty-three from dad. At the completion of fertilization, the egg and sperm come together to form the single-cell zygote, which has forty-six chromosomes, made up of twenty-three pairs, and contains all the genetic material needed for further development. Scientists have numbered the chromosomes from the largest (c. #1) to the smallest (c. #22); these are called the autosomes. There are also two chromosomes, which have been given the letters X and Y; these are the sex chromosomes. In their somatic cells, a female has forty-four autosomes and two X sex chromosomes, while a male has forty-four autosomes, one X sex chromosome, and one Y sex chromosome. In their germ cells, females have twenty-two autosomes and an X chromosome, and males have twenty-two autosomes and an X or Y chromosome. Chromosomes consist of strands of DNA that twist and coil up like a ball of string. Each bead of DNA is a gene that has a specific location on the chromosome. Genes come in pairs, with the exception of the genes on the sex chromosomes. Thousands of genes make up each chromosome (though this varies among sex chromosomes).

Each gene is a different packet of information that has a particular job in terms of directing how our bodies develop and work, as well as how we look. The information in the genes is in the form of a chemical (DNA) code, often referred to as the genetic code. Genes issue instructions to the cells by these chemically coded "messages." This is why the DNA that makes up the genes is often called "coding DNA," whereas the DNA string between the beads of genes is called "noncoding DNA," as it does not contain messages that the cells use. Interestingly, genes comprise only 2 percent of the human genome; the remainder consists of noncoding DNA.

There are four basic "building blocks" (nucleotide bases) that make up DNA: adenine (A), guanine (G), thymine (T), and cytosine (C). DNA is made up of long chains of these bases. The bases pair up to form the rungs of a "ladder" twisted into the now-famous double helix structure. The pairing of the bases follows strict rules: A with T, and G with C. The DNA message is made up of three-letter "words" composed of combinations of these letters A, G, T, and C. A gene can therefore be thought of as a coded message that the body understands. There may be hundreds or even thousands of letters in each gene message; a significant aspect of the HGP is that it has figured out the sequence of these letters. The DNA message in the genes tells the cell to produce particular proteins, which are large, complex molecules made up of smaller subunits called amino acids. The sequence of three-letter words in the gene enables the cells to assemble the amino acids in the correct order to make up the protein. Although genes get a lot of attention, the proteins perform most life functions and even make up the majority of cellular structures.

The body has many different types of cells (e.g., skin, muscle, liver, and brain), all of which contain the same genes. However, not all genes are active in every cell because only certain genes are required for the cell to function correctly. Therefore, different genes are active in different cell types, tissues, and organs, producing the necessary specific proteins for proper cellular function. Sometimes genes can be altered or have mutations, causing a change in the message sent from the gene to the cell and thus affecting protein production. Most of the time genetic mutations do not cause any problems or manifest as a genetic disorder. In fact, everyone is born with several gene mutations, and sometimes these can even be beneficial because they allow us to adapt to our environment (e.g., there is a faulty hemoglobin gene that can protect us from malaria).[13] However, genetic mutations can be harmful in at least three different ways: (1) mutations can lead to a genetic disorder; (2) mutations can make us a carrier of a disorder, which we can pass on to our offspring; or (3) mutations can predispose us to a disorder, thereby increasing our risk of being affected by a specific genetic disorder. Of course, with new knowledge comes new technologies, and one of the primary tasks of health care ethics as we understand it is to ensure that new technologies serve the good of the human person and help to restore right relationships. It has not always been the case that genetic knowledge and technology have been used in the service of human good.

A Cautionary Tale: The Slippery Slope to Eugenics

Genetics did not start with the Human Genome Project. Questions concerning how traits are inherited or handed down from one generation to the next go back to the beginnings of human history. In 1865 an Augustinian monk named Gregor Mendel found that individual traits are determined by "discrete factors," later known as genes, which are inherited from parents. By analyzing purebred and hybrid pea plants, Mendel also found each trait (e.g., seed color) has two alternative forms (e.g., yellow or green) and each alternative form of a trait is expressed by alternative forms of a gene. Although Mendel's work was done on pea plants, the knowledge gained was shortly thereafter applied to humans. The study of family pedigrees affected by disorders provided many of the first examples of Mendelian inheritance in humans.

Building on the knowledge gained from the scientific field of genetics, Francis Galton (1865), hypothesized that the human race could be bettered if we multiplied desirable traits and minimized undesirable ones. Positive eugenics (the promoting of desirable traits through reproductive choices) gave way gradually in the early 1900s to negative eugenics (the "breeding out" of undesirable traits by preventing reproduction, either voluntarily or otherwise).[14] Rooted in social Darwinism, the idea of negative eugenics was accepted in the United States and other "developed" countries and was endorsed by prominent scientists who thought it could eliminate the "feeble-minded" (a blanket term used in the early 1900s to describe the mentally ill, the cognitively impaired, slow learners, uneducated, and those considered morally suspect).[15] The idea was to provide no support to the "feebleminded" and not to allow them "to propagate their unfit kind" by forcing sterilization; there were also attempts to limit the immigration of "inferior races."[16] Several states adopted laws authorizing compulsory sterilization of the "feebleminded" but were checked by constitutional challenges, except for a Virginia statute upheld by the U.S. Supreme Court in the notorious case of *Buck v. Bell* (1927).

The case of *Buck v. Bell* involved Carrie Buck, an 18-year-old cognitively impaired woman who resided at the Virginia State Colony for Epileptics and Feebleminded. In 1924, just months after Virginia adopted a statute allowing for the compulsory sterilization of the "feebleminded" for negative eugenics purposes, the superintendent of the institution sought to have Carrie sterilized because she represented a "genetic threat to society." Carrie was herself the daughter of a woman with cognitive impairments. After being raped by her adopted mother's nephew, Carrie had given birth to a baby deemed "feebleminded," which most likely prompted Carrie's institutionalization. After two lower courts upheld the request for the sterilization, the case eventually made its way to the U.S. Supreme Court, which, in an eight–one decision, ruled that it was in the state's interests to have Carrie sterilized. Writing the majority opinion, Justice Oliver Wendell Holmes Jr., stated,

We have seen more than once that the public welfare may call upon the best citizens for their lives. It would be strange if it could not call upon those who already sap the strength of the State for these lesser sacrifices . . . in order to prevent our being swamped with incompetence. . . . Three generations of imbeciles is enough.

The ruling reinforced Virginia's compulsory sterilization statute and encouraged other states to write similar statutes. Fortunately, explicit negative eugenics began to fall out of favor in the wake of the horrible consequences of the Nazi quest for racial purity, which led to the deaths of hundreds of thousands of "inferiors." It was further subverted as new knowledge about human nature and disease was gained, leaving scientists to conclude the eugenics description of human life was too simplistic and ultimately unconvincing. Simple dominant/recessive schemes did not fully explain complex behaviors and mental illness, which we now know involve many genes, nor did they account for environmental effects on human development. Still it would be a bit too optimistic to presume the eugenics mind-set does not persist today in the form of the new quest for the "perfect child" with the "right traits," the "right gender," and so on. Our current techniques may be a bit more sophisticated than compulsory sterilizations and our language may be more politically correct, but reproductive technologies, prenatal and preimplantation diagnosis, selective abortion, and the like can and have been used for eugenic purposes.

As explicit bias and bigotry were largely supplanted by hard science, new breakthroughs in genetics resulted. It is evident from these advances that genomics does indeed hold great promise. However, with great promise can come great peril. Genomic medicine could further the divide between the "haves" and the "have-nots" within an already unjust health care system. For example, if diagnoses can lead to prevention through presymptomatic predisposition profiling, those who can afford such profiling (either personally or through their health care coverage) would be at a significant advantage insofar as they could access therapies or cures. Another danger is that knowledge about genomics could lead to genetic reductionism (the idea that the complexity of the human person can be explained solely via genetics). The limits of privacy and confidentiality could be tested as caregivers are confronted with genetic information that has wider implications. Genetic information could be mishandled and used to discriminate for work or insurance purposes.[17] Moreover, if genetic enhancement becomes a part of medicine, those who can get access to such interventions could reap significant advantages in the areas of physical size, less need for sleep, aging, intellect, and personality disposition. However, the peril that genomics may pose does not necessarily mean we should turn away from its promise. Rather, it means we have to proceed carefully and govern ethically our new-found power over the human genome. We must not let technological progress outpace ethical reflection. History has shown us what will come of us if we let this happen.[18]

The ethical issues raised by current and future genetic technologies, however, are complex and there are few clear-cut answers. Consider, for example, Case 8C. Does the mandatory newborn screening and gene therapy program constitute eugenics? If so, would you consider this positive or negative eugenics? Does such a program constitute a morally appropriate public policy aimed at noble ends or is there something morally objectionable about such programs? The ethical issues associated with the promise and peril of genetic technologies, however, are not limited to future hypothetical possibilities but are equally relevant to many current uses of this technology. A current application of genetic technology that exemplifies both the promise and peril is genetic testing (GT), which is by far the most significant and immediate spin-off of the advances made in genomics. For this reason we consider genetic testing and the associated ethical issues before exploring the possibilities associated with gene therapy and genetic enhancement.

Discussion: Ethical Issues and Analysis

GT is the examination of a person's chromosomes, the protein product of a gene, or DNA. GT is used to predict risks of disease, screen newborns for disease, identify carriers of genetic disease, establish prenatal or clinical diagnoses or prognoses, and direct clinical care. GT can be done using many different biological samples, including blood, amniotic fluid (from which fetal cells are obtained), or individual embryonic cells.

In the past, GT was used to detect or confirm rare genetic disorders that have a specific inheritance pattern. More recently, however, tests have been developed to detect genetic mutations with links to multifactorial disorders (such as cardiovascular disease and breast, ovarian, and colon cancer), the effects of which generally do not appear until later in life. GT has generally been reserved for individuals who have a family history of a disease; in the future, though, GT will likely be offered to individuals without a family history. At present, there are 614 laboratories testing for 1,355 diseases.[19]

The following are some specific types of genetic tests:

- newborn screening
- diagnostic testing
- predictive testing
- presymptomatic testing

Newborn Screening (NS)

NS is performed in newborns as part of state public health programs so that certain genetic disorders can be detected soon after birth and early intervention or therapy can begin. Through NS programs, more than four million newborns in the United States are tested each year for diseases such as phenylketonuria (PKU), hypothyroidism, sickle-cell disease, and cystic fibrosis. All states, the District of Columbia, Puerto Rico, and the U.S. Virgin Islands now have their own mandatory NS programs. Because the federal government has set no national standard, however, screening requirements vary from state to state and the comprehensiveness of these programs varies as well. States routinely screen for anywhere from two to thirty disorders, with the average state program testing from four to ten disorders.[20]

NS is done within the first two or three days of life by pricking the baby's heel and drawing a small sample of blood that is then applied to a card (called a Guthrie card after the scientist who developed a blood test for screening newborns for PKU). In general, consent to screening is not required; however, parents can refuse screening if they notify the health care provider in advance. Most states have identified a state or regional laboratory to which hospitals send the samples for analysis. Although NS is designed to detect infants with metabolic illnesses, certain tests can identify the infant as a carrier who may be clinically asymptomatic. Such information is important for the family in terms of planning future pregnancies and could be important to the infant when he or she reaches reproductive age.

Ethical Issues. More than four million newborns are screened in the United States each year. The intention of newborn screening as a public policy is prevention of serious illness where parents may not even be aware of genetic risk. The ethical issues in the area of newborn screening, therefore, are many. Matters of informed consent, access, confidentiality and privacy, adequacy of social support services, and resource allocation highlight the complexity and multidimensional array of ethical issues involved in newborn screening. Difficulties associated with obtaining adequate informed consent in this area are compounded by the difficulties involved with any issue within the context of labor and delivery and its associated anxieties and pressures. Furthermore, the disorders for which a child is screened may depend on the place the child happens to be born. Once knowledge of a disorder is gained, ethical reflection shifts to adequacy, availability, and access to social support services to help families with children in whom a disorder is discovered. This raises corollary ethics questions concerning resource allocation: (1) what tests should society consider in light of its ethical aims and (2) what criteria do we use to select the disorders for which we test, given issues of access and availability of resources in the local community?[21]

Privacy and confidentiality in the area of newborn screening takes on special significance because third parties have some legitimate interests regarding reimbursement or insurance. Newborn screening may have implications for further access to health care services. Given that the genetic information gleaned from newborn screening will follow the person throughout his or her entire life, agencies and health care institutions must ardently guard the privacy of this information.

Diagnostic Testing/Predictive Testing

Two forms of genetic testing are used to identify or predict diagnoses. Diagnostic testing is used to identify or confirm the diagnosis of a disease or condition in an affected individual. It may also be useful to help predict the course of a disease and determine the choice of treatment. Predictive testing is used to determine the probability that a healthy individual with or without a family history of a certain disorder might develop that disorder (e.g., mutations to BRCA1, BRCA2, or both genes are associated with an increased risk of breast and ovarian cancer). Predictive testing that leads to the detection of a mutated gene provides the person with an increased risk estimate rather than certainty that he or she will develop a particular disorder later in life.

Presymptomatic testing is used to determine if a person has a particular genetic mutation that will lead to a certain disorder later in life, though the person is not yet experiencing any symptoms. Presymptomatic testing is available for several neurodegenerative diseases, such as Huntington's disease, and some forms of bowel cancer. A key difference between presymptomatic testing and predictive testing is that discovery of a genetic mutation through presymptomatic testing indicates that the likelihood of developing the disorder is very high, whereas detection of a mutated gene through predictive testing indicates an increased risk of developing the disorder.

Ethical Issues. In addition to many of the previously discussed ethical issues related to differing forms of genetic testing, there are ethical issues unique to these three types of genetic tests. In the area of diagnostic testing, ethical issues raise concerns about whether there is a duty on the part of the patient who may be diagnosed with a genetic disease to disclose information to family members. Other concerns relate to the usefulness of the information. That is, are there curative or preventive measures available? Will having the information provide psychological relief? Who should decide for minors, and on what grounds? And so on.

In the area of predictive testing, there are concerns about false positives and false negatives of the tests. In other words, a patient may incorrectly test positive for the disease, experience the psychological burden associated with such knowledge, and perhaps disclose the genetic disorder to other family members, but not actually have the genetic disorder. Genetic discrimination or stigmatization because of the diagnosis is also possible. Issues of social justice must also be raised; namely, is there fairness in testing and equitable distribution of the benefits and burdens?[22]

Because genetic testing is never without risk, counseling must always be coupled with such testing for it to respect the human dignity of the patient. That is, risks may be associated with the psychological uncertainty, interpretation of results, and implications of results, including effect on future health coverage, privacy of information obtained, and duty to tell family members. Consider again Case 8A in which the neurologist recommends a predictive test for Jeb, who has a family history of Alzheimer's disease and has begun experiencing possible symptoms, though these may also be the result of chemotherapy he has been undergoing for stomach cancer. The ethical issues raised in this case include whether the test should be offered in the first place, given that there is no treatment of Alzheimer's disease, the question of whether Jeb has an obligation, after discovering the results, to inform his children of their risk, and the risks and harm associated with having a 75-percent chance of developing the disease. After all, the course of treatment will likely be the same for Jeb if the symptoms persist, whether or not they are due to his chemotherapy or Alzheimer's disease. Still, there may be some psychological benefit in knowing the symptoms will eventually subside if they are due to the chemo. Yet even if he does not have the gene for Alzheimer's disease, there is still the possibility he could develop a different form of Alzheimer's (i.e., the noninheritable type).

Beyond Testing: Gene Therapy and Genetic Enhancement

Gene Therapy

Although testing and screening are by far the most prevalent applications of genetic technology today, gene therapy is another application that many believe holds great promise. Generally, gene therapy is a technique for reversing, reducing, or eliminating diseases that have a genetic basis by correcting defective genes that are responsible for the development of the disease. Gene therapy accomplishes this through a variety of methods. Most commonly, a normal gene may be inserted into the genome to replace a nonfunctioning or malfunctioning gene. In some cases, a mutated gene could actually be exchanged for a normal gene using a technique called homologous recombination. Another method is to introduce genetic material into a gene so as to correct or repair that gene to its normal function through selective reverse mutation. Finally, a mutated or malfunctioning gene could simply be "turned off," so it is no longer producing the undesired effect. All of these techniques are accomplished by using a carrier molecule, referred to as a vector, to deliver the therapeutic gene to the patient's target cells. These vectors are usually comprised of retroviruses or adenoviruses, which are capable of propagating themselves and recombining their DNA with that of existing cells within the body.[23] These vectors can be used to target and treat either somatic (i.e., nonreproductive) cells within the body or germ-line cells, the sperm or egg cells in which any modification to the genome would be passed down to the next and all subsequent generations of offspring.

The development of somatic cell gene therapy has been an on-again, off-again affair. There has not been significant technological advancement since the first gene therapy trials took place in 1990. In the beginning, it seemed as though gene therapy would become one of the most rapidly growing fields of medical research. Five years after the first FDA-approved gene therapy trial, there were 100 studies under way targeting such diseases as various cancers, HIV, rheumatoid arthritis, peripheral artery disease, arterial stenosis, and a host of genetic diseases including cystic fibrosis, Gaucher's disease, SCID, Fanconi anemia, Hunter syndrome, and several others.[24] However, in 1999, gene therapy suffered a major setback when 18-year-old Jesse Gelsinger died from multiple organ failure only four days after starting a gene therapy trial. His death was believed to be the result of a severe immune response to the vector used to deliver the treatment gene. Another major setback came in 2003, when the FDA stopped all gene therapy trials using retroviral vectors after learning that two children in a French gene therapy trial to treat SCID had developed a leukemia-like disease as a result of the treatment.[25] Though the FDA lifted this ban later that same year, the safeguards and restrictions under which human trials involving retroviral vectors can be undertaken were significantly tightened. Today, somatic cell gene therapy trials are generally limited to enrolling the most severely ill patients suffering from conditions for which there are no other existing therapies.[26]

Along with the safety risks, gene therapy faces several scientific or logistical obstacles that have kept it from becoming an effective, mainstream treatment. First, most gene therapies last for only a short while due to the nature of cell division. The short-lived nature of gene therapy treatments means patients have to undergo multiple rounds of therapy to achieve a lasting effect. Second, as seen in the case of Jesse Gelsinger, gene therapy can stimulate unknown immune responses that not only result in safety risks but also can make it difficult to repeat gene therapy as required by its short-lived nature. Third, problems with viral vectors, including effectiveness and safety, remain. Finally, gene therapy appears to be most effective in treating single-gene disorders, although most diseases are caused by variations in multiple genes.[27] Thus, the usefulness of gene therapy is currently limited to a confined set of relatively rare diseases. Still, as of 2007, 1,340 clinical trials involving gene transfer were either completed, ongoing or approved worldwide.[28]

Ethical Issues. Early in the history of gene therapy, it was assumed that something was inherently different about the nature of somatic cell gene therapy from other types of medical interventions. However, as time has passed, somatic cell gene therapy has come to be viewed as a natural and logical extension of current techniques for treating disease.[29] Consistent with this reasoning, most of the ethical issues regarding somatic cell gene therapy today are the same as those regarding any experimental medical technology and human subject research. For example, the primary ethical issues around gene therapy today involve questions regarding whether there are alternative interventions that are equally as effective, safe, and inexpensive as the experimental gene therapy; whether the potential harm outweighs the potential benefit; fairness in selecting the participants for the trials; the adequacy of informed consent and the voluntariness of subject participation; and how the privacy and confidentiality of subjects will be protected. These ethical issues are not distinctive to gene therapy but are similar, if not the same, to those ethical issues that must be addressed when considering any experimental intervention as part of human subjects research.

The ethical issues begin to take on a different hue, however, when one considers the possibility of germ-line gene therapy. Again, germ-line gene therapy is the technique of modifying genes within the reproductive system so that both the individual on whom the therapy is initiated and all of his or her offspring and all subsequent generations of offspring will have the same altered genes. Germ-line gene therapy could be undertaken on the gamete of an affected individual in conjunction with an in vitro fertilization (IVF) procedure, so that the genetic disease-causing mutation would not be passed on to any offspring. Alternatively, the corrected genes could be introduced at the very earliest post-fertilization stages of human development, that is, in zygotes or preimplantation embryos, in which case it would be performed in conjunction with preimplantation genetic diagnoses (for more on PGD, see chapter 6).

Advocates for germ-line gene therapy have asserted several possible advantages over somatic cell gene therapy. First, because it would be performed at the very earliest stages of human development, before cell division, the properly functioning gene could be added to the entire genome in one fell swoop in conditions that would otherwise require multiple separate somatic cell gene therapy procedures. Second, because it would be performed at such an early stage, it could prevent the damage to the cells that would be caused by defective genes in embryo development from occurring in the first place, whereas somatic gene therapy can only reverse or reduce damage that has already occurred. This, some might argue, is more in keeping with the preventive goals of medicine. Finally, germ-line gene therapy brings with it the prospect of reducing or eliminating the incidence of certain inheritable diseases from the human gene pool altogether. Thus, from a social, economic, and public health perspective, the proponents argue, germ-line gene therapy would be a more efficient and cost-effective model of disease prevention and health promotion than somatic cell gene therapy. Some have even argued that, if it is ever proven safe and effective, germ-line gene therapy would be more in keeping with the medical profession's moral obligation to prevent harm. There are, however, risks similar to those with somatic cell gene therapy; only in the case of germ-line gene therapy, any adverse effects would affect not only the individual receiving the initial gene modification but all of his or her future offspring, as well as all subsequent generations. For this reason, there is some consensus that the risks of manipulating the genes through germ-line interventions far exceed the potential benefit and, thus, should not be attempted.[30]

In addition to the risks outweighing the potential benefit, several interrelated arguments against attempting germ-line gene therapy arise from our normative framework. A foundational concern has to do with the inherent dignity of all human life from its beginning. Extensive experimentation using human embryos would have to occur in the development of germ-line gene therapy techniques to prove its effectiveness. As human subjects trials with somatic cell gene therapy has shown us, there would inevitably be many trials and errors that would occur through this experimental phase. Inevitably, many human embryos would be destroyed through this process. Ultimately, the destruction or other harm to preimplantation embryos that would be required would be incompatible with the respect owed to those embryos according to our normative framework. Another concern is the effect such therapy would have on societal attitudes toward already existing individuals who suffer from genetically based disease. Can we attempt to eradicate certain genes from the gene pool without also implying those who have those genes are somehow less worthy of our care and resources, and even that the world would be a better place if they were not part of it? Thus, we might ask whether such an undertaking is compatible with the virtue of solidarity and fostering the types of social relationships that contribute to the advancement of human well-being generally. And what about those who could not afford the intervention? Or, more precisely, would not those who have the means to afford the intervention have a greater advantage? It would at least seem that such technology would be accompanied by an even greater disparity between the haves and have-nots than seen under the current health care system. Finally, how would society determine which genetic traits should be eliminated from the genome?

Genetic Enhancement

Back in 1989, W. French Anderson wrote a keystone article in which, to ensure that resources are directed toward exploring new ways to combat life-threatening and severely disabling medical conditions, he advocated for drawing a line between gene therapy aimed at curing or preventing disease and genetic interventions intended to enhance or improve the capacities of healthy human beings.[31] More recently, genetic enhancement has been defined as "improving human traits that without intervention would be within the range of what is commonly regarded as normal, or improving them beyond what is needed to maintain or restore good health."[32] As we have already alluded, the primary areas of human capacity that would be open to genetic enhancement include physical size, reducing the need for sleep, slowing the aging process, increasing memory and cognitive ability in general, and to some extent modifying behavior, especially aggression. Indeed, genetic technologies are already being used for enhancement in the areas of physical performance, memory and learning, and physical appearance.[33] The question of where to draw the line between therapy and enhancement is not easily answered. Consider, for example, our Case 8B. Does short stature, as in the case of Mark, constitute a disability or disease for which the use of HGH is an appropriate therapeutic intervention? Or does the use of HGH to regulate height constitute an enhancement? Does it make a difference whether in Mark's case his parents choose to use HGH so he will grow to average height or to a height greater than average, which might give him a certain advantage, say, as a college basketball player? This case illustrates that the line between therapy and enhancement is anything but clear. Yet how we answer these difficult questions could have significant implications for how we walk the line between improving the human condition and falling back into a social eugenics movement. Short of that, how we answer these questions has direct implication for where we draw the line between healing and enhancing the genetic makeup of the human person, and thus where we dedicate our valuable societal resources.

Ethical Issues. The argument in favor of genetic enhancement is generally twofold. First, advocates purport there is nothing fundamentally new or different about genetic enhancement techniques compared with other types of enhancement efforts that human beings already commonly employ. For example, Robert Sade, MD, among others, has argued using genetic enhancement intended to reduce susceptibility to disease is not really any different from using vaccines to prevent polio and other diseases. Similarly, using genetic enhancement to improve cognitive performance and reduce the need for sleep isn't any different from using coffee or other stimulants to do the same. Moreover, even though risks and possible harms may be associated with genetic interventions intended for the purpose of enhancement, many of the environmental and physiologic enhancement interventions already employed today are also harmful.[34] Likewise, just as genetic enhancement interventions have the potential to increase existing inequalities, so do environmental interventions aimed at enhancement, such as sending one's children to a private school.[35] Thus, the argument goes, genetic enhancement is really no different than any number of actions human beings already undertake to enhance their own capabilities, as well as those of their children. This argument, then, is often coupled with a libertarian ethical framework that focuses on maximizing the freedom of parents to choose different ways of influencing the genetic development of their children so as to maximize their prospects for a good life.[36]

Although we would not necessarily rule out the possibility that genetic enhancement could be morally acceptable *in principle*, our normative framework calls us to take a more cautious approach on several grounds. First, within our normative framework, we are called to give special consideration to the least well-off in society, especially regarding resource allocation. We cannot see how society could justify the expense and use of resources that would be required for the development of genetic enhancements when so many struggle to access even the most basic care, not to mention life-saving treatments. As in the case of stem cell research (see chapter 7), we believe society's medical resources should be dedicated to purposes more aligned with the principles of the common good, solidarity, and the preferential option for the poor than to the purposes of improving and expanding the capacities of already healthy individuals. Thus, our normative framework leads us to agree with W. French Anderson that society should draw a hard line—though that line may at times be in part the result of arbitrary social consensus—between therapy and enhancement to ensure its resources are dedicated first to the development of therapies that will benefit larger percentages of the population.

Second, given that our health care environment today is and will continue in the foreseeable future to be largely unregulated and market-driven, we cannot see how genetic enhancements distributed primarily through market mechanisms would result in much else besides a widening of the gap between the most and the least well-off in society. Although it is undeniable that many existing inequalities are the result of environmentally and socially based enhancement initiatives undertaken by individuals of their own initiative, there does seem to be a morally significant difference between these types of inequalities and those that would arise from genetic enhancement. In particular, environmental and socially based enhancements (for example, the use of coffee and other stimulants, vaccines, private education, physical training, and so on) improve our ability to actualize our capabilities within a characteristically human range, while genetic enhancements would likely improve the innate range or extent to which we are capable of functioning in a certain way, as well as our ability to actualize that capability. In an extreme scenario, genetic enhancement could even be used to introduce new capabilities. Thus, there seem to be certain limits to the extent to which capacities built into the human genome can be actualized, and with those limits come inherent constraints on the degree of inequality that results from environmental and socially based enhancements. Genetic enhancements, however, would seem to carry the possibility of expanding the range of those capacities and create the possibility for even greater advantage for those who could afford to purchase them over those who could not. Though this concern might be adequately accounted for, if adequate guarantees regarding procedural fairness or justice could ensure the same enhancement opportunities are available to everyone and the least well off would be given priority with regard to the distribution of those opportunities, we see no evidence of such procedural justice in our current health system and have no reason to believe it would be achieved regarding genetic enhancement.[37]

This potential for even greater inequality with regard to the range and ability to actualize certain human traits and capabilities is directly related to our third reason for taking an extremely cautious approach to genetic enhancement. Specifically, individuals with highly valued societal characteristics, such as a pleasant disposition, attractive physical appearance, and athletic ability, are rewarded with position, respect, and financial gain, as well as a number of other social advantages.[38] By espousing or endorsing genetic enhancement as a socially acceptable practice, society would be increasing the value it already places on these traits and capabilities. Although this is not in itself morally wrong, it would likely lead to greater disparities regarding social position, respect, and financial benefit, insofar as those who already have these valued traits and capabilities would be those who could access the enhancements in the first place, as discussed in our previous concern. Moreover, such social initiatives would seem to be inconsistent with a view of the moral worth of persons as being intrinsic, arising solely from their human nature as made in the image and likeness of God, rather than of dignity as attributable to particular individuals in light of their possessing some socially valued traits. In a worst-case scenario, the societal reinforcement of these socially recognized values through genetic intervention carries with it the dangers of eugenics, both negative and positive, and potentially places society on the slippery slope of our past.

Conclusion

Although many issues will likely surface in the legal and public policy discourse on applications of future genetic technologies, the current focus is largely on the privacy of genetic data and on the safety of human subject research in gene therapy. Concerns regarding future applications center on germ-line interventions and enhancement techniques. Of particular relevance in these areas are issues of procedural justice, fairness, equality, and nondiscrimination. Ethics must be at the front of these debates, as questions must be raised about access and distributive justice; attempts to eradicate certain genetic diseases and traits from the human genome altogether; the desire to maximize socially valued characteristics, which stem from an extrinsic view of dignity and moral worth; and whether people are likely to be stigmatized by genetic information. As political scientist Francis Fukuyama reminds us, "Denial of the concept of human dignity—that is, of the idea that there is something unique about the human race that entitled every member of the species to a higher moral status than the rest of the natural world—leads us down a very perilous path. We may be compelled to take this path, but we should do so only with our eyes open."[39] Even though our human nature may be growing more and more malleable, we must always keep our eyes trained on our constant and immutable telos, our ultimate good: human flourishing understood as loving God in right relationships through which we fulfill the second commandment to love our neighbor.

Additional Case Studies

Case 8D

In May 2002 the Burlington Northern Santa Fe Railroad (BNSF) agreed to pay $2.2 million to settle charges of illegally testing workers for genetic defects. BNSF had performed genetic tests on more than thirty employees who sought worker's compensation and medical attention for carpal-tunnel syndrome. The employees claim they did not give consent for or have knowledge of the genetic tests at the time blood samples were taken. They also contended that BNSF conducted the tests to avoid the medical care costs associated with the syndrome.

The BNSF employees filed a complaint with the Equal Employment Opportunities Commission (EEOC), who in turn filed suit against BNSF on the grounds that the railroad violated the American's with Disabilities Act (ADA). The EEOC asked the court for an order directing BNSF to (1) halt its policy requiring genetic testing for track worker employees who file worker's compensation claims related to carpal tunnel syndrome and (2) halt disciplinary action or termination of employees who refused to submit a blood sample for genetic tests.

BNSF settled out of court and agreed to stop testing employees. It also agreed to destroy all blood samples from workers who were already tested and delete the genetic results from their employment record. Finally, BNSF agreed to promote efforts to create federal legislation prohibiting genetic testing related to employment.

Discussion questions. Should BNSF have settled out of court, or did it have an ethical basis on which to justify testing? There are often restrictions on certain types of jobs that require minimal levels of strength, endurance, or ability; why should BNSF's claim be any different? Is there something different about attempting to seek a perceived genetic basis for carpal tunnel syndrome in order not to be required to provide worker's compensation for a work-related injury?

Case 8E

Henrietta Lacks has been dead for more than 60 years, yet some of her cells live on. Henrietta died of cervical cancer in 1951. Shortly after her death, scientists using cells taken from her tumor discovered the cells continued to survive and grow in the lab. These cells, now known as Hela cells, became the first immortal human cell line. Her cells have since been used in countless scientific and medical research experiments. In fact, it is estimated scientists have grown twenty tons of her cells and almost 11,000 patents are related to the use of her cells. However, Henrietta's cells had been taken without consent and her family never knew of this until more recently, when scientists began contacting the family to get more of the family's genetic makeup and history. In essence, Henrietta's cells had launched a multimillion dollar industry selling human biological materials, yet her family never saw any of the profits.

Discussion questions. Who owns genetic material? Should private interests be able to patent someone else's genetic material and information? Should people who have donated genetic material or information that leads to patents be entitled to some of the profits? Beyond requiring informed consent, should the government regulate the commercial use of such genetic material and information?

SUGGESTED READINGS

Clayton, E. W. "Genomic Medicine: Ethical, Legal, and Social Implications of Genomic Medicine." *New England Journal of Medicine* 349 (2003): 562–9.

Collins, F. C. "Shattuck Lecture: Medical and Societal Consequences of the Human Genome Project." *New England Journal of Medicine* 341 (1999): 28–37.

Ensenauer, R. E., V. V. Michels, and S. S. Reinke. "Genetic Testing: Practical, Ethical, and Counseling Considerations." *Mayo Clinic Proceedings* 80 (2005): 63–73.

Keenan, James F. "What Is Morally New in Genetic Manipulation?" *Human Gene Therapy* 1 (1990): 289–98.

McCormick, Richard A. "Moral Theology and the Genome Project." In *Controlling Our Destinies*, edited by Philip R. Sloan, 417–28 (Notre Dame, IN: University of Notre Dame Press, 2000).

MULTIMEDIA AIDS FOR TEACHERS

Gattaca. Directed by Andrew Niccol. Starring Ethan Hawke. Rated PG-13. 1997. This movie depicts a future world where genetic technology has run amock.

Rabbit-Proof Fence. Directed by Phillip Noyce. Starring Everlyn Sampi. Rated PG. 2002. This movie depicts the tragedy that befalls an aboriginal family caught in the web of a eugenics-minded Australia in the 1930s.

A Question of Genes: Inherited Risks. Public Broadcasting System. 1997. This two-hour television special follows the personal journey of individuals and families who confront questions about genetic testing. For more information on purchasing the VHS, see *http://www.backbonemedia.org/genes/educator/44_video.html*.

"Trial and Errors: A Family's Quest for Answers." *Dateline NBC*. 2002. The story of Jesse Gelsinger's life, his involvement in gene therapy trials, and his father's efforts to find out what happened to his son and improve the oversight of human subject research, especially gene therapy trials.

"Against All Odds." *48 Hours*. CBS. 2000. This program focuses on people struggling with difficult health circumstances. David Bailey has a brain tumor. Eight-year-old Katie Mahar has XP, a rare and often fatal disease. The section of the tape entitled "Saving Amy" profiles Amy Frohnmayer, who has the rare genetic disease called Fanconi's anemia. This segment also discusses gene therapy and research into genetic diseases. Paul Gelsinger, the father of teenager Jesse Gelsinger, who died while enrolled in a gene therapy clinical trial, is also interviewed. Available at CBS Online Store.

ENDNOTES

1. Francis Collins, "Shattuck Lecture: Medical and Societal Consequences of the Human Genome Project," *New England Journal of Medicine* 341, no. 1 (July 1, 1999): 28–37.

2. Lily E. Kay, "A Book of Life? How a Genetic Code Became a Language," in *Controlling Our Destinies*, ed. Philip Sloan (Notre Dame, IN: University of Notre Dame Press, 2000), 99–124.

3. Collins, "Shattuck Lecture," 30.

4. Timothy Lenoir and Marguerite Hays, "The Manhattan Project for Bio-Medicine," in *Controlling Our Destinies*, ed. Philip Sloan (Notre Dame, IN: University of Notre Dame Press, 2000), 29–62.

5. Willard Gaylin, "The Frankenstein Factor," *New England Journal of Medicine* 297 (September 22, 1977): 665–7.

6. J. Jin, "An Evaluation of the Ethical, Legal, and Social Implications Program of the U.S. Human Genome Project," *Princeton Journal of Bioethics* 3, no. 1 (2000): 35–50; and E. M. Meslin, T. J. Thomson, and J. T. Boyer, "The Ethical, Legal, and Social Implications Research Program at the National Human Genome Research Institute," *Kennedy Institute of Ethics Journal* 7, no. 3 (September 1997): 291–8.

7. For a substantive listing of single-gene disorders, see "Online Mendelian Inheritance in Man at Johns Hopkins University," *http://www.ncbi.nlm.nih.gov/entrez/query.fcgi?db=OMIM*.

8. J. G. Shaw, "Cancer and Genetic Medicine: A Medical View," *Health Progress* 86, no. 5 (2005): 31–5; and C. Bayley, "Cancer and Genetic Medicine: An Ethical View," *Health Progress*, 86, no. 5 (2005): 35–7.

9. See "Genetics Home Reference," *http://ghr.nlm.nig.gov*.

10. F. S. Collins and A. E. Guttmacher, "Genetics Moves into the Medical Mainstream," *JAMA* 286, no. 18 (2001): 2322–4; and P. R. Billings et al., "Ready for Genomic Medicine? Perspectives of Health Care Decision Makers," *Archives of Internal Medicine* 165, no. 16 (2005): 1917–9.

11. Adapted from LeRoy Walters and Julie Gage Palmer, *The Ethics of Human Gene Therapy* (New York: Oxford University Press, 1997), 87.

12. Graphics of different DNA structures can be found in the illustrated glossary provided at the GeneTests Web site, *www.genetests.org*. GeneTests is funded by the National Institutes of Health.

13. For an understanding of the relationship between faulty hemoglobin gene and malaria, see "Malaria and the Red Cell" at the Information Center for Sickle Cell and Thalassemic Disorders Web site, *http://sickle.bwh.harvard.edu/malaria_sickle.html*.

14. It is important to note a possible link between the widespread promotion of birth control and racism. Historically, this link was most evident in the appearance of new government-funded clinics in the 1970s that seemingly targeted African Americans. At that time, many religious leaders in the African American community accused family-planning clinics of "genocidal"

intentions. See Linda Gordon, *Women's Body, Women's Right: Birth Control in America*. (New York: Penguin Books, 1976); Ellen Chesler, *Woman of Valor: Margaret Sanger and the Birth Control Movement in America* (New York: Simon & Schuster, 1992).

15. Jael Silliman et al., *Undivided Rights: Women of Color Organize for Reproductive Justice* (Cambridge, MA: South End Press, 2004).

16. Douglas S. Diekema, "Involuntary Sterilization of Persons with Mental Retardation: An Ethical Analysis," *Mental Retardation and Developmental Disabilities Research Reviews* 9 (2003): 21–6.

17. For information on introduced legislation on genetic nondiscrimination, see the National Human Genome Research Institute, *http://www.genome. gov/media.*

18. A number of other sources may be important to the reader: Martin S. Pernick, "Define the Defective: Eugenics, Esthetics, and Mass Culture in Early-Twentieth-Century America," in *Controlling Our Destinies*, ed. Philip Sloan (Notre Dame, IN: University of Notre Dame Press, 2000), 187–208; Arthur L. Caplan, "What's Morally Wrong with Eugenics?" in *Controlling Our Destinies*, ed. Philip Sloan (Notre Dame, IN: University of Notre Dame Press, 2000), 209–22; Philip Kitcher, "Utopian Eugenics and Social Inequality," in *Controlling Our Destinies*, ed. Philip Sloan (Notre Dame, IN: University of Notre Dame Press, 2000), 229–62.

19. This information is provided at the site for GeneTests, *www.genetests.org.*

20. T. S. Raghuveer, V. Garg, and W. D. Graf, "Inborn Errors of Metabolism in Infancy and Early Childhood: An Update," *American Family Physician* 73, no. 11 (January 2006): 1981–90; S. R. Rose, "Update of Newborn Screening and Therapy for Congenital Hypothyroidism," *Pediatrics* 117 (2006): 2290–303; R. I. Raphael, "Pathophysiology and Treatment of Sickle Cell Disease," *Clinical Advances in Hematology and Oncology* 3, no. 6 (June 2005): 492–505; D. Paul, "Contesting Consent: The Challenge to Compulsory Neonatal Screening for PKU," *Perspectives in Biology and Medicine* 42 (1999): 207–19.

21. T. Lewens, "What Is Genethics?" *Journal of Medical Ethics* 30, no. 3 (June 2004): 326–8; B. Wicken, "Ethical Issues in Newborn Screening and the Impact of New Technologies," *European Journal of Pediatrics* 162, Supplement (December 2003): S62–6; M. J. McQueen, "Some Ethics and Design Challenges of Screening Programs and Screening Tests," *Clinica Chimica Acta* 315, no. 1–2 (January 2002): 41–8.

22. M. Harris, I. Winship, and M. Spriggs, "Controversies and Ethical Issues in Cancer-Genetics Clinics," *Lancet Oncology* 6, no. 5 (May 2005): 301–10; J. P. Mackenbach, "Genetics and Health Inequalities: Hypotheses and Controversies," *Journal of Epidemiology and Community Health* 59, no. 4 (April 2005): 268–73.

23. Jonathan Kimmelman, "Recent Developments in Gene Transfer: Risk and Ethics," *British Medical Journal* 330 (2005): 79–82.

24. Walters and Palmer, *The Ethics of Human Gene Therapy*, 101–7.

25. U.S. Department of Energy, "Human Genome Project Information," *http://www.ornl.gov/sci/techresources/Human_Genome/medicine/genetherapy.shtml.*

26. Kimmelman, "Recent Developments in Gene Transfer," 79.

27. U.S. Department of Energy, "Human Genome Project Information," *http://www.ornl.gov/sci/techresources/Human_Genome/medicine/genetherapy.shtml.*

28. M. Edelstein, M. Abedi, and J. Wixon, "Gene Therapy Clinical Trials Worldwide to 2007: An Update," *Journal of Genetic Medicine* 10 (2007): 833–42.

29. Robert Sade and George Khushf, "Gene Therapy: Ethical and Social Issues," *Journal of the Southern Carolina Medical Association* 94, no. 9 (1998): 406–10.

30. Centre for Genetic Education, "The Australasian Genetics Resource Book," Fact Sheet 27 (2007), *http://www.genetics.edu.au.*

31. W. French Anderson, "Human Gene Therapy: Why Draw a Line?" *Journal of Medicine and Philosophy* 14, no. 6 (1989): 681–93.

32. Mark Frankel, "Inheritable Genetic Modification and a Brave New World: Did Huxley Have It Wrong?" *Hastings Center Report* 33, no. 2 (2003): 31–6.

33. See M. Kiuru and R. Crystal, "Progress and Prospects: Gene Therapy for Performance and Appearance Enhancement," *Gene Therapy* 15 (2008): 329–37.

34. R. Sade, "Enhancement Technology, Ethics, and Public Policy," *Journal of the Southern Carolina Medical Association* 94, no. 9 (1998): 411–5.

35 See, A. Buchanan, D. Broch, and N. Daniels, *From Chance to Choice: Genetics and Justice* (New York: Cambridge University Press, 2000), 159–61.

36. For a review of arguments in favor of genetic enhancement based on the "expansion of liberty" view, see J. Borenstein, "The Wisdom of Caution, Genetic Enhancement, and Future Children," *Journal of Science and Engineering Ethics* 15 (2009): 517–30.

37. Regarding procedural justice as part of the ethics of genetic enhancement, see J. Harris and S. Chan, "Understanding the Ethics of Genetic Enhancement," *Gene Therapy* 15 (2008): 338–9.

38. Kiuru and Crystal, "Gene Therapy for Performance and Appearance Enhancement," 330.

39. F. Fukuyama, *Our Posthuman Future: Consequences of the Biotechnology Revolution* (New York: Farrar, Straus and Giroux, 2002), 160.

CHAPTER 9

Medical Research on Humans and the Pharmaceutical/Device Industry

Mark Repenshek

Balancing Scientific Inquiry and Human Dignity

The book *Institutional Review Board: Management and Function* includes a foreword by Paul Gelsinger, whose 19-year-old son, Jesse, died as a result of a gene therapy protocol. The relevance of the case here rests in Paul Gelsinger's final plea to the institutional review board (IRB):

> I supported these doctors for months, believing that their intent was nearly as pure as Jesse's. They had promised to tell me everything. Even after the media started exposing the flaws in their work, I continued to support them. I discovered that federal oversight was woefully inadequate, that many researchers were not reporting adverse reactions, and that the FDA was being influenced into inaction by industry.
>
> Please remember Jesse's intent when you review studies or when you make policy. You are professionals and you know the issues. I ask—and life itself demands—that you take the time and energy to review each protocol as if you were going to enroll your own child. Please use Jesse's experience to give you the strength to say no or the courage to ask more questions.

If researchers, industry, and those in government apply Jesse's intent—not for recognition, not for money, but only to help—then they will get all they want and more. They'll get it right.[1]

Revealed in this quote is the powerful tension that can arise when the desire to pursue scientific inquiry is pitted against the protection of individual human beings. This tension is inescapable when experimentation and research are carried out on humans. Yet ethics demands that we never allow scientific inquiry to trump the interests and inherent value of the irreplaceable human beings who altruistically enroll in such research. Historical challenges to this norm, and seminal works that have resulted from such challenges, will be considered in this chapter.

Gelsinger's letter rightly alludes to the significance of the work and the mission of an IRB to protect the rights and welfare of human research participants. This is another critical area in medical research and one that we take up here by elaborating the ethical principles that ought to guide such bodies. We also expand on some of the basic topics related to human research, namely, (1) the distinction between research and therapy; (2) the ethics of randomized clinical trials, especially the use of placebos in research; (3) impartiality and consent in selecting research subjects; (4) potential areas of conflict of interest in clinical research, including industry influence; and (5) special concerns related to research involving vulnerable populations.

Our goal for this chapter is to raise your awareness about the ethical issues central to research on human beings and to consider these issues from our normative basis. We especially want you to understand "Jesse's intent" better, because this gets to the true meaning and ethics of research on humans. Let us consider the following case to illustrate some of these issues:

Case 9A

On October 14, 1984, a baby was born in a community hospital in Southern California with a heart malformation known as

cont.

Case 9A *cont.*

hypoplastic left-heart syndrome (HLHS). This essentially means the child was born with an underdeveloped mitral valve or aorta on the left side of the heart. Therefore, only the right side of the heart functions properly. The occurrence of this disease affects roughly 300 to 2,000 children a year. At the time of this case, most babies suffering from HLHS died within weeks of birth; today, however, survival rates are significantly better because surgical techniques have improved.

Baby Fae, as she was known to the public, was taken to Loma Linda University Hospital Center. There, Baby Fae was given a heart transplant with a baboon heart. This first-ever baboon-to-infant transplant was performed by Dr. Leonard Baily. Baby Fae died twenty days later.

Setting the Context: Basic Concepts and Definitions in Research on Human Beings

Throughout history, research on human beings has been central to the practice of medicine. Advances in medicine cannot occur without the involvement of human beings in research. This presents a difficulty when one attempts to distinguish between clinical practice and medical research. Take, for example, the case of Baby Fae: is this experimental research or clinical practice? The distinction is essential in determining how processes are reviewed and the degree to which people are therapeutically engaged. In a seminal work on the ethics of research on human beings, Jay Katz observed, "Drawing the line between research and accepted practice . . . (is) the most difficult and complex problem."[2] Thomas Chalmers adds, "It is extremely hard to distinguish between clinical research and the practice of good medicine. Because episodes of illness and individual people are so variable, every physician is carrying out a small research project when he diagnoses and treats a patient."[3] Yet, we must work with a standard definition of research on human beings, so we will define it here as research on human beings in carefully designed protocols, conducted so as to gain and analyze knowledge with the intent to contribute to the greater good of science and humanity.

One can see from this definition that a number of issues come to the fore. In contrast to the practice of good medicine, which intends to benefit or heal the patient, research on human beings is truly research. That is, its benefit to the subject is unknown. This raises the following key questions, which we address in this chapter: How do we ensure people receive enough information to adequately consider whether to enroll in a protocol that may provide little or no direct benefit to them? How does one weigh contributing to the good of humanity against a potential risk to oneself? How does a review board ensure principal researchers will not inappropriately influence people to enroll? Ought research participants, in certain circumstances, be compensated for their participation? If so, what would prevent such compensation from having a coercive effect on decisions to enroll? Is it appropriate for a physician to be a care provider and a researcher for a patient/subject? To what extent should physicians be compensated for their willingness to serve as principal investigators? What amount constitutes a conflict of interest?

Individual versus Social Good

These questions lead us to the tension inherent in all research on human beings: the polarity between the common good and the individual good. Animals often fulfill the role of experimental subject in research, but to determine the effects of a therapy on humans, ultimately research on humans is needed. We are convinced the following norm must be upheld in all considerations of research on human subjects: the desire to pursue scientific inquiry must never be allowed to trump the interests and inherent value of the irreplaceable human beings who enroll in such research. Our normative basis calls us to respect the inherent dignity of all human beings because it is essential for right relationships and ultimately human flourishing. Therefore, in research, we hold that humans must never be treated as a means to an end and that research must never subject humans to unethical protocols. But what does it mean for a protocol to be unethical?

Many have turned to the process of informed consent to resolve the question of what is an ethical protocol, but this resolution is not entirely satisfactory. Might there be research that ought never be done, even if some people provide their informed consent? Further, if only autonomous adults can give truly informed consent, is research with all others inherently unethical? Is it truly possible for any research subject to give adequately informed consent, given both the competing interests in human research and the knowledge differential between researcher and subject?

Turning to a model where the common good may take precedence, however, begs questions regarding the inherent dignity of the individual human and that individual's interest in protecting his or her own person from violation. History offers examples of the dangers of weighing the interests of the many above those of the few (some of which are noted below). Yet this same argument—that the interests of the many outweigh the interests of the few—is widely supported as a general philosophical principle, even though no one person would desire, presumably, to be the one whose sacrificed interest can be justified for the greater good.

Unfortunately, individuals' dignity, rights, and interests have often been violated in pursuit of generalized scientific knowledge. The Nuremberg Tribunals on German war crimes following World War II referred to atrocities that must never be forgotten, carried out on innocent human beings in Nazi concentration camps:

> In every single instance appearing in the record, subjects were used who did not consent to the experiments; indeed, as to some of the experiments, it is not even contended by the defendants that the subjects occupied the status of volunteers. In many cases experiments were performed by unqualified persons; were conducted at random for no adequate scientific reason, and under revolting physical conditions. All of the experiments were conducted with unnecessary suffering and injury and but very little, if any, precautions were taken to protect or safeguard the human subjects from the possibilities of injury, disability, or death. In every one of the experiments the subjects experienced extreme pain or torture, and in most of them they suffered permanent injury, mutilation, or death, either as a direct result of the experiments or because of lack of adequate follow-up care.

Manifestly human experiments under such conditions are contrary to the principles of the law of nations as they result from the usages established among civilized peoples, from the laws of humanity, and from the dictates of public conscience.[4]

Though the Nazi atrocities awakened the world to the potential for abuses in research, abuses continued to occur, even in the United States, where individual autonomy and liberty typically outweighed the interests of the state. The withholding of newly discovered penicillin from African Americans in the U.S. Department of Public Health's Tuskegee syphilis study, noted in chapter 1, is but one among many examples: In the Willowbrook hepatitis experiments, children who were profoundly cognitively delayed were used as experimental subjects. Some were deliberately infected with the strain of the hepatitis virus prevalent at Willowbrook, using highly questionable methods for obtaining informed consent from some parents. At New York City's Jewish Chronic Disease Hospital, live cancer cells were injected into patients without their knowledge. During the cold war, experiments were conducted on people ranging from pregnant women to prisoners, who, without their consent, received high doses of radiation and injections of plutonium. From 1946 to 1956, nineteen children with cognitive disabilities were fed radioactive iron and calcium in their breakfast oatmeal at a residential school in Fernald, Massachusetts—the consent form mailed to parents failed to mention radiation.[5]

In response to such violations of human dignity resulting from research on human beings in the United States, numerous sets of guidelines were established by different entities that incorporated and even expanded on the principles set forth in the Nuremberg Code. These formal statements include (1) the Belmont Report from the Department of Health, Education, and Welfare, Office of the Secretary, concerning Ethical Principles and Guidelines for the Protection of Human Subjects of Research, issued in 1979, and (2) the Declaration of Helsinki from the World Medical Association, issued in 1964, and most recently revised in 2000.[6] These documents, along with other seminal works, have offered sets of principles to govern the ethics of research on human beings. The ethical principles for the evaluation of research on human subjects presented in these groundbreaking efforts include the principle of human dignity (core to all research involving human subjects), the principle of free and informed consent (a corollary to human dignity but grounded in human freedom and the development of a well-formed conscience), and the principle of totality and integrity (relevant to therapeutic experiments).[7] These principles should be familiar from our normative basis (see chapter 2).

Though these principles provide a general framework for ethical reflection on what constitutes legitimate human subjects research, they need to be further defined as norms that ground such reflection. To this end, Benedict Ashley and Kevin O'Rourke propose six norms consistent with our normative basis and supported by the Belmont Report, the Declaration of Helsinki, and the Nuremberg Code. To this list we wish to add three more essential norms, items 7–9, below.

1. Knowledge sought through research must be vital and obtainable by no other means, and the research must be conducted by qualified people.
2. Appropriate experimentation on animals and cadavers must precede human experimentation.
3. The risk of suffering or injury must be proportionate to the good to be gained.
4. Research candidates should be selected so that risks and benefits will be distributed equitably among all members of society.
5. To protect the integrity of the person, free and informed (voluntary) consent must be obtained.
6. At any time during the course of research, the subject (or the guardian who has given proxy consent) must be free to terminate the subject's participation.
7. Research that is methodologically flawed may never be performed even if people are willing to provide free and informed consent.
8. Where a standard-of-care therapy exists, a placebo control arm requires a high threshold for justification when used in a research protocol.[8]

9. As soon as a protocol's research shows conclusive evidence of a study drug or device's therapeutic efficacy, the research must be suspended and the investigated drug or device should be offered as therapy.

Norms 1–3 and 7 are necessary in view of the principle of human dignity. From the perspective of our normative basis, therefore, human research cannot proceed unless these four norms are met. Norm 3, the benefit–burden analysis, is perhaps the most operative when the other three norms have been met. Our unwavering commitment to the inherent dignity of all humans requires that principal investigators explain to the potential subject, as accurately as possible, the level and nature of the risk from any potential research protocol, even though this can be difficult to calculate. The more true this process, the better further norms will be met in terms of free and informed consent and the ability of the research subject to terminate his or her involvement at any time during the protocol.

Returning to the core tension raised earlier in this chapter, individual good versus social good, the norms listed above provide an absolute norm related to the risk a person can incur in light of the social good achieved through research. In other words, scientific inquiry must never be allowed to trump the interests and inherent value of the irreplaceable human beings who are enrolled in such research. Experiments may be beneficial in terms of scientific progress, but when they proceed at the expense of human beings, such experiments violate human dignity and are therefore unethical. In other words, the individual must not be sacrificed for "the interests of the state or for scientific progress."[9]

We have noted the fundamental principles and norms necessary to guide research on human subjects. In light of these guiding principles and norms, we now turn to the functions required to evaluate human research protocols. We understand most readers may not serve on an IRB or even be aware of the process of reviewing human subjects research. However, because much of the ethical analysis on human research in the United States is performed by these groups, it is important for readers to be aware of the IRB and understand some of the issues it works through in evaluating human research protocols.

Discussion: Ethical Issues and Analysis

Institutional Review Board

The Department of Health and Human Services Code of Federal Regulations regarding the Protection of Human Subjects outlines numerous requirements for review of research on human beings. Before human participation in any research can occur, federal regulations mandate that IRBs must review and approve all clinical research protocols. Review and approval of research protocols ensures (1) the protocol is consistent with sound research design and does not expose participants to excess risk, (2) risks to research participants are reasonable in relation to possible benefits, and (3) informed consent will be obtained and documented from all potential enrollees before participation in the research.[10] Additionally, in actual practice IRBs review the protocol, the informed consent documentation, and supporting information. In certain cases, IRBs also review any amendments and continuing protocol review reports.

The work of the IRB as it relates to the Code of Federal Regulations is merely the beginning in terms of ethics review. Although the federal regulations are deeply rooted in the ethical principles set forth in the Belmont Report, the Declaration of Helsinki, and the Nuremberg Code, they are designed to be the starting point for IRB review. In other words, IRBs are free, and encouraged, to move beyond these ethical principles to incorporate the values and principles unique to an institutional or a particular normative framework, or a particular cultural milieu of a community. Additionally, institutional values, mission statements, and simple administrative capacity also determine whether research is suitable for a particular institution. For example, a cancer research protocol designed by a cooperative research group through the National Institutes of Health might wish to enroll participants at a community hospital. Let's presume the IRB has reviewed and approved the protocol. Despite IRB approval, the hospital may decline to enroll subjects for reasons related to the mission of the community hospital or simply because the hospital is unable to staff an oncology unit to meet the requirements of the protocol. It is also important to note that an institution may not implement a research protocol if that institution's IRB has found the protocol unacceptable for research on human beings.

Internal or external audits of the IRB files, minutes, and documents can verify whether the IRB is meeting the requirements set forth in the federal regulations. A far greater challenge is determining whether the IRB is meeting the requirements intended in the overarching documents: the Belmont Report, the Declaration on Helsinki, and the Nuremberg Code. Here, a greater deal of trust must be placed in the competency and level of commitment of the IRB to carry out a prudent review of human research protocols. The difficulty of attaining this threshold of review can be understood when one examines the complexity of the research environment today.

The Research Environment

The research environment has attained a level of complexity not present in 1974 when IRBs came into existence. First, new technology across all disciplines of medicine have added a level of intricacy to new research protocols that only a few specialists in the field in question may completely understand. The ability of an IRB to understand the details of the research protocols and their effect on the human subject may be severely constrained, therefore, even when it is able to seek outside counsel from experts in the field. Second, institutions have become the new recruiting grounds for for-profit companies seeking to test new medical devices and drugs. The increasing pressure over the past thirty years from health care institutions seeking to have a robust research program (and thereby establish a new lucrative revenue stream) has added the potential for conflict of interest. Third, there seems to be an increasing blur between research and therapy. That is, the medical device industry and the pharmaceutical industry seem to be targeting medical professionals directly with the goal of enrolling patients in human research. Thirty years ago institutions were very aware of the research being carried out by a few medical practitioners. Today, with the size of medical staffs, the desire to have a nationally recognized research program, the pressure for tenure within academic medical centers, and the increasing flow of research dollars into an institution, institutions are far less aware of the research that is occurring within their walls and are therefore potentially ignorant of the interface between the institution's patients and medical research. Here, the IRB may not even be involved in review of research protocols due to such ignorance or to claims made by the manufacturer that the protocols have already been reviewed by the manufacturer's own IRB. As noted earlier, this is not an acceptable level of review, as the federal regulations mandate an institution's IRB review and approval of human research protocols.

As the level of research becomes more complex and the potential for conflicts of interest increase, the IRB must maintain itself as a well-educated and authoritative body within the institution. IRBs must continue to protect human subjects in research and have the courage and wherewithal to challenge, question, and sometimes reject research proposals that do not meet the requirements of federal regulations or the ethics that govern research protocols.

Let us now return to the case of Baby Fae (Case 9) presented at the beginning of this chapter. Although Baby Fae was not the first to receive such an organ transplant, questions arise immediately about the legitimacy of the experimental procedure on several levels. Should a human donor have been ruled out before using the heart of an animal? This question is grounded in the justification for research that relates to our primary norm. Recall that we stated IRBs are never to allow scientific inquiry to trump the interests and inherent value of the irreplaceable human beings enrolled in such research. This norm requires that (1) the knowledge sought through research must be vital and obtainable by no other means and the research must be conducted by qualified people, and (2) appropriate experimentation on animals and cadavers must precede human experimentation. Using the Loma Linda case as our context, our principles would suggest that although a baboon-to-infant heart transplant may have offered great potential for Baby Fae, its experimental nature requires us to ensure the baboon heart is truly the method of last resort for Baby Fae. Also it suggests the transplant surgeon and his or her team must carefully discern the extent to which their desire to be the first to achieve this medical feat played a role in their decision to use such a procedure. Finally, because Baby Fae could not voice her own interests, the difficulty of surrogate decision making was in play. We discussed this at some length in chapter 6 with regard to the care of critically ill newborns. The same ethical issues are relevant here: who decides, and by what criteria? The relational best-interests standard we offered in chapter 6 applies here as well: is such a procedure worth the risk, if it were to allow Baby Fae to achieve a level of human flourishing proportionate to her inherent human dignity?

Further complicating the ethical analysis here is the existence of the Norwood procedure, available in Boston and Philadelphia, which could have been used on Baby Fae, although the procedure is invasive and repetitive (continued surgical interventions are required as the child grows and develops).[11] Was the potential for research or experimentation placed before the well-being of the patient? Was there an obligation to use the Norwood procedure before attempting to use an animal organ? Recall our norms for evaluating research protocols, especially number 3 (the risk of suffering or injury must be proportionate to the good to be gained). Certainly, curing Baby Fae's heart anomaly (by means of an animal organ transplant) would be preferable to continued invasive procedures throughout her lifetime (Norwood procedure). Yet the notion of proportionality suggests that although most children with this heart condition die within a few weeks, great caution should have been used lest Baby Fae become an object of experimentation.

One strategy for preventing such exploitation is to observe the principle of informed consent. Examining the principle of informed consent using our normative basis raises further questions. Even if informed consent were obtained from the parents, could the parents ethically offer their child for such experimental procedures if a known alternative exists? In other words, might the parents have been so persuaded by the potential cure the procedure offered that true informed consent was not obtainable, given the emotional factors at play, namely, the high rate of morbidity and mortality related to the illness, the desire to have the child live at all costs, and the inability to sort the balance between risk and benefit. This is not to say emotional factors should be irrelevant in such decisions, but parents and health care providers must recognize the limitations such emotions can place on the principles traditionally used to assess and protect patients against unwarranted procedures or experimental therapies.

Human Research: The Protocol

Recall the definition of research on human beings used in this chapter: research on human beings in carefully designed protocols, conducted so as to gain and analyze knowledge with the intent to contribute to the greater good of science and humanity. Since an IRB must review all human research protocols within the IRB's institution, it is important that we briefly review the areas of accountability for protocol review. These areas include the rationale, objectives, procedures, outcomes of interests, experimental design, protection for human subjects to minimize risk, methods of analysis of data, endpoints of protocol, and method for review and monitoring of adverse events. Additionally, the IRB is charged with assessing the qualifications of the principal investigator in light of the research proposed. In what follows we cover the substantive areas of IRB review for research on human beings, intermingled with case studies to illustrate each concept.

Before examining each of these areas, it is important to understand that there are four distinct phases of research involving human subjects as classified by the Code of Federal Regulations:

Phase I. Human subjects research open to a small number of individuals (or sample set) and designed solely to test safety or toxicity of a pharmaceutical and gain early evidence of effectiveness. Data from animal models usually forms the substantive basis for understanding the effect of the investigational drug at a signal introductory dose or the investigational device with a potential for clinical benefit.

Phase II. Human subjects research open to a larger number of subjects and designed to test toxicity thresholds of a drug for particular indications in patients with the disease or condition under study. Data from Phase I trials is incorporated into informed consent and forms the substantive basis for understanding the preliminary safety and efficacy of the research.

Phase III. Human subjects research using a still larger number of subjects to meet the thresholds required to establish statistical significance of research efficacy. At this point the safety profile is well understood. If research proceeds to this point, it is usually the case that the information gathered is fleshing out the risk–benefit calculus for potential future patients.

Phase IV. Human subjects research open to large sample sets, typically post marketing. These trials are designed to further test hypotheses over long periods of time after a drug or device has already been approved for treatment. The information gathered may help clarify uncertainties or test outlier adverse events in the broader patient population [12]

Regardless of the phase of the clinical trial, the IRB is accountable to review each protocol in light of the experimental design, selection of human subjects, qualifications of the investigator, worth of the research, and clinical research and informed consent.

Experimental design. A significant issue in experimental design is the use of a placebo such as a sugar pill in research studies. A placebo-controlled clinical study may be justified when no satisfactory treatment exists for the disease being investigated. Norm 8 (in the beginning of this chapter), however, states that where standard-of-care therapy exists, a placebo control arm requires a high threshold for justification. If scientific and medical practice indicate there is a standard-of-care treatment for a disease, people may be enrolled in only a protocol that exposes them to no additional risk; the use of a placebo in such cases requires significant scrutiny of the experimental design and therefore protocols with a placebo arm should be reviewed by an IRB with expertise in the relevant clinical area.

Some protocols randomly place human subjects into either an intervention group or a placebo group with neither the researcher nor the subject knowing which group the subject is in; these are called randomized, double-blind, placebo-controlled clinical trials. For various reasons many researchers and manufacturers prefer this experimental design. Such protocols raise a number of ethical issues in addition to that cited in the preceding paragraph. A case study may help to illustrate this point.

Case 9B

A physician at your health system submits a protocol to the IRB. In that protocol he has created two arms for research purposes and will use a randomized, double-blind, placebo-controlled trial as the experimental design. The physician argues that the

cont.

Case 9B *cont.*

hypothesis he is trying to test is the effectiveness of a new lipid-lowering drug for high cholesterol. The drug has gone through animal and safety phase I and II trials and is now looking for efficacy in a phase III trial. The principal investigator notes that his group has designed the placebo to be indistinguishable from the investigational drug. People who will be selected for the study must have a cholesterol level significant enough to require a 35–45-percent reduction in bad cholesterol. The physician explains potential subjects will be told they will be participating in an experiment to test the efficacy of a new lipid-lowering drug and the drug will not hurt them. In fact, he adds, they may see a lowering of their cholesterol while in the study.

You tell the principle investigator you feel the research design is problematic because patients will not be told they may receive a placebo when there is already a known therapy for high cholesterol, although perhaps slightly less efficacious. The physician responds by noting a placebo-controlled trial is the best way to determine whether the drug is effective and therefore this type of trial is required. He also feels he has adequately informed the research subject because the phase I and II trials were sufficient for moving to phase III and the participant will not be harmed. The principal investigator ends by saying, "We usually have no trouble recruiting for studies. Patients want access to the latest and greatest drugs. I feel this is the next step in the progression of lipid-lowering drugs. I would really like to see this study approved."

Would you recommend approval for this study? If so, on what grounds would you recommend it? Recall our proposed norm: where a standard-of-care therapy exists, a placebo control arm requires a high threshold for justification when used in a research protocol. Given that the drug's safety has been tested on animals and a small number of human beings, the principal investigator (PI) claims the drug is essentially safe. He also asserts potential subjects only care about whether they will be harmed. The PI feels it will be ethical to proceed to phase III testing of the drug because its safety has already been determined.

Ethical concern, however, requires a more robust discussion as to whether there are problems with the design of the study; it may be unethical to enroll people in the trial, because the study is flawed. Even if the test drug is essentially safe, potential research subjects should not be exposed to a placebo when standard therapies already exist for lowering one's cholesterol. This argument, based on honoring the human dignity of the potential research participant, finds the phase III trial unethical in its present design, regardless of the drug's safety.

If you answered no to the question about whether to recommend approval for the study, an interesting follow-up question might be: How would you challenge the PI's use of placebo in this trial? You might also discuss ways to structure the phase III trail so it meets the ethical principles and norms presented in this chapter.

Again, our normative basis calls into question competing claims against human dignity, such as those of the manufacturer concerned about dollars or time lost as the investigational study drug or device remains in clinical research. These are valid concerns, and some (consequentialist) ethical theories could be made to override the concern of the human subject. The primary consideration of our normative basis, however, is human flourishing. From this perspective, research trials are unethical when they attach more weight to benefit to the researcher or manufacturer than to concern for human beings.

Selection of Human Test Subjects. In recruiting human subjects for research, risk must be distributed equitably across the study population, and the matter of inducement must be carefully evaluated by the IRB. Studies typically involve some level of monetary compensation to participants; however, compensation may not be an incentive to enroll in the research or maintain the initial enrollment through phases of the study design. Costs directly related to the study and the drug or device being tested are typically included for potential participants in the research protocol. In studies where participants are compensated for volunteering, the IRB must ascertain that the amount offered is not coercive and that payments are not tiered so that participants would need to complete the entire study to receive compensation. No specific federal guidelines exist for this evaluation. Nevertheless, the possibility that the potential study population might be exploited or induced to participate must be seriously considered by the IRB.

Coercive inducement is not necessarily limited to monetary payment. Ethical questions arise when researchers, for reasons of convenience, wish to enroll their staff, colleagues, students, or other personnel. Such participants may fear to refuse to participate lest they incur the displeasure of their employer or colleague, or may feel that participation would enhance their prospects of future employment or promotion. An IRB has an obligation to remove such potential conflicts of interest. The difficulty here is for the IRB to protect potential research subjects from coercion in whatever form without being overly paternalistic. Consequently, anonymous solicitation of potential enrollees is generally preferable because it rules out numerous potential ethical problems. A case study may help to illustrate this point.

Case 9C

You are a student in a college-level psychology class studying behavior modification through reward mechanisms. It is well known on campus that the professor of the class often uses his students in research studies—usually only surveys—to test her hypotheses on behavior modification. The same holds true the semester you enroll: an expectation of the course is to either design a research study and enroll fellow classmates in the hypothetical research design or to participate in one instructor-led research protocol.

You decide to enroll in an instructor-led research protocol. Given what you know about research methodology to date, and given that this is a simple survey protocol, you see little harm in participating.

Unfortunately, due to the demands of your other courses, you postpone completing this requirement until well into the latter stages of the semester. You decide a couple weeks before finals to complete the online survey. Reading through the survey, you notice several background questions asking whether you have experienced mood changes or have had episodes of clinically diagnosed depression; whether you have been treated for depression; and (for females) whether you have ever taken

cont.

Case 9C *cont.*

any medication that may affect hormone changes. Although you understand that these questions are basic background questions for the survey that are needed to categorize subjects and that the data gathered are completely anonymous, you remain concerned about completing the survey. You decide to hold off until you have a chance to talk with your professor about the survey.

Unfortunately, in putting off taking the survey you realize the end of the semester is approaching and you have not yet had the courage to approach your professor regarding the survey content. You do not have time to design a research protocol yourself and are now left with the choice of either completing the survey or suffering the consequences on your grade for lack of participation in a course requirement. You wonder whether your feelings of "being trapped" signal some ethical problems with the course requirement. You wonder whether these feelings are well grounded or just end-of-semester jitters.

This case raises several significant ethical issues. Most notable is the vulnerability of the study population. Given that participants in this case are students of the professor, some may enroll simply to meet a course requirement. On the other hand, some may feel compelled to answer questions to please the professor by participating in her research study, or more problematic, enroll as a subject in the research survey due to a perception that the student is obligated to answer all questions or suffer consequences to his or her grade. Here the IRB may also wish to consider whether a grade demonstrates a perverse incentive to complete or participate in the professor's research protocol without the true ability of the participant to withdraw at any point. In this context the IRB should evaluate the position in which the students are placed and whether the vulnerability of student to professor sets up conditions that make this type of research inherently ethically problematic.

Ethical arguments not based on our comprehensive normative basis might suggest that so long as informed consent is achieved, people should be free to enter whatever research protocols they want as a matter of human freedom and respect for autonomy. Although our normative basis does not deny the importance of these principles, it argues that human flourishing supersedes all other goals—it is the goal to which all others should be directed. Therefore, despite the fact that the good grades are important for success in the class and perhaps future success in the program, the relevant question is whether enrollment in the research protocol offers you the possibility of living a good life, a life in which you flourish as an individual in relation to others. Notice that in this case "others" would be those who might truly be served by the outcome of the research.

Finally, consider that participants will receive their "compensation" (i.e., their grade) only upon completion of the study. We have already noted that contingencies can be ethically problematic in human testing. In this case, the contingency is that research subjects will not receive "compensation" until completion of the study. One of the norms for ethical research offered at the beginning of this chapter notes that at any time during the course of research, the subject (or the guardian who has given proxy consent) must be free to terminate the subject's participation in the experiment. In this case study, will participants truly feel free to drop out at *any time* given that either the student participates in the professor's research or designs his or her own protocol per the course requirements? Such a design has clear advantages to the PI, as it helps guarantee a solid and stable cohort throughout the duration of the study. It would shorten the time needed for the study because it would decrease the likelihood that new subjects would need to be enrolled or high dropout rates would need to be accounted for. Yet our normative basis calls into question such a practice. Given that the primary consideration of our normative basis is human flourishing, the IRB should minimally require the students' participation in the research not be linked to their grades. Any participation in such research should be for the sake of the knowledge gained regarding research design and participant experience. This would ensure the effect of fear of a negative grade would not coerce students to maintain enrollment when, for whatever reason, they might wish to withdraw from the study.

Qualifications of the Investigator. The IRB has the responsibility to ensure the PI is qualified to carry out the proposed research protocol. Is the PI trained in the areas of clinical expertise required in the protocol? Is the PI's institution well versed in the procedures or medication described in the protocol? Is the PI trained in performing clinical research?

There are obvious areas the IRB should examine with regard to the qualifications of the PI, namely, whether he or she is board-certified in the area of specialty required by the research protocol, and also whether the hospital has granted privileges to the PI with regard to the investigational drug, procedure, or device. Determining that a clinician is trained in performing clinical research may be difficult. Many institutions require that clinicians who are interested in carrying out human research receive training in ethics and compliance for human research either through federally sponsored training programs or institution-specific training programs. This has gone a long way to familiarizing researchers with ethical and legal issues related to human research. However, such training is not standardized and great variability exists in the level of researchers' competency. Data safety monitoring boards—external boards designed to monitor a research protocol for participant safety—may be essential for the protection of human research subjects.

Worth of the Research. IRBs are also charged with evaluating the worth of the proposed research protocol. Research protocols can be designed so as to be statistically significant and methodologically sound but still not worth performing because the small amount of knowledge to be gained does not justify the risks.

For the IRB to determine whether the research is worthwhile, the project objectives must be explicit in the research protocol. The IRB may also need to know the external agency funding the research; the competition for such research is significant and may imply the level of worth. This rationale must be scrutinized lest funding and market share become the primary motives. A third method to determine worth of research may include the commitment of the institution to cancer research, for example, wherein a protocol is related to maintaining the institution's center of excellence standing. Again, the IRB should carefully evaluate the potential conflict of interest between the desire to be a part of such research and the true worth of the project. Finally, an IRB should be receptive to its required community members in this area. That is, the community members on the IRB should help decide whether such research is significant and worth pursuing for those for whom the protocol will be directed. Perhaps a case study will help to flesh out these criteria.

Case 9D

Leah is a member of an independent IRB that reviews protocols for the military. The particular protocol in question relies on the data gathered from the Nazi altitude experiments. The protocol is funded by NASA and is designed to determine the necessary oxygen requirements in a rescue mission to return a shuttle flight crew safely to Earth in the event of an emergency. A flight simulator will be used to gather the data that will simulate oxygen levels at certain altitudes. Only high-altitude Air Force pilots who are familiar with safety precautions will be allowed to enroll in the study.

Leah is aware the Nazi altitude experiments took prisoners from concentration camps against their will and flew them to extreme altitudes without the benefit of oxygen to determine what would happen to the human body when exposed to such high altitudes. This would shed light on whether, for example, a pilot should bail out at high altitude. She recalls the horrors of such experiments as recounted to her by her grandmother, who was a concentration camp survivor. She argues the knowledge gained from such atrocities should not be memorialized in this way and recommends the study be rejected, given that it uses knowledge gained from exploitive and unethical research.

In this case we face an interesting question regarding the worth of research.[13] In this proposed protocol, the data gathered from the Nazi altitude experiments helps protect research participants from unnecessary harm. If these data are protecting human subjects in the proposed protocol, how can use of this knowledge be ethically problematic? None of the principles and norms put forward in this chapter seems to directly relate to this question. Recall chapter 3, however, where we mentioned a principle called *solidarity* under the broad category of *justice*. This principle was defined as "the responsibility we have to stand with our fellow human beings in times of need." One might suggest Leah is acting from a position of solidarity with those who were exploited in Nazi human experimental atrocities. Out of a position of solidarity, Leah wishes to reject any research that builds on data gathered from such an abuse of human beings. Alternatively, Leah is suggesting that out of a responsibility to the *common good*, she cannot allow the voices of those who were so exploited to be muted by permitting the use of such data, even if beneficial.[14]

On the other hand, one could argue Leah fails to consider the additional dangers researchers are likely to face if the experiments do not draw on the knowledge gained from the Nazi experiments. The principle of solidarity in this case might require that the potential research subjects not be exposed to unnecessary harm. In this way, one could suggest that although the data were obtained in a completely unethical manner, the use of the data might actually provide an important good. In other words, in certain circumstances good may come out of something horribly evil.

Given the relevant considerations raised by the principle of solidarity in both instances, a proper reading of our normative basis would suggest the latter use of solidarity is not faithful to its context, namely human dignity. Recall that the principle of solidarity is to be understood in the context of human flourishing and right relationships with God and neighbor. In this way, solidarity with those who were at the most extreme end of vulnerability and completely exploited to obtain these data tends to rule out the use of the data completely, regardless of the circumstances. In other words, as Henry K. Beecher noted, it would seem "this loss . . . would be less important than the far reaching moral loss to medicine if the data were to be published." The principles of human dignity and solidarity demand we memorialize those people not through use of the data garnered via experiments that denied their dignity, but rather by halting research that attempts to use such data. In this way we have not "conferred a scientific martyrdom on the victims," but rather recognized such violence against human beings should never be permissible regardless of what good may someday come of it.[15]

This section sought to highlight some of the relevant factors IRBs are to consider when evaluating the ethical legitimacy of a proposed human subject research protocol. It should be evident the responsibilities of an IRB member include the protection of human beings from potentially harmful research, and extend far beyond simply examining the process of informed consent. Nevertheless, informed consent remains a significant component of the work of the IRB.

Clinical Research and Informed Consent. After an IRB has considered all of the above elements and found the human research protocol is ethical and meets compliance standards, it still must consider the issue of informed consent. The Department of Health and Human Services Code of Federal Regulations (often referred to simply as 45 CFR 46) requires the following eight elements:[16] (1) a statement that the study involves research along with an explanation of the purposes and procedures, duration of participation, and identification of experimental elements; (2) a description of risks; (3) a statement of benefits to the individual or to others who may reasonably be expected to benefit from the research; (4) alternatives to participation; (5) provisions for confidentiality; (6) medical treatments and compensations available in the event of research-related injury; (7) identification of individuals or groups that may be contacted for answers to questions about the research, for information about a research-related injury, and for information about the rights of research subjects; and (8) assurance that participation is voluntary and that participants may discontinue participation at any time without penalty or loss of benefits. All IRBs must meet these regulatory standards for informed consent. IRBs must also see that informed-consent language is appropriate to a broad audience and understandable to the potential participant.

The consent document is the most important piece of the protocol review process for the IRB. As such, many IRBs require that investigators adapt their documents to templates created by the IRB. In this way IRBs can ensure that essential elements have been properly addressed by the principal investigator. Additionally, the use of such templates helps the IRB to establish a set of guidelines that each PI is required to meet. This can minimize pressure on an institution from an influential investigator or company looking to offer particular research at its institution. A problem with templates, however, is that these documents are not standardized and may vary greatly among institutions. Lack of standardization becomes especially problematic in the case of cooperative multisite studies. Using such templates requires a great deal of "template language" that is nonnegotiable if the researcher or manufacturer wishes to perform research at that particular institution. This can lead to lengthy consent documents with exhaustive lists of risks and benefits that become, at best, unclear to the potential participant.

The IRB, therefore, must provide to potential research subjects the information they need to make a truly informed choice as to whether to participate in the proposed research protocol. Minimally, the consent documents should be written at a sixth- to eighth-grade reading level, contain no technical language, and rank risks and benefits in accordance with likelihood of occurrence. It must be noted, however, that simply having an adequate form does not make informed consent. The informed-consent process should be a dynamic process between researcher and potential subject wherein the form acts as a starting point for further discussion to evaluate whether the research is appropriate for the individual considering participation. Here it is important to note that it is within the scope of the IRB to review the entire informed consent process, not just the consent documents. IRBs may wish to consider random review of the informed consent process where there may be areas of concern.

This leads to a final point about presentation of informed consent to potential participants. Certain research protocols, by virtue of their design, require approaching a potential research participant in the midst of medical treatment. In such cases, it is not appropriate to allow for only a limited parameter for participants to consider involvement (i.e., the patient encounter in the office or during an acute care stay), especially when concurrent with another medical procedure. Furthermore, the vulnerability of the patient population must be considered insofar as participants in emotional or acute pain may not be appropriate for participation in research. In such circumstances, assuming the research is considered ethically appropriate, therapy and research must be clearly distinguished so as not to allow for therapeutic misconceptions in the research. That is, there must be no misperception on the part of the patients (research subjects) that their involvement will benefit them personally in the form of a cure or relief of symptoms.[17]

Conflict of Interests

Lastly, the question of conflict of interest or the perception of conflict of interest is relevant for clinical trials with human subjects. A conflict of interest may take various forms but exists when there is a divergence between an individual's or institution's private interests and the professional obligations to administer or monitor clinical research in an objective manner. This divergence occurs in such a way that an independent observer might reasonably question whether the individual's or institution's professional actions or decisions might be influenced by considerations of gain, financial or otherwise, for the individual, his or her immediate family members, or institution.

A financial interest means anything of monetary value that may benefit the principal investigator or research site and hence could affect the clinical research. Examples include the following:

- salary or other remuneration for services (e.g., consulting fee or honoraria) in excess of some predetermined value (e.g., $10,000)
- equity interest (e.g., stocks, stock options, or other ownership interest) in excess of some predetermined value (e.g., $10,000) and represents more than some percentage (e.g., 5 percent) of the ownership interest in the sponsor of the clinical study during the time of the study and some length of time after the study
- proprietary or other intellectual property rights (e.g., patents, copyrights, royalties, or licensing agreement) in the item being studied

It is important to note that there is nothing intrinsically unethical about a conflict of interest; these conflicts are virtually ubiquitous in clinical trials because so many trials are funded privately. The ethical issue concerns the nature of the conflict of interest as related to potential risk of scientific misconduct. An example might serve well at this point.

Case 9E

Dr. Smith is the PI for a phase II, randomized, placebo-controlled, double-blind study with approval for research by the Food and

cont.

Case 9E *cont.*

Drug Administration for a particular primary indication. The sponsor of the study is Drug Company Z—a large pharmaceutical company whose stock is publicly traded. Dr. Smith is interested in seeing the study drug through its approval phase, as it is a drug for a disease for which no current therapy exists. Although Dr. Smith has worked as a consultant for the sponsor of the study regarding the development of protocols for large cooperatives studies, she has not done so for this particular study or drug. In this advisory role, Dr. Smith has received annual compensation in the amount of $10,000 and also sits—in a voluntary capacity—on the sponsor's scientific advisory board. Dr. Smith also serves as a clinical research advisor for a number of competing drug companies and as such feels the potential for conflict of interest to negatively affect this protocol is limited to nonexistent. Dr. Smith has no stock interest in the company nor does she have any patents or personal interest in the drug other than the potential benefit for her patients.

In this case study, Dr. Smith has a financial interest in the sponsor of the study, albeit $10,000. Given that the study is randomized, placebo-controlled, and double-blind, do you see any potential for conflict of interest negatively affecting the clinical research? What factors might either change your decision or further reinforce your determination? Would changing the scenario in the following ways alter your decision?

Case 9E modification A: What if Dr. Smith received $100,000 a year for her work with Drug Company Z, and this was her primary source of income as she rarely sees patients any longer and largely serves as a consultant?

Case 9E modification B: What if Drug Company Z was founded in part by Dr. Smith? What if it was a small, private company, a hopeful startup, and this phase II drug was its leading source of potential revenue for years to come?

It is important to clarify your determination of conflict of interest as you answer these questions, including the modifications. When considering conflicts of interest, what constitute thresholds that move your decision from recognizing the case as permissible versus too conflicted? Are those thresholds relevant to all studies of this nature? Should conflict of interest be assessed on a case-by-case basis? If so, are there any baselines that can be established that represent a conflict of interest that is unethical in all cases?

Let us assume for the sake of examination that the IRB has reviewed this particular protocol and has recommended the following to the PI:

> Given the design of the study, it seems that Dr. Smith's $10,000 advisory role will not compromise the integrity of the research as long as this potential conflict of interest is disclosed to the research subjects in the informed consent document.

However, IRB members have also raised the following questions. How might you answer these?

1. Should we require the PI to terminate all consulting activities during the course of the study?
2. Should we inquire as to the PI's stock portfolio to verify no holdings?
3. If holdings exist, should we require the stock to be sold before approving the drug?
4. Should we require that the PI be removed from subject selection, recruitment, and data analysis?
5. Should we appoint a data safety monitoring board (DSMB) of our choosing to review the data to ensure there are no creeping study biases?

As you can see, the questions raised propose an array of potential issues that an IRB may need to discuss thoroughly beyond the scope of the informed consent and above-mentioned protocol review. The purpose of an examination of conflicts of interest is to promote and ensure the objectivity in the conduct of all clinical research through

the diligent investigation, monitoring, and resolution of all conflicts of interest, actual or apparent. In so doing, the integrity of the
research is maintained.

Conclusion

Human research continues to increase in complexity. This has been
the case since 1974 when formal IRBs were first formed to review
such research. IRBs must continue to place the protection of human
beings at the forefront of their responsibilities when reviewing proposed human research protocols. To that end, IRBs must continually
strive to ensure the informed-consent process is accurate, truthful,
and understandable to the potential participant.

IRBs must also have a profound sense of humility that allows
them to ask questions and seek answers where necessary. They
must also have the courage to table, suspend, or reject studies that
do not meet the requirements set forth by legal and ethical norms
for human research. All IRBs must know the federal regulations
(45 CFR 46) for human research and require them of the protocols
they review. However, applying the ethical principles and norms
put forth in this chapter and those outlined in the Belmont Report,
the Nuremberg Code, and the Declaration of Helsinki is not easily accomplished. IRBs will need to debate these principles and
determine each principle's relevance for the protocol before them.
Appropriate training and education must be required for all IRB
members, especially the IRB chairperson. The IRB will do well to
remember their primary goal is the protection of human beings in
research protocols. The IRB will do even better if it has a clear
sense of the norm we have posited in conjunction with the goal
of human flourishing, namely, never to allow scientific inquiry to
trump the interests and inherent value of the irreplaceable human
beings enrolled in such research. In this way, as Paul Gelsinger, the
father of Jesse quoted at the outset of this chapter, notes, "researchers, industry, and those in government" will get it right—"not for
recognition, not for money, but only to help."

Additional Case Studies

Case 9F

In the early 1980s it was discovered from a suit filed in Illinois that patients of a state-operated mental health facility underwent "therapeutic surgery" in the 1950s and 1960s, possibly without consent. The surgery, intended to relieve or ameliorate symptoms of schizophrenia, involved removing the subjects' adrenal glands. A theory put forward at the time surmised removal of the adrenal gland might correct a hormone imbalance some psychiatrists believed to be a cause of schizophrenia.

The investigation that ensued as a result of the suit found the surgery did not lead to improvement in any of the patients. It was also unclear whether the patients had given informed consent. All of those who had their adrenal glands removed required injections of cortisone for the rest of their lives to compensate for the loss of function of their adrenal glands.

Case 9G

In the early 1990s, research on Parkinson's disease focused on ways to ward off the diminishment or disappearance of specific brain tissue. It was thought, in certain cases, Parkinson's assault on the central nervous system could be ameliorated or significantly lessened if there were ways to stimulate redevelopment of specific brain tissues. One method to do so would be to deliver fetal tissue to desired locations within the brain through holes drilled in the skull.

To determine whether this therapy might work, a control of some sort would be needed. Given that in the early 1990s no good treatments were available for severe Parkinson's, it seemed the best study model would be to have a group of people with Parkinson's serve as a control. The control group would not receive the delivery of fetal tissue. However, to eliminate study bias by the research subjects, all of the people enrolled in the study would need to have the holes drilled in their skulls. This would mean some of the study participants would be required to have holes drilled in their skulls without any intention of delivering fetal tissue.

SUGGESTED READINGS

Vanderpool, Harold Y. "An Ethics Primer for Institutional Review Boards." In *Institutional Review Board: Management and Function*, edited by Elizabeth A. Bankert and Robert J. Amdur, 3–8. Boston, MA: Jones and Bartlett, 2006.

The World Medical Association Declaration of Helsinki. June 1964. *http://www.wma.net/en/30publications/10policies/b3/index.html.*

MULTIMEDIA AIDS FOR TEACHERS

Deadly Medicine: Creating the Master Race. Exhibition. Susan Bachrach, curator. According to the U.S. Holocaust Memorial Museum, this work "inspires reflection on the continuing attraction of biological utopias that promote the possibility of human perfection. From the early twentieth-century international eugenics movements to present-day dreams of eliminating inherited disabilities through genetic manipulation, the issues remain timely." *http://www.ushmm.org/museum/exhibit/online/deadlymedicine/.*

Miss Evers' Boys. Directed by Joseph Sargent. Starring Alfre Woodard. Rated PG. 1997. This movie documents the true story of the U.S. government's Tuskegee study of untreated African Americans with syphilis. It provides a powerful example of how research subjects can be abused. It is available on DVD or VHS through retailers.

Steven Spielberg Film and Video Archive. U.S. Holocaust Memorial Museum. A collection of video footage documenting the Holocaust and World War II. Available through *http://www.ushmm.org/research/collections/filmvideo.*

Cases on Clinical Trials for Teachers

The following case can be used to illustrate new ethical quandaries posed by genomic-based human subject research. Critics of a clinical trial of drug PLX4032 for a particular melanoma suggest that when potential benefit is demonstrably better, even in initial stages of a protocol, the control arm should be suspended, allowing participants to get the drug under investigation. Others suggest that to preserve integrity of the data gathered in the clinical trial, a control arm is necessary, otherwise future use of the drug will come with only hypothetical benefit at best. For more information, see *http://www.nytimes.com/2010/09/19/health/research/19trial.html?_r=2&pagewanted=1.*

The following is a link to an article excerpted from Carl Elliott's book *White Coat, Black Hat: Adventures on the Dark Side of Medicine.* The article discusses in depth the ethical questions raised when physicians serve as a consultants to drug companies. See *http://chronicle.com/article/article-content/124335*.

The following link provides a list of fines levied against Pharma for improper marketing and other infractions. The largest for a single drug was Eli Lilly with three fines totaling more than $1.4 billion (Zyprexa). The largest settlement by a maker goes to Pfizer and totals $2.3 billion for a host of drugs. See *http://www.fiercepharma.com/special-reports/big-pharma-behaving-badly-timeline-settlements*.

ENDNOTES

1. Paul Gelsinger, "Jesse's Intent," in *Institutional Review Board*, ed. Elizabeth A. Bankert and Robert J. Amdur (Sudbury, MA: Jones and Bartlett, 2006), xi–xix.

2. J. Katz, *Experimentation with Human Beings* (New York: Russell Sage Foundation, 1972).

3. T. C. Chalmers, "The Clinical Trial," *Milbank Memorial Fund Quarterly* 59 (1981): 324–39.

4. Trials of War Criminals before the Nuremberg Military Tribunals under Control Council Law, no. 10, vol. 2, Nuremberg, October 1946–April 1949. Washington, DC: U.S. GPO, 1949–1953, 181–2.

5. Baruch A. Brody, *The Ethics of Biomedical Research* (New York: Oxford University Press, 1998), 31–6.

6. World Medical Association Declaration of Helsinki: Recommendations Guiding Medical Doctors in Biomedical Research Involving Human Subjects. Adopted by the 18th World Medical Assembly, Helsinki, Finland, 1964, and as revised by the 52nd WMA General Assembly, Edinburgh, Scotland, October 2000, with note of clarification on paragraph 30 added by the WMA General Assembly, Tokyo, Japan, 2004.

7. Kevin O'Rourke and Benedict Ashley, *Health Care Ethics: A Theological Analysis* (Washington, DC: Georgetown University Press, 1997), 346.

8. This is notably a more rigid position than that of the Declaration of Helsinki. In the clarifications of paragraph 29 (added in 2002 at the WMA General Assembly in Washington), it states, "The WMA hereby reaffirms its position that extreme care must be taken in making use of placebo-controlled trial and that in general this methodology should only be used in the absence of existing proven therapy. However, a placebo-controlled trial may be ethically acceptable, even if proven therapy is available, under the following circumstances: (a) where for compelling and scientifically sound methodological reasons its use is necessary to determine the efficacy or safety of a prophylactic, diagnostic or therapeutic method; or (b) where

a prophylactic, diagnostic or therapeutic method is being investigated for a minor condition and the patients who receive placebo will not be subject to any additional risk of serious or irreversible harm." We believe, however, in general this principle does hold and for the purposes of this work, the general principle serves the reader well.

9. Pius XII, "Allocution to the First International Congress of Histopathology (1952)," in *The Human Body: Papal Teachings,* selected and arranged by the Monks of Solesmes (Boston: Daughters of St. Paul, 1960), n. 349; John Paul II, "Medicines at the Service of Man," (October 24, 1986).

10. Department of Health and Human Services, Protection of Human Subjects, Title 45, Code of Federal Regulations, Part 46.111.

11. O. Jonasson and M. A. Hardy, "The Case of Baby Fae" (letter), *Journal of the American Medical Association* 254 (1985): 3358–9.

12. National Institutes of Health. "Understanding Clinical Trials." Found at *http://clinicaltrials.gov/ct2/info/understand#Q19* (accessed on April 16, 2011).

13. David Bogod, "The Nazi Hypothermia Experiments: Forbidden Data?" *Anaesthesia* 59, no. 12 (December 2004), 1155–6.

14. For a similar argument, see H. K. Beecher, "Ethics and Clinical Research," *New England Journal of Medicine* 274 (1966): 1354–60.

15. Baruch C. Cohen, "The Ethics of Using Medical Data from Nazi Experiments," *Jewish Virtual Library, http://www.jewishvirtuallibrary.org/jsource/Judaism/naziexp.html#1* (accessed June 12, 2011).

16. Department of Health and Human Services, Protection of Human Subjects, Title 45, Code of Federal Regulations, Part 46.116.

17. G. Sreenivasan, "Informed Consent and the Therapeutic Misconception: Clarifying the Challenge," *Journal of Clinical Ethics* 16, no. 4 (2005): 369–71.

CHAPTER 10

Forgoing Treatment at the End of Life

Michael Panicola

An Ethically Complex Issue

Forgoing treatment at the end of life is one of the most documented issues in health care ethics. Clinicians, theologians, philosophers, lawyers, and others have written extensively on it. Even though well-established medical, ethical, and legal guidelines have been in place for several decades, decisions about forgoing treatment at the end of life frequently raise ethical concerns for families of dying patients and the caregivers who attend to them. This is one reason why ethics committees in long-term care facilities and hospitals consult on this issue more than any other. To help navigate the ethical complexities involved in decisions regarding forgoing treatment, we begin with a framework, a set of moral considerations that offer perspective for understanding and thinking through such decisions. This framework supplies the backdrop against which we will consider two pressing issues around forgoing treatment at the end of life: artificial nutrition and hydration (ANH) and medical futility.

Setting the Context: Framework for Decisions to Forego Treatment

Before we begin outlining the framework, however, we need to clarify a few things. First, when we refer to "treatment" at the end of life, we are referring to all treatments that could be employed in an effort to prolong a patient's life. This includes, among other interventions, breathing machines (mechanical ventilation), kidney machines (dialysis), cardiopulmonary resuscitation (CPR), surgical interventions, various medications and antibiotics, and feeding tubes (ANH). In considering the ethics of forgoing treatment, all treatments are evaluated in the same way and with the same ethical criteria, which we discuss below. Medications and ANH in and of themselves, for example, are no more obligatory than breathing machines or surgical interventions, though we will see in the discussion below on forging ANH that not everyone agrees with this position.

Second, we use the word *forgoing* to mean either withholding or withdrawing treatment. As has been established in the law and is widely agreed on among health care ethicists, we make no moral distinction between refusing or not initiating treatment (withholding) and removing or stopping treatment (withdrawing). Both can be permissible depending on the circumstances. Some people, however, including a fair number of health care professionals, do make such a distinction by presuming that withholding treatment is more acceptable morally than withdrawing treatment because they believe withdrawing causes the death of the patient. In some cases this may be true; in most it is not. The fact is we cannot make this determination without considering each case individually in light of the overall situation of the patient.

Distinguishing between withholding and withdrawing treatment is not only wrong morally but can be extremely dangerous and irresponsible clinically. On one hand, it can lead to overtreatment, in which the patient is kept alive with medical technologies well beyond what is medically and morally reasonable because one fears that withdrawing treatment will kill the patient. On the other hand, it can lead to undertreatment, where patients who might meaningfully benefit from treatment do not receive it because one fears once treatment is started it may not be stopped. Admittedly there is a physical difference between withholding and withdrawing treatment: in one case we are doing something, in the other we are not. There can also be an emotional difference: for some people, removing feels different from not starting. But there is no moral difference, at least none that can be determined *in advance* or apart from a consideration of the patient's overall situation. The only way we can judge whether an act of withholding or withdrawing is right or wrong morally is by considering the benefits and burdens of treatment and evaluating the intention of the one performing the action.

Third, there is a moral difference between an act of killing a patient (say, with a lethal drug injection) and allowing the patient to die by forgoing treatment that is not beneficial or excessively burdensome. Although some try to collapse this distinction, particularly those in favor of physician-assisted suicide and euthanasia, an honest evaluation leads to a different viewpoint. The result of the two actions may be the same (the patient dies) but the cause and intention are different in morally significant ways. In the first scenario, the patient dies because of the lethal injection, and the intention, at least in part, is to bring about this result. In the second scenario the patient dies because of his or her underlying condition after medical technologies are removed because they have been found not to provide a meaningful benefit or they impose undue burdens. Unlike the act of giving a lethal injection, the intention here most often is not to cause death but to stop a treatment that simply is not in the patient's best interests. The person making the decision, whether a family member or caregiver, usually would like nothing more than for the patient to get better but decides the likelihood of this happening is slim.

We are obviously into a debate that borders on the theoretical. There is, however, one very good practical reason why we should maintain the distinction between killing and allowing death. If we were to give up this distinction, think how much more difficulty families and caregivers would have forgoing treatment at the end of life. In many instances they are already reluctant to forgo treatment because they fear they will be causing the death of the patient, even when it is clear the treatment is not benefiting the patient or is even harming the patient. We could only imagine that their fear would be much worse, to the detriment of patients, if the distinction were collapsed and every act of forgoing treatment was equated with or lumped into the same category as killing. Since most people have a moral aversion to killing, patients would be left to linger, unduly suffering, while their bodies gave out on medical technologies.

With this background we can now move toward constructing a moral framework that can guide decision making in the end-of-life context. Much of what we will discuss here has already been said or implied in earlier parts of this book. Still, there is good reason to pull it all together specifically for purposes of looking at the issue of forgoing treatment at the end of life. Although many religious traditions and secular medical associations have examined the issue of forgoing medical treatment at the end of life, the Catholic tradition has examined this issue for literally hundreds of years. What we outline below is taken largely from the insights of that tradition, insights that have played an important part in debates over forgoing treatment at the end of life. We will discuss the duty we have to preserve our own lives, the criteria we use for making end-of-life treatment decisions, and the meaning of benefit and burden in the end-of-life context.

The Duty to Preserve Life[1]

The basis for our moral framework on forgoing treatment at the end of life is found in the basic Christian understanding of life and death. As Christians we believe human life is a great good that has been given to us freely out of love by God. It is through life on earth that we are able to enter more fully into communion with God by loving others as God loves us. For these reasons, we have a strong moral duty to protect and to preserve our lives. Yet this duty is not absolutely binding under all circumstances because our ultimate end lies not in this life but in eternal life with God. To hold otherwise would be to deny a central Christian belief: namely, through death we rise to new life.

This balanced view of life and death is important because it stakes a middle ground between two extreme views often present in debates on forgoing treatment at the end of life. On one side are those who claim or imply we have complete authority over our lives and as such we can decide to do with it what we will, even ending our lives if we so choose. This argument, often cited in support of physician-assisted suicide and euthanasia, is problematic when considered in light of our duty to preserve life and the effect of our decisions on others, including society at large. On the other side are those who claim or imply life is an absolute good and must be preserved at all costs regardless of a person's condition or prospects for recovery. This argument is equally problematic because it limits human choice and could hold us hostage to the many medical technologies available today that have the ability to stave off death while also imposing significant burdens and increasing patient suffering. A more balanced Christian view holds neither extreme to be true, recognizing both a duty to preserve life and reasonable limits to this duty.

Criteria for Making Decisions

Just what these limits are is a question that has been given considerable attention in medical, legal, and especially religious circles, most notably the Catholic moral tradition. It has been widely accepted among Catholic theologians since the sixteenth century, and subsequently by others in the fields of medicine, ethics, and law, that one is only morally obligated to use medical means that offer a proportionate hope of benefit without imposing an excessive burden or an excessive expense on one's family or the community (this is what is meant by "ordinary" or "proportionate" means). One is not morally obligated, however, to use medical means that either fail to offer a proportionate hope of benefit or impose an excessive burden or expense on the family or the community (this is what is meant by "extraordinary" or "disproportionate" means).

In determining one's duty to preserve life with medical means, the Catholic tradition has always held that treatment must be considered in light of factors *relative to the person* and her or his total circumstances (e.g., physical, spiritual, financial, familial, social, and so on). Only then can one get a true sense of the benefits and burdens of treatment and decide whether it is proportionate and hence morally obligatory, or disproportionate and hence morally optional. That this is true can be seen in the most comprehensive historical study of the topic, the 1958 doctoral dissertation of Archbishop Emeritus Daniel A. Cronin (Hartford, Connecticut) entitled *The Moral Law in Regard to the Ordinary and Extraordinary Means of Conserving Life*. In his study, Cronin reviewed the work of virtually every theologian who had commented on the issue to date and had this to say about the importance of relative factors in determining the proportionality of treatment:

> In summary, therefore, we may say that the notion of proportionate hope of success and benefit is an essential part of

the nature of ordinary [or proportionate] means. Without this hope of benefit, a means is hardly an ordinary [or proportionate] means and therefore is not obligatory. In determining the presence of this hope of success and benefit, one must consider not only the *nature of the particular remedy or means involved*, but also *the relative condition of the person* who is to use this means. *Then, and then only,* can the moral obligation of using such a means be properly determined. [emphasis added][2]

The importance of relative factors is also seen in recent authoritative Catholic Church documents. For instance, in the 1980 "Declaration on Euthanasia" issued by the Congregation for the Doctrine of the Faith (CDF), we read, "It will be possible to make a correct judgment as to the means by studying *the type of treatment* to be used, its *degree of complexity* or risk, *its cost* and the possibilities of using it, and comparing these elements with the *result* that can be expected, taking into account the *state of the sick person* and his or her *physical and moral resources.*"(emphasis added).[3] Likewise, Pope John Paul II stated in his 1995 encyclical letter *Evangelium vitae* (Gospel of Life): "Certainly there is a moral obligation to care for oneself and to allow oneself to be cared for, but this duty *must take account of concrete circumstances*. It needs to be determined whether the *means of treatment* available are objectively *proportionate to the prospects for improvement*" (emphasis added).[4]

In practice, this means the determination of one's duty to preserve life with medical means is a personal moral assessment that must be done on a case-by-case basis. The implication is we can never say *in advance* that a breathing machine or feeding tube, for instance, is proportionate and hence morally obligatory, or disproportionate and hence morally optional. In actual clinical situations, this could result in one patient deciding against a treatment that is painful, expensive, and only likely to prolong life for a short time, while another patient with the same condition opts for the treatment because, among other things, she or he is willing to endure the pain for a slightly longer life. Although some people may be uncomfortable with the leeway afforded in this approach, the genius of it morally is it does not simply default to what is medically indicated or technologically possible.

Rather, it allows us to consider treatment options in light of personal circumstances and ultimately decide for or against treatment based on how it will affect us holistically as well as how it will affect our family and the community. The wisdom of this approach, which allows room for consideration of personal factors, has served the Catholic tradition well for hundreds of years and has been adopted by and integrated into contemporary medicine and health care ethics.[5]

The Meaning of Benefit and Burden

If benefits and burdens are the main criteria for assessing whether treatment is proportionate and thus morally obligatory in view of our duty to preserve life, we need to know what these concepts mean and how they are applied *morally* to treatment decisions at the end of life. This is perhaps the most challenging question in this chapter, because so many personal and contextual factors go into deciding the benefits and burdens of any treatment. Before further discussing benefits and burdens, we would like you to reflect on how you might understand these concepts personally if faced with a serious illness. In the following scenarios, which build on one another, put yourself in the shoes of the patient and reflect on the questions following each scenario.

> **Scenario A:** Two years ago, you were diagnosed with congestive heart failure, or CHF, a chronic, debilitating condition in which the heart cannot pump enough blood to the body. In addition, you have had diabetes (a chronic disease marked by high blood sugar levels) for more than five years but have managed to control it fairly well. Your overall quality of life has been pretty good since you were diagnosed with CHF, especially because you made some wise lifestyle changes (better diet, more exercise, quitting smoking, etc.). Although you have been able to do most things as always in recent months you often become short of breath with moderate exertion. More recently, you have been feeling lightheaded, weak, and tired. As such, you go see your physician, with whom you have a long-standing relationship. After conducting numerous tests, she informs you that your heart failure has worsened and that the cause of your lightheadedness and

other symptoms is a very rapid, irregular heartbeat. Because she is concerned that in time you could go into sudden cardiac arrest (failure of the heart to pump blood to the body), she suggests surgery to implant a cardioverter defibrillator, or ICD (a small battery-powered electrical impulse generator that detects and corrects abnormal heart rhythms by delivering a jolt of electricity) in your chest. Would you agree to have the ICD implanted? Why or why not? What factors would you consider in reaching this decision?

Scenario B: You have been living with the ICD now for more than a year but your overall condition has slowly worsened. Now you become short of breath with minimal activity and have significant swelling in your ankles, feet, legs, and abdomen due to fluid buildup. You visit your physician frequently but are mostly confined to your home with your spouse, who is still relatively healthy and active. The fluid buildup has caused considerable weight gain and you have developed a cough, which is worse at night when you are lying down. Just last night the coughing was so bad you felt as though you could not breathe and your spouse called 911; an ambulance took you to the emergency department (ED) of the local hospital where you were treated for acute pulmonary edema (abnormal build-up of fluid in the lungs). In the ED you receive oxygen via a nasal cannula (a device with two prongs inserted in the nostrils to provide supplemental oxygen), which helps relieve your symptoms somewhat. Because your breathing is still labored, the ED physician suggests you go to the intensive care unit (ICU) and be placed on a mechanical ventilator or breathing machine, hopefully for just a couple of weeks, until they can decrease the fluid in your lungs and get you breathing normally again on your own. Would you agree to be placed on the breathing machine and admitted to the ICU? Why or why not? What factors would you consider in reaching this decision?

Scenario C: You were released from the hospital after more than three weeks, with most of that time spent in the ICU. Since then, you have been mostly inactive and have not left your home. You are unable to do virtually anything that requires minimal exertion. Even going to the bathroom or getting something from the refrigerator has become quite a chore. During your most recent visit with your physician, she emphasizes that your condition is grave and that, to have any chance of living more than a year, you will need major surgery to implant a heart pump, or left ventricular assist device, which is inserted into the abdomen and attached to the heart to help it pump. She also suggests putting you on the transplant list to receive a healthy heart from a donor as she is not sure how long the heart pump will reduce the severity of your symptoms. Would you have the surgery for the heart pump and agree to be placed on the transplant waiting list? Why or why not? What factors would you consider in reaching this decision?

The point of these scenarios is to get you to reflect on the factors you would consider important in deciding for or against treatment, because these factors are at the heart of the meaning of benefit and burden. Keeping in mind these factors, let us consider the meaning of benefit and burden in more detail. In the medical context, we tend to think of treatment as *beneficial* when it restores health, relieves pain and suffering, improves physical function and mental status, restores consciousness, enables communication with others, prolongs life, and so on; and we tend to think of treatment as *burdensome* when it causes pain and suffering, emotional distress and anxiety, physical complications (e.g., nausea, diarrhea, constipation, unconsciousness, difficulty breathing, infection, pressure sores), is not easily accessible, confines one to a hospital or bed, is prohibitively expensive, and so on.

All of these factors may qualify as benefits and burdens from a *medical perspective* in that they are positive and negative effects of treatment. However, we can reach a moral determination about the proportionality of treatment only by considering the totality of these effects, not just one, on the person in view of her or his total circumstances (e.g., physical, spiritual, financial, familial, social, and so on). In the third scenario above, for instance, a positive effect of the heart pump is its potential to prolong the person's life beyond one year. This positive effect, however, does not necessarily mean the heart pump offers a proportionate hope of benefit because many other factors would need to be considered before the person arrives at this judgment. This is important to remember, especially in our technological age in which a treatment may be considered morally required simply because it might achieve some positive effects, considered quite apart from the person holistically. However, in using our normative basis as the backdrop for considering benefit and burden from a *moral perspective*, a treatment is generally deemed proportionate and hence morally obligatory when it enables one to pursue goods bound up with human flourishing, especially human relationships, and other personal goods one finds important, at least at a minimal level, without imposing excessive burdens or excessive expenses on the family or community.

There is perhaps no better way to demonstrate this than by sharing a personal story. Janice, the mother of one of the authors, was diagnosed with ovarian cancer just shy of her thirty-second birthday, after nearly a year of nondescript symptoms that her physician insisted were simply side effects of stress and "life changes." Upon diagnosis, Janice was informed by her oncologist (cancer specialist) from the local university hospital that the cancer had spread to other parts of her body and, of most concern, to her liver. The good news, as he put it, was that through a combination of surgery, chemotherapy, and radiation, they could "beat the cancer."

First came the surgery, which Janice reluctantly accepted because it meant she would never again be able to have children. Then came months of chemotherapy and radiation, which also took their toll. Janice lost considerable weight, as well as her long hair, and frequently experienced intense pain and violent bouts of vomiting. Despite her oncologist's optimism, the treatments did not put the cancer into remission or shrink the tumor in Janice's liver. Unphased, the oncologist advocated a second round of chemotherapy, combined again with more radiation. This time, though, they would use a different cancer-fighting agent for a longer time, which could, he cautioned, worsen Janice's previous symptoms. As before, Janice agreed to the treatments, but once again they failed to have their desired effect.

For much of the second round of treatments, Janice was hospitalized so they could manage her complications, especially the anorexia (loss of appetite) and recurrent buildup of fluid in her abdomen that made her appear as though she were in the late stages of pregnancy. As she became further removed from the chemotherapy and radiation treatments, Janice began to feel somewhat more like herself, but she was still dealing with persistent pain, which at times was so excruciating, her cries could be heard throughout the hospital wing she shared. About two months after the treatments ended, Janice's oncologist informed her the tumor in her liver had grown to such proportions there was a good chance it would cause her liver to burst, in which case she would die. Janice's only hope, he said, was to submit to even more toxic levels of chemotherapy drugs, "investigational doses" were his precise words, so they could shrink the tumor. Rather than acquiescing to the treatment as she had before, Janice wanted to know how much pain she would have; whether her insurance would cover the costs; how her relationships with her only child and other loved ones would be affected; how much time she would have to spend in the hospital; if she would be physically able to work, which she needed to do for financial reasons; and if she would feel well enough to do some of the things she loved such as drawing and painting.

If the positive effect of sustaining life were all that mattered in determining proportionate hope of benefit, Janice would have jumped at the chance to receive more chemotherapy. However, Janice knew intuitively what we are saying here, that treatment is truly beneficial insofar as it enables one to pursue goods bound up with human flourishing and other personal goods that are important, at least at a minimal level, without imposing excessive burdens or an excessive expense on one's family or the community. For Janice, and we suspect for most of us (think again about what you decided in the scenarios above and why), these goods included things such as pursuing personal interests, engaging loved ones, deepening her relationship with God, and contributing to her family and society. In questioning the doctors, what Janice really wanted to know was whether treatment would give her a fighting chance to pursue these goods, or whether she would be profoundly frustrated in her pursuit of them as she struggled to stay alive. Janice ultimately decided for the treatment but, significantly, length of life was not her only consideration, perhaps not even the most important. She wanted to know what type of life she would be able to live in the time she had left. This story captures both the meaning of benefit and burden from a moral perspective and how one determines proportionality of treatment in actual clinical situations.

We close this section by listing moral norms that can serve as useful guidelines for treatment decisions at the end of life:

- Human life is a basic good and as such one, has a strong moral obligation to protect and preserve it; however, this obligation is not absolute: there are limits to this duty.
- The moral obligation to preserve life with medical means is a personal moral assessment that must be made on a case-by-case basis, taking into consideration one's total circumstances (e.g., physical, spiritual, financial, familial, social, and so on).
- One should be able to make treatment decisions for oneself; if one is unable to do this, then a person who is best suited to apply one's sense of personal goods and values should make these decisions (often called a "surrogate" or "durable power of attorney for health care").
- Generally, one is morally bound to preserve life with medical means if it enables one to pursue goods bound up with human flourishing, especially human relationships, and other personal goods one finds important, at least at a minimal level, without imposing excessive burdens or an excessive expense on one's family or the community.
- Generally, one is *not* morally bound to preserve life with medical means if (1) it will merely sustain one's life for a short time and thereby prolong the dying process; (2) it cannot improve one's condition to the point of being able to pursue goods bound up with human flourishing, especially human relationships, and other personal goods one finds important, even at a minimal level; (3) it only maintains one in a condition in which one will be profoundly frustrated in the pursuit of these goods; or (4) it imposes an excessive expense on one's family or the community.
- When serious doubt exists as to the benefits and burdens of a particular medical means, such doubt should be resolved by deciding in favor of its use.

These norms and the framework from which they arise apply to all treatment decisions at the end of life, regardless of the type of treatment. In the next section, we use them as a lens through which to consider the issues of artificial nutrition and hydration (ANH) and medical futility.

Discussion: Ethical Issues and Analysis

Artificial Nutrition and Hydration

Perhaps the most challenging of all forgoing treatment decisions are those that involve feeding tubes, or what clinicians sometimes refer to as artificial nutrition and hydration (ANH). Although feeding-tube decisions are or should be driven by the same moral considerations as other treatments, they tend to be much more emotionally complex because ANH is often attached to the symbolic meaning that eating food and drinking water have for us, thus conjuring up indelible memories and emotions and making its use seem morally obligatory. Further complicating such decisions is that they are often made for individuals who no longer have the ability to decide for themselves and are thus more vulnerable to abuses than other patients. Given these factors, families and caregivers sometimes ask, "How can we withhold 'food' and 'water'?," believing that forgoing ANH is tantamount to starvation. Consequently, it is important to demystify some of the perceptions around ANH so that decisions about its use can be made in the person's best interests and overall well-being.

Clinical Features of ANH

For ANH, feeding tubes are used in place of the natural processes of eating: chewing, swallowing, and digestion.[6] Patients who need ANH have difficulty performing these natural tasks because of their medical condition. ANH is therefore a technological method or medical means of getting nutrients to individuals whose nutritional needs cannot otherwise be met, temporarily or permanently, due to their medical condition. There are several indications for using ANH. Whatever the condition, the point is to get enough nutrients into the body to help in the recovery process. ANH is often used in patients who have neurological deficits such as brain trauma, including coma, persistent vegetative state, stroke, or brain tumors that disrupt the natural processes involved with eating. In advanced and critical illness, ANH is often used because individuals can be too debilitated to eat. In dementia-type illnesses, ANH is often used because people have forgotten how to eat. In psychiatric illnesses, ANH is often used because some people have an eating disorder of some type that prevents adequate nutritional intake. ANH is also used to prevent aspiration, which occurs when food, gastric contents, or oral secretions such as saliva enter the lungs. Aspiration can cause pneumonia and can be very serious. ANH does not prevent aspiration in some patients, such as chronically ill, debilitated individuals.

ANH should not be used when it cannot be absorbed or assimilated by the body or when there is an obstruction in the gastrointestinal tract. ANH is not indicated for patients with severe kidney, liver, or heart failure who cannot metabolize or break down the actual contents of the feeding. Those who are imminently dying (i.e., within hours) are going through natural, physiological processes and one of these processes is the complete and final cessation of eating and drinking. Using ANH in these individuals can cause fluid overload, severe breathing problems, and edema—all of which are very uncomfortable and make the dying process more difficult for the patient and the patient's loved ones.

Depending on the indications for its use, caregivers will determine what kind of feeding tube to use. Nasogastric feeding tubes are inserted through the nostril, into the nasopharnx, down the esophagus, and into the stomach or duodenum. Nasogastric tubes are ideally used on a short-term basis because they can cause ulcers in the nostril or pharynx, sinus blockage, and infection if used beyond two weeks. Patients with dementia on nasogastric feeding tubes often try to pull them out because of the discomfort they experience.

Gastrostomy feeding tubes are inserted directly into the stomach and are used on a more long-term basis. The tube is inserted in a special procedure done by a surgeon or gastroenterologist called a percutaneous endoscopic gastrostomy. This is referred to as a PEG procedure. In a similar procedure, feeding tubes can also be inserted into the jejunum. PEG tube placements are normally well tolerated if used in the right population of patients. PEG tube placement requires sedation, so patients who are critically ill and those with breathing problems have increased risks during placement. Though serious complications of PEG tube placement are rare, medical professionals need to watch for perforations in the gastrointestinal tract that can cause bleeding and infections either at the site of PEG tube placement or inside the abdominal cavity.

Irrespective of the route of transmission, all tube feedings have a formula that is designed to meet the nutritional needs of the patient. Registered dieticians and pharmacists will typically evaluate and then determine the specific needs of the patient. The feeding mixture is a commercial product that contains the right balance of nutrients for the patient. ANH can be burdensome, although patients' experiences vary. Common complications can include diarrhea, blockage of the tube, site infections, aspiration pneumonia, and the use of restraints to keep individuals from pulling out their feeding tubes. Thus careful monitoring by skilled caregivers is required.

Contrary to what many outside of health care believe, forgoing ANH in seriously ill and dying patients does not necessarily result in a painful death. In actuality, death can be quite mild and relatively peaceful. Dying patients often naturally quit eating and drinking and do not experience hunger or thirst. In the absence of nutrition and hydration, the body tends to draw on endorphins or endogenous opioid peptides that can comfort or palliate the patient. Furthermore, diminished bodily fluids can lead to reduced urinary output, relief of pulmonary and peripheral edema or swelling, reduced pulmonary secretions with less coughing and congestion, and relief from choking. Nausea and vomiting also tend to be minimized with less gastric fluids. Patients may, however, still experience or appear to be in discomfort. As such, continued nursing care is important, such as moistening the patient's mouth to relieve any sensation of thirst, putting lotion on the body and running a humidifier to prevent the patient's skin from becoming excessively dry and breaking down, and providing palliative morphine to relieve any residual pain or discomfort.

Consensus and Controversy

Despite the emotional complexity involved in decisions to forgo ANH, a solid medical, ethical, and legal consensus has developed over the last several decades that ANH should be viewed as any other medical treatment subject to a benefit–burden analysis by the patient (or surrogate) and that ANH can legitimately be withheld or withdrawn, especially for patients at the end of life for whom the benefits of ANH are questionable and the burdens sometimes considerable.

Yet even with this consensus, people still seem conflicted about forgoing ANH. This was clear from the way people reacted during and in the years since the highly publicized case involving Terri Schiavo, the Florida woman who was in what is called a persistent vegetative (or unconscious) state (PVS) for more than fifteen years and who died on March 31, 2005, after her husband "won" the legal right over her parents and siblings to have her feeding tube removed. PVS is characterized by the loss of all higher brain functions, with either complete or partial preservation of hypothalamic and brainstem autonomic functions. Given the absence of higher-brain activity, patients in a PVS are completely unaware of themselves and their environment and are unable to interact with others. Yet because lower-brain function is relatively intact, such patients exhibit periodic wakefulness manifested by sleep–wake cycles and have the capacity to achieve a wide range of reflex activities. Death for patients in a PVS is commonly brought on by an infection in the lungs or urinary tract, respiratory failure, or sudden death of unknown cause. The length of survival depends in part on how aggressively such complications are treated. The life expectancy of such patients is greatly reduced, with the average ranging from two to five years, and survival of ten years unusual.

Numerous courts, politicians, heath care professionals, theologians, ethicists, and ordinary citizens weighed in on the Schiavo case, often on national newscasts and in local and major newspapers. The Schiavo case exposed a rift in public thinking over the removal of feeding tubes as people lined up on both sides and everywhere in between, thus suggesting there is anything but consensus on this contentious issue. Curiously, many Catholics, including priests and high-ranking Catholic Church officials, argued against removing Terri Schiavo's feeding tube and described it as murder by starvation. Their position was based on the view that ANH is food and water and therefore basic care (as opposed to medical treatment) that should never be withheld or withdrawn from a patient or only in very limited circumstances, namely, (1) when the patient is imminently dying or (2) when the patient cannot physically assimilate ANH. Without getting into more of the specifics surrounding the Schiavo case, what is curious about this position is it leaves little or no room for personal circumstances and one's personal sense of the goods bound up with human flourishing to factor into decisions about ANH. Instead, it seems to rely strictly on medical indications in determining one's obligation to preserve life with ANH.

This is a significant departure from the thought of traditional theologians, who resisted the temptation to set requirements around the use of any means, including nutrition and hydration, which in earlier times meant ordinary food and fluids, not feeding tubes surgically placed and medically administered. Archbishop Cronin again makes this clear in summarizing traditional views on the issue:

> It is hardly possible *to establish categorically* that a particular means will always offer proportionate benefit under all circumstances and to all people. In other words, it is *difficult to establish an absolute norm* when determining the required hope of success and benefit in *any procedure* designed to conserve life. . . . Even the older moralists teach that such a purely ordinary and common means of conserving life as food, *admits of relative inconvenience and difficulty.* Furthermore, they point out that this very common means, food, sometimes *can offer no proportionate hope of success* relative to a particular individual. [emphasis added][7]

For the traditional theologians, the decisive moral question in determining one's duty to preserve life with nutrition and hydration was not whether the means is a basic element of care versus a medical treatment, or even if the person is imminently dying or can physically assimilate the nutrients and fluids. Rather, it was whether the means offers a proportionate hope of benefit considered in light of the person and her or his total circumstances (e.g., physical, spiritual, financial, familial, social, and so on).

The Pope Speaks

An interesting development occurred at the peak of the Schiavo debate in March 2004 when the late Pope John Paul II weighed in on the issue of nutrition and hydration as he addressed participants at a conference on life-sustaining treatments and the vegetative state. The pope seemed to give credence to the more restrictive position on forgoing ANH outlined above, at least as it applied to patients in a PVS. One part of the pope's address (or allocution) is particularly important for our purposes. However, before getting to it, we would like to provide a thumbnail sketch of the contents of the allocution. In his comments, the pope emphasized that patients in a PVS have an inherent dignity that is not lost because of their illness; that caregivers, families, and society have a duty to care for and protect these patients; that caregivers should be careful in diagnosing this condition because there are reports of misdiagnosis; that appropriate rehabilitative services should be provided to these patients because their condition is not necessarily hopeless; that the term *vegetative* is not appropriate because it suggests these patients are less valuable than other persons; and that we can never remove treatment from these patients with the intention of killing them, as to do so would be a form of euthanasia.

If this were all the pope had said, we probably would not be talking about the allocution because such comments are insightful, important, and noncontroversial. However, the pope made additional comments that apply directly to our discussion here, the most noteworthy of which are the following:

> The sick person in a vegetative state, awaiting recovery or a natural end, still has the right to basic health care (nutrition, hydration, cleanliness, warmth, etc.), and to the prevention of complications related to his confinement to bed. . . . I should like particularly to underline how the administration of water and food, even when provided by artificial means, always represents a *natural means* of preserving life, not a *medical act*. Its use, furthermore, should be considered, *in principle*, *ordinary* and *proportionate*, and as such morally obligatory, insofar as and until it is seen to have attained its proper finality, which in the present case consists in providing nourishment to the patient and alleviation of his suffering.[8]

In this passage the pope makes a general comment about nutrition and hydration and applies it specifically to patients in a PVS. The general comment is that nutrition and hydration, including ANH, should be considered, "in principle, ordinary and proportionate, and as such morally obligatory, insofar as and until it is seen to have attained its proper finality." This is a departure from the tradition in that it elevates ANH to a special class of means of preserving life that must be considered ordinary and proportionate, in principle, apart from personal circumstances. One cannot find such a way of thinking about any means in the tradition. At most we have an "in principle" obligation to preserve our lives, but not to use a certain means. If true of nutrition and hydration, why not oxygen provided by a breathing machine or filtered blood provided via dialysis? Importantly, though, the pope does not say ANH is always ordinary or proportionate and hence absolutely required. This he makes clear by saying ANH is obligatory "insofar as and until it is seen to have attained its proper finality." Thus, in the pope's opinion, ANH is required morally only if or to the extent that it attains its proper finality.

What is the "proper finality" of ANH? The pope only gives us the answer for patients in a PVS, for all others he leaves it open-ended. This he does by saying, "in the present case [by which he presumably means PVS] consists in providing nourishment to the patient and alleviation of his suffering." Thus, according to Pope John Paul II, nourishment and alleviation of suffering are the proper finality of ANH for patients in a PVS. If ANH is achieving these ends, then, in the pope's opinion, it is ordinary and proportionate and hence morally obligatory. This may seem benign and the pope may have been hoping to protect vulnerable PVS patients from careless-ness or malice. Nonetheless, it is a break from the tradition in that *he* and not the PVS patient or an appropriate surrogate defines what the benefits and burdens are in light of the circumstances surrounding the patient.

Catholic Ethical and Religious Directives

Despite criticisms of the pope's comments, the essential features of his address, particularly those related to the passage above, have been accepted by the U.S. Conference of Catholic Bishops (USCCB) and incorporated in their *Ethical and Religious Directives for Catholic Health Care Services* (ERDs). The ERDs is an official document pub-lished and approved by the (USCCB) to which all Catholic health care organizations must adhere. The ERDs provide specific guidance on issues that arise in the context of delivering health care, includ-ing forgoing ANH. The ERDs were changed or revised in 2009 to reflect the pope's comments and incorporate feedback from the CDF to questions posed by the bishops themselves. ERD 58, which deals specifically with ANH, now reads,

> *In principle*, there is an obligation to provide patients with food and water, including medically assisted nutrition and hydration for those who cannot take food orally. This obligation extends to patients in *chronic and presumably irreversible conditions* (e.g., the "persistent vegetative state") who can reasonably be expected to live indefinitely if given such care. Medically assisted nutrition and hydration become morally optional when they cannot *reasonably be expected to prolong life* or when they would be "excessively burdensome for the patient or [would] cause significant physical discomfort, for example resulting from complications in the use of the means employed." For instance, as a patient draws close to inevitable death from an underlying progressive and fatal condition, certain measures to provide nutrition and hydration may become excessively burdensome and therefore not obligatory in light of their very limited ability to prolong life or provide comfort. [emphasis added][9]

Although the new version of ERD 58 basically reiterates the key features of the passage quoted above from the pope's allocution, there are two particular items that stand out and bear mentioning. The first is that the new ERD 58 maintains, as the pope did in his allocution, there is an "in principle" obligation to provide ANH to patients. In addition to departing from the tradition, this is problematic from a practical medical standpoint in that not all patients who are unable to take food orally are situated alike. While one *might* be able to make a case for an "in principle" obligation to provide ANH to PVS patients because of their presumed vulnerability, the same cannot be said of certain patient populations, such as those with end-stage cancer or advanced dementia. For these patients, ANH can be medically contraindicated because the burdens far outweigh any benefits.[10] As such, an "in principle" obligation seems misplaced insofar as it could result in such patients being subjected to ANH and its burdens when they should not. Significantly, though, the new ERD 58, like the pope in his allocution, does not absolutely require the use of ANH for these patients, or for PVS patients for that matter, so good sense can still prevail in actual clinical situations.

The second item that bears mentioning is considerably more weighty than the first: The new ERD 58, similar to the pope's allocution, attempts to define the benefit of ANH in the abstract and apart from factors relative to the person and her or his total circumstances. Unlike traditional formulations that refer to "proportionate hope of benefit" and leave it to the patient to decide what this means, the new ERD 58, without ever uttering the word *benefit*, sets the terms for how benefit should be understood when it comes to decisions about ANH by stating that ANH becomes "morally optional when [it] cannot *reasonably be expected to prolong life*" (emphasis added). This limited understanding of benefit is not the way the concept developed in the tradition nor how traditional theologians understood it. As we have noted, the simple fact that a means is capable of prolonging life does not necessarily mean it provides a proportionate hope of benefit and is thus morally obligatory. This is because the notion of benefit is a broad human judgment that encompasses factors that include but go beyond prolongation of life. The great Dominican theologian Francisco de Vitoria, writing in the sixteenth century, makes this point clear in stating,

> One is not held to lengthen his life, because he is not held to use always the most delicate foods, that is, hens and chickens, even though he has the ability and the doctors say that if he eats in such a manner, *he will live 20 years more*; and even if he knew this for certain, he would not be obliged. [emphasis added][11]

This passage may be dated when it comes to the means being discussed (hens and chickens). Nevertheless, the main point still applies, perhaps even more forcefully in our age of highly technological medicine: prolonging life alone or in and of itself does not exhaust the meaning of "proportionate hope of benefit."

So where does this leave us in the debate over forgoing ANH, especially from a Catholic perspective? For individual Catholics (patients, families, and caregivers), as well as Catholic health care organizations, the new ERD 58, while problematic in parts when compared against the tradition, does not require a change in philoso-phy or practice. At the end of the day, Catholic teaching still holds that human life is a basic good; we have a strong moral obligation to preserve life; there are limits to this obligation when it comes to using medical means, including ANH; and these limits are deter-mined by considering the benefits and burdens of the means rela-tive to the person and her or his total circumstances (e.g., physical, spiritual, financial, familial, social, and so on). As in the past, this still requires decisions about ANH or any other medical means be made on a case-by-case basis. This is how Catholics can and should approach such decisions as well as others who want to do so in an ethically balanced way.

Medical Futility

Medical practice must distinguish among (1) known beneficial treat-ments or therapies, (2) innovative but still experimental treatments, and (3) treatments that have empirically failed to show realistic ben-efit.[12] Here we deal with the third class of treatments, which are often called nonbeneficial or futile treatments. The practice of requesting, initiating, or continuing such treatments is commonly referred to as medical futility. Medical futility is best understood as any effort to initiate or continue a treatment when it is highly unlikely to succeed in achieving its desired ends or when its rare beneficial exceptions cannot be systematically explained or reproduced.[13]

Requests for futile treatment usually arise in the context of pro-viding medical care to patients who are critically ill, unable to make decisions for themselves, and living with an underlying serious illness that is not likely to respond to medical interventions. The overall treatment goal for this class of patients is less about cure and more about comfort. Consequently, requests for futile treatment, which usually come from family members, can be problematic because the goals of care in such cases may not call for aggressive, curative therapy. It is one thing to intervene aggressively with patients who can both withstand and benefit from the therapy; it is another thing to intervene aggressively with patients who, because of their underly-ing illness and poor prognosis, will not proportionately benefit from curative therapies.

An Ethical Issue

Medical futility is an important ethical issue in contemporary medicine for several reasons. The first is that it raises important questions about decision-making authority in the end-of-life context. What are the goals of therapy and who determines these goals: the physician, the patient, the family, or some combination thereof? Should physicians have the authority to make unilateral decisions about the appropriateness of certain medical interventions? What happens if a patient or family member disagrees with the physician's assessment about what constitutes a burden or benefit? When pressured and threatened, should physicians pursue treatments they know will not work and could even harm? Should patients, families, or loved ones have the right to request or, indeed, demand nonbeneficial life-sustaining treatments be initiated or continued? Today's medical practice has widely adopted a shared approach to decision making, but because of this approach, more voices seek to be heard. Each voice brings its own particular conception of goods, personal history, and set of experiences to the conversation, which makes it difficult at times to reach consensus about the goals of care for a particular patient. Appreciating diverse points of view is both a necessity and challenge in today's health care environment. This is particularly true in the end-of-life setting where human life is at stake and emotions tend to be high.

A second reason why medical futility is an important ethical issue for contemporary medicine is that it requires us to be more mindful of—and clear about—the implicit moral meaning and significance that the goals of medicine can have for decision making in concrete cases. A common list of the goals of medicine would include (1) relieving pain and suffering, (2) prolonging life, (3) promoting health and preventing disease, and (4) engaging in research.[14] An important ethical subtext to these goals of medicine is the notion of benefit. In this respect, medicine is explicitly tied to human flourishing. Its organizing moral force is to intervene for the overall well-being of the patient. Therefore, when patients or families request treatment deemed to be futile, they are essentially asking caregivers and health care institutions to consider a course of action that may be contrary to the overall mission and purpose of medicine. Requests to initiate or continue futile treatment can be particularly disturbing when the intervention in question is likely to be harmful. As we mentioned in the section on ANH, for example, there is good evidence that using artificial means to feed and hydrate people with advanced dementia is not only nonbeneficial but also harmful in certain situations.[15] Yet it is commonly requested and used in patients for whom it is contraindicated.

A third reason why medical futility is an important ethical issue for contemporary medicine is that it raises important social questions about the just and equitable distribution of limited health care resources (human, technical, and financial). As became clear in the national debate on health care reform in 2009, health care costs in the United States have reached or will soon reach unsustainable levels that are detrimental to the well-being of our nation. Whether we want to accept it or not, managing health care costs will require, among other things, setting limits and being more prudent in how we use our resources. Every time we intervene with a futile treatment in the end-of-life setting—say, with a breathing machine, dialysis, or feeding tube that may prolong life for a time but ultimately does nothing to alter or improve a patient's underlying illness or prognosis—we are using valuable resources that could go to others and are increasing the overall costs of health care.

Reasons Underlying Requests

There are many reasons underlying requests for futile treatment. One reason is different people have different ideas of what is beneficial when it comes to treatment. For one person simply prolonging life with medical means when individuals are severely ill with little hope of recovery might not be a benefit, but for another it might be. This is why it is so difficult to achieve consensus on a precise definition of futility. A second reason is that communication is often poor in settings such as intensive care units where difficult, end-of-life decisions must be made. Families tend not to be informed "early enough" about the seriousness of the patient's condition and are not given sufficient time to reconcile with this reality before they are asked to forgo life-sustaining treatments. What is more, families are often given only bits and pieces of information about the patient's condition or progress and sometimes conflicting information is presented by the various caregivers, as no single caregiver is designated as the primary contact person. A third reason is physicians and other caregivers often do not communicate among themselves effectively and do not meet to coordinate the patient's care. Moreover, goals of care and specific care plans are often not established for patients and important issues sometimes go unaddressed (e.g., code status, pain and symptom management needs, patient preferences).

A fourth reason underlying requests for futile treatment is physicians tend to present all treatment options as equal and leave it to families to decide what they want without providing much direction as to what course of treatment might best promote the patient's well-being under the circumstances. In addition, physicians tend to shy away from having difficult conversations with families, do not address inappropriate requests for treatment up front, and practice defensive medicine to protect themselves from legal liability. A fifth reason is that deciding to forgo treatment at the end of life is perhaps the most agonizing decision a family member or loved one will ever be asked to make. We are never truly prepared for it, and our desire to avoid the pain and loss can sometimes outweigh our desire to do what is best for the patient. A sixth, but by no means final, reason for requesting futile medical treatment is often that there is conflict, anger, or guilt in and among the family members responsible for decision making. When this occurs, it is easy for family members to forget that the patient's needs are of central importance. Concern for the patient can also be a motivating factor for requests for futile treatment as families sometimes feel decisions to limit treatment will result in the patient being abandoned and not receiving the fullest level of care and attention.

Case Illustration

To illustrate the ethical dimensions of medical futility and the reasons underlying requests for futile treatment, we invite you to reflect on the following case. An 81-year-old female patient was admitted to the hospital more than two months before the request for an ethics consultation for an elective surgery to repair an abdominal aortic aneurysm (large blood vessel that supplies blood to the abdomen, pelvis, and legs that is abnormally large or balloons outward). Endovascular aneurysm repair (minimally invasive surgery performed via major blood vessels), which was originally planned, proved too difficult and so an open surgical repair was performed. The patient initially seemed to be recovering well in the intensive care unit (ICU), but around two weeks postsurgery, she developed multiple complications, including ischemic bowel (damage to or death of part of the large intestine due to inadequate blood supply), necessitating surgery to remove part of the colon; blood stream infection requiring antibiotic therapy; multiple pneumonias leading to tracheostomy (surgical opening in the trachea to insert a catheter or tube) and use of a breathing machine; ischemic stroke (death of part of the brain tissue caused by inadequate supply of blood and oxygen) resulting in paralysis on the left side and cognitive deficit (decline in brain function); disseminated intravascular coagulation, or DIC (bleeding disorder that results in abnormal clotting), which caused significant bleeding requiring frequent administration of platelets and fresh frozen plasma; and acute kidney failure, for which dialysis would be necessary. At the time of the ethics consultation, the patient was still in the ICU on a breathing machine at 100-percent oxygenation, still on antibiotics, receiving blood products every other day for the DIC, had a feeding tube for nutritional support, was mildly sedated for pain and rest, and had not moved from her left side. Despite repeated attempts by the intensivist to persuade the family to limit some forms of treatment given the patient's overall medical condition, the family insisted the patient continue to receive ventilation, tube feedings, blood products, and surgery as needed, and that dialysis be initiated.

The family dynamics and physician interactions with the family were remarkable in this case. The patient's immediate family consisted of her husband, a daughter who lived out of town, and a son who visited every day. The husband was very quiet, hesitant to speak up, and often deferred to his children, especially the daughter, when decisions needed to be made. He really only expressed that he wanted his wife to get better and that he did not want her to suffer. The daughter, on the other hand, was very vocal and uncompromising when it came to what she thought was best for her mother. Participating by phone for most discussions and visiting once from out of town, the daughter repeatedly insisted that "everything be done" and that the hospital or the physicians could not stop anything unless she or the family consented. The daughter talked often about "firing" certain physicians, especially the intensivist, and mentioned frequently the possibility of a lawsuit. The son, who sat by the bedside of his mother every day for hours on end, was initially insistent everything be done but began to moderate his stance as time went on, except when in discussions where his sister was involved.

The physicians involved were all in agreement that the patient had virtually no hope of recovering but they were not uniform in what they communicated to the family. The intensivist, who had been overseeing the patient's care for much of her stay in the ICU, was straightforward with the family early on about the seriousness of the patient's condition and her poor chances of recovering. In fact, about three weeks before the ethics consultation, he engaged the family in earnest about stopping blood products and writing a do-not-resuscitate (DNR) order should the patient stop breathing. The vascular surgeon, who performed the original procedure, remained active in the patient's care and often communicated to the family that they "should not give up hope," even though he told his colleagues the patient "did not have much of a chance." The general surgeon, who performed the colon resection, also remained active in the patient's care but, like the intensivist, believed limiting some forms of treatment was in the patient's best interests. Yet she also told the family she would be willing to perform exploratory surgery to determine the source of the patient's bleeding if they wanted that. The infectious disease specialist, who had been called in to treat the patient's pneumonia, expressed to the family her belief that further antibiotic therapy was futile and that the patient had no reasonable hope of recovery. The nephrologist, who was consulted soon after the patient's kidneys started to fail just before the ethics consultation, informed the family that the patient was not a viable candidate for dialysis and recommended comfort measures only.

Because of the intractable conflict that developed between the family and the physicians, especially the intensivist, an ethics consultation was requested. The consultation was successful in that it provided a forum where all the primary caregivers could come together with the family and all involved in the consultation were allowed to express their viewpoints. As far as developing a realistic care plan, however, the only item the family agreed to was to make the patient a DNR. The end result was that the patient remained in the ICU for two more weeks, receiving all current therapies as well as the addition of dialysis three times per week, until her heart finally gave out and she died. Not a single person involved in the patient's care felt right about continuing with the aggressive care plan and one nurse in particular requested to be reassigned because she could not in good conscience carry it out. Meanwhile, the family left angry and throughout the remaining weeks following the consultation grew increasingly detached from and mistrustful of the caregivers and the hospital in general. By all accounts it was a bad outcome, both in process and result.

Three Generations of Medical Futility

Attempts to address the issue of medical futility and the reasons behind requests for futile treatment go back well over twenty years. Despite this it seems that little progress has been made in preventing, reducing, or successfully resolving these situations. Jeffrey Burns and Robert Truog, in a 2007 article in *Chest,* help structure the debate by describing three generations of efforts to deal with medical futility.[16] The first is characterized by attempts to define futility. One author proposed seven clinical conditions for which further treatment should not be provided.[17] Another proposed a distinction between "qualitative" futility (based on a quality-of-life judgment) and "quantitative" futility (involving a judgment about what is a reasonable likelihood of the treatment's success).[18] Yet another recommended limiting the concept of futility to treatments that are "physiologically" futile, that is, they are unable to attain their physiologic goal or therapeutic end.[19] Burns and Truog note that there are serious difficulties inherent in each of the definitional approaches and that they were largely unsuccessful in resolving the more challenging cases. For these reasons, clinicians and ethicists, by the late 1990s, abandoned this attempt and sought alternatives.

This led to the second generation of the futility debate, which consisted in the development of procedural guidelines to resolve disputes over medically futile treatment. A consortium of Houston-based hospitals offered the first such procedural approach; the approach quickly gained in popularity and spread to other areas of the country.[20] In 1999 it was endorsed by the American Medical Association.[21] Many policies in hospitals across the country reflect this approach. Typically, the procedural guidelines are invoked as a last resort and attempt to ensure all voices are heard by the ethics committee. They also usually identify options for moving forward.

Texas, along with a few other states, has incorporated the procedural approach into law.[22] In addition to embodying the elements typical of procedural approaches, the Texas Advance Directives Act (1999) mandates a 10-day waiting period between a decision by the ethics committee affirming medical futility and the actual withdrawal of treatment. The Emilio Gonzales case in 2007, however, revealed weaknesses in the procedural approach, especially in legislated form. The case sparked a statewide, often contentious, debate about the legislation. Right-to-life and disability groups in particular advocated for changes in the legislation that have not yet occurred.

Burns and Truog maintain that neither first- nor second-generation attempts to address the matter of medical futility have been successful. What they propose as an alternative is better communication between clinicians and patients or their families and the use of mediation techniques to resolve differences when disputes arise. The goal, they say, is to "mitigate conflicts as they arise but before they become intractable."[23] Underlying their approach is the belief that most futility cases are the result of breakdowns in communication and trust. Hence, they urge improvement in communication skills among caregivers and suggest a four-step approach to negotiation.[24] Recognizing that good communication and attempts at negotiation do not always work, they suggest going to court to seek appointment of another surrogate if the patient is being harmed by a family member's decisions. Short of that, they recommend acquiescing to familial requests for futile treatment.[25] Because of the potential negative impact on the morale of caregivers, toleration of requests for treatment deemed to be futile should be accompanied by support for those who continue to care for these patients rather than trying to overrule requests for medically inappropriate treatments. The authors consider their approach to the problem to constitute the third-generation approach to medical futility.

Burns and Truog's approach has an opportunity to succeed where definitional and procedural approaches have failed because it emphasizes communication and negotiation as opposed to passive acceptance or domination/oppression. As such, the approach seems better suited to address some of the reasons underlying requests for futile treatment in the first place. By way of summary, and in an effort to further the approach presented by Burns and Truog, we present the following guidelines for physicians and other caregivers.

A. Communicate early and often with patients and families.

Patients and families need to be informed early on about the patient's diagnosis, prognosis, and treatment options. They also need to be updated frequently about any new developments in the care and condition of the patient, such as progress, setbacks, effectiveness of current treatment modalities, alternate treatment options, and necessary changes in the goals of care. Too often patients and families are left in the dark, informed too late about the patient's true condition, or receive inconsistent information from the various physicians and other caregivers. As a result, they may form unrealistic expectations and misinterpret insignificant physical signs in the patient as genuine signs of improvement. Clear, consistent, and frequent communication with patients and families in language they can understand goes a long way in preventing this from happening.

B. Communicate early and often with other physicians and caregivers.

Physicians and other caregivers often do not communicate effectively or frequently among themselves. Not only can this lead to problems in the care of the patient but it can also be a significant source of confusion for patients and families as they are told different things by different caregivers. Physicians should be sure to talk often among themselves and with other caregivers about the patient's situation so they can better coordinate the patient's care. To avoid sending conflicting messages, it is often best to designate a single physician (e.g., the attending or primary treating physician) to communicate *on a routine basis* with the patient and family and, as appropriate, to relay the sentiments of the various caregivers back to them. This not only enables more effective and consistent communication but also lends itself to a more fruitful and trusting relationship with patients and families. For care conferences (see below), however, it is essential that most, if not all, of the physicians and other caregivers treating the patient be involved.

C. **Determine the goals of care and evaluate routinely.**

Setting clear and realistic goals of care with patients and families and evaluating them frequently is critical for all patients, especially those who are seriously ill. Only when this is done can a care plan be developed that corresponds to the present reality of the patient's situation and her or his particular wishes and values. Additional benefits are that patients and families gain a better understanding of what can reasonably be hoped for through the care provided, and physicians and other caregivers are able to come together in establishing a more holistic and coordinated care plan.

D. **Make time for and participate in care conferences.**

One tried-and-true method for enhancing communication and coordinating care for seriously ill patients is to conduct a care conference early in the patient's admission and as needed throughout the patient's stay. Care conferences allow the patient (if able), family members, physicians, and other caregivers to come together to discuss important issues, such as reasonable treatment options; patient and family values, beliefs, and special needs; pain and symptom management; transition or discharge plans; code status; palliative and hospice care options; and so on. Unfortunately, care conferences are not a standardized, routine practice in medicine and are often conducted only when conflict has already manifested. The main reasons for this are that care conferences are seen by some as too time consuming, and it is difficult to get the various physicians and other caregivers together at the same time. Health care facilities that do care conferences routinely, however, have found them to be beneficial, as time spent up front is often time and heartache saved in the end. Moreover, clinical data from recent studies indicate care conferences help to improve communication with patients and families, and among caregivers; achieve consensus around reasonable goals of care; and avoid intractable conflict. Palliative care physicians and nurses, case managers, and social workers, among others, are typically well trained to facilitate care conferences, and physicians should use their expertise. In some cases involving prolonged hospitalization, it may be necessary to have more than one care conference, and time should always be allowed for the patient and family to come to terms with what is discussed, no matter how many care conferences are held.

E. Exercise care in offering or discussing treatment options.

Too often patients and families are offered every treatment option possible and asked to decide what they want. Fortunately, this approach works most of the time as patients and families tend to make reasonable decisions after being given this inordinate amount of power. When the patient or family requests treatment that seems inappropriate or unreasonable, however, physicians object despite the fact they offered the option in the first place. Not only is this a poor medical practice founded on the false idea that patients should have absolute autonomy and physicians must honor any request no matter how impractical, it also puts the patient and family in a difficult position as all the responsibility for treatment decisions shifts to them. A better practice, one built on the concept of shared decision making, is for physicians to offer only those treatment options that are reasonable and realistic in light of the patient's overall condition and the agreed-on goals of care. With this comes the responsibility for physicians to engage in honest dialogue about why such treatment options might benefit the patient and why other options will not.

F. Address unreasonable requests up front and candidly.

Patients and families have a right to participate in treatment decisions and to make requests for treatment. However, physicians are *not* legally or ethically bound to meet every request made by a patient or family. This is particularly true if the request for treatment will extend or increase the suffering of the patient without conferring a proportionate benefit, is medically contraindicated because the treatment will be ineffective, violates generally accepted medical standards of care and is inconsistent with professional experience, or any combination of these. Too often in the end-of-life context, physicians acquiesce to unreasonable requests for treatment for fear of legal liability. This is not only an abdication of physicians' responsibility to their patients, it can also result in harm to the patient, moral distress in physicians and other caregivers, and an inappropriate use of limited health care resources. In addition to exercising care in offering treatment options, physicians need to address unreasonable requests up front and candidly, accepting the responsibility that comes with their role as a medical professional and an advocate for the patient.

G. Ensure nonabandonment and quality end-of-life care.

When discussions are held about treatment options for seriously ill patients, it is important for physicians to assure patients and families that the patient will receive high-quality end-of-life care and not be abandoned if the decision is made to forgo treatment. Patients and families often think that once they decide against a more aggressive approach to treatment, the care of the patient will be compromised and they will be left on their own to attend to the needs of the patient. Unfortunately, this is sometimes the case in modern medicine, and it is one reason why patients and families are inclined to press on with treatment against their better judgment. Physicians should be aware of end-of-life care resources available to them, such as pain-management experts, palliative care and hospice providers, chaplains, and bereavement-support specialists. They should call on these resources not only to assist them in caring for the patient but also as a sign that the patient will continue to receive appropriate care designed to promote comfort, dignity, and emotional and spiritual support. Though it is important to enlist the help of others at this time, nothing can replace the presence and compassionate care of the attending or primary treating physician.

H. Once the decision has been made . . .

If the decision has been made to forgo treatment, and it is likely the patient will die rather soon while in the hospital or other health care setting, physicians and other caregivers should observe the following:

- Be sure everyone involved in the patient's care is aware of the decision.

- Be appropriately present to the patient and family.
- Attend to any requests of the patient and family that can be accommodated.
- Address questions of organ and tissue donation as appropriate.
- Discontinue monitors and alarms.
- Cease any unnecessary treatments and assessments.
- Move the machinery away from the bed.
- Remove encumbering or disfiguring devices.
- Have pain medications readily available so they can be provided as needed.
- Attend to the psychosocial and spiritual needs of the patient and family.
- Allow time and space for family and other loved ones to be present to the patient.
- Prevent any unnecessary intrusions and noise in and around the patient's room.

Conclusion

As we have seen, deciding whether to forgo treatment at the end of life can be and often is a complex process. We have attempted to provide some insight into the ethical dimensions of these decisions by outlining a framework and moral norms and applying these to two particularly challenging issues, namely, ANH and medical futility. This framework and the moral norms do not provide clear-cut answers to every treatment decision at the end of life and do not eliminate the emotional complexity that often arises for patients, families, and caregivers faced with these tough decisions. However, they do provide a helpful backdrop against which we can better determine when treatment is proportionate, and thus morally obligatory, or disproportionate and thus morally optional in light of our duty to preserve life. To further your understanding of the framework and moral norms, we invite you to apply what you have learned in this chapter to the following cases.

Case Studies

Case 10A

Mrs. Neil is a 58-year-old school teacher. She had a stroke six weeks ago that left her with some severe deficits. Her doctor has told her family that because of her injury, she will not be able to walk on her own, feed herself, or be independent from full assistance for the rest of her life. Currently, she is still in the hospital and has not communicated with her family since her stroke. She is breathing on her own but will most likely experience unpredictable bouts of respiratory distress for the rest of her life, requiring future mechanical ventilation. She is receiving nutrients through a feeding tube, which has been inserted surgically in her stomach. Her husband wants the doctor to remove the feeding tube and allow the effects of the stroke to take their natural course. He is sure this is what his wife would want, especially given the grim diagnosis. He knows this not only from what she has told him in the past but also because of her free and independent character. She would not want to live like this. The doctor has told the husband that she does not feel comfortable removing the feeding tube because she believes it is necessary to sustain his wife's life.

Discussion questions. Do you think the husband's request is reasonable? What do you think about the doctor's response? If you were the husband, how would you proceed? Do you think you can remove this feeding tube and still honor the sanctity of Mrs. Neil's life?

Case 10B

Ms. Right is 79 years old and has end-stage renal disease and liver failure. She also has congestive heart failure and pneumonia and has been on and off the breathing machine during her four-week stay in the ICU. She is very sick, and her medical situation is critical. She was admitted with mental status changes, namely, confusion, memory loss, and loss of alertness. Her doctor has been talking with her and her family about whether CPR

cont.

Case 10B *cont.*

would be appropriate should she stop breathing or her heart stop beating. Her doctor believes she is not a candidate for CPR. Given her medical situation, she is not likely to survive the resuscitation attempt. The family, however, wants the doctor to attempt resuscitation. One night, late on his shift, the doctor is called to Ms. Right's room because she has gone into pulmonary arrest. Against the family's wishes, he does not proceed with CPR.

Discussion questions. Are you comfortable with the doctor's decision? Did he make the right choice? What would you say to him if you were Ms. Right's son or daughter?

Case 10C

Mr. Stanley is 83 years old. His cancer has recently spread to his brain. He has been admitted to the ICU with respiratory distress and pneumonia. He has been hospitalized four times in the past two months for similar reasons. Given his overall medical condition and very poor prognosis for a meaningful recovery, his doctor recommends forgoing mechanical ventilation in favor of an approach directed toward comfort. Mr. Stanley's wife disagrees with this plan. She wants everything done to keep him alive. She tells the doctor that it is criminal to suggest not using a breathing machine to keep her husband alive. She threatens to file a lawsuit against the hospital and the attending physician if they refuse. Knowing that a breathing machine will only prolong Mr. Stanley's death and will not offer any overall benefit to the patient, the doctor wants to deny Mrs. Stanley's request.

Discussion questions. Can the doctor do this? Should the doctor do this? How should doctors handle requests for treatments they know will not benefit patients?

Case 10D

Bob, a 38-year-old business executive, suffered a ruptured aorta in a car accident nearly eight years ago. The lack of oxygen

cont.

Case 10D *cont.*

to the brain that Bob sustained as a result of the injury left him in what is defined as a persistent vegetative state (PVS). Though Bob was unconscious and unable to communicate, he has been kept alive by a feeding tube medically inserted into his gastrointestinal tract that provides the nutrients and fluids needed to maintain life. After being treated in an acute care facility and two rehabilitation hospitals with no improvement in his overall condition, Bob was transferred to a Catholic nursing home where he has been now for more than five years. He continues to receive medical care, including artificial nutrition and hydration and other treatments as needed to manage the numerous complications that routinely arise, such as aspiration pneumonia, bed sores, urinary tract infection, and so on. Bob's wife of fourteen years, Lola, and their two children, Michael, 13, and Lilly, 11, visit him nearly every day. Bob's parents visit just as often and are supportive of Lola and the children.

Recently, Lola and Bob's parents approached Bob's physician and requested that he remove the feeding tube "keeping Bob's body alive." Lola said that this is what Bob would have wanted and that everything he did in life suggested he would never want to be "confined to a broken body" without any hope of recovery. She also noted that the constant vigil over Bob with no hope in sight was taking a tremendous toll on her, the children, and the rest of the family and that the costs of Bob's nursing home care were too much to sustain even with the help of Bob's parents and others. The physician agreed it was acceptable to remove the feeding tube from Bob but informed Lola he would have to check with administration to see if they could do it at the nursing home given recent Church statements on the issue of withdrawing nutrition and hydration from patients in Bob's condition.

Case 10E

Samuel Lions is an 84-year-old with end-stage lung cancer, progressive kidney disease, and severe dementia. He has been in the ICU for sixty-eight days on mechanical ventilation, dialysis (3 times per week), and a PEG tube. Several times the treating

cont.

Case 10E *cont.*

physician has tried to get the family to withdraw these aggressive treatments and enroll Samuel in a hospice program. Each attempt has failed as the family insists "everything should be done." Finally after having resuscitated Mr. Lions following his cardiac arrest, the treating physician informs the family he will longer acquiesce to their wishes because, in his words, "it is not in Mr. Lion's best interests, is causing a lot of distress among the nursing staff, and is not the best use of limited community-serving resources." The family objects and requests an ethics consult.

Case 10F

Josie, a 69-year-old woman with a long history of chronic obstructive pulmonary disease (COPD) and progressive dementia, is admitted to your hospital from a nursing home for post-seizure shortness of breath. For the last three months, she has been non-ambulatory and nonverbal and has been hospitalized twice, with a decline in function with each visit. On her last admission, her daughter, Susan, who is her durable power of attorney for health care, authorized a DNR order. However, upon receiving a call from the medicine intern in the ED where Josie was admitted, Susan refused to confirm her mother's DNR status and told the intern, "Do everything for her. Intubate her if you have to, just keep her alive." Josie was subsequently intubated and put on a ventilator. She was admitted to the ICU with a diagnosis of acute COPD exacerbation and treated. Five days later, with Josie showing no sign of improvement, the medical director of the ICU approached Susan and suggested she might want to consider taking her mom off the ventilator and allowing her to die. Susan broke down crying and stated she did not really know her mom's wishes and felt she would be killing her mom if she decided to "take her air away." She asks for an ethics consult to sort through the issues.

Case 10G

Mr. Z is a 79-year-old man with a history of diabetes and heart disease. He has been in and out of the hospital for the last eight

cont.

Case 10G cont.

months. On his last admission, it was discovered he had an infected left hip that required the removal of the hardware from his previous hip replacement surgery and aggressive antibiotic treatment to stem the infection that had developed. After being home for nearly four weeks, Mr. Z was brought back to the hospital by his son because of a high fever. The physicians found that the infection had reoccurred and that his leg, on the same side as the hip complications, was gangrenous. Further antibiotic therapy proved unsuccessful as the infection was resistant to the medications. Mr. Z subsequently had a stroke that left him unconscious, and he developed pneumonia and a severe infection in his blood. When asked by the attending physician about the future course of treatment, the son, who is Mr. Z's durable power of attorney for health care, said he wanted "everything done to keep my father alive," including, if necessary, amputating the gangrenous leg with partial pelvic removal, starting mechanical ventilation, and inserting a feeding tube. The attending physician was dismayed and told the son that what he was asking to be done was tantamount to torture. The son did not relent, however, and insisted that everything be done or else he would bring suit against the physician and the hospital as well as go to the local papers and tell them how the hospital wants to kill his father because of racial bias and financial concerns. The attending physician did not know what to do so she called for an ethics consult.

Case 10H

Josephine Stewart, a 78-year-old Caucasian woman with no family support, has lived for more than ten years with diabetes and, what she has called, "pretty painful" arthritis. In addition to these medical problems, Josephine had a pacemaker inserted nearly six years ago because of her severe arrhythmia. Yet despite all this, she remained very active: she was a regular volunteer at her parish, attended bingo with friends religiously, and even worked more than thirty hours a week at the Walmart near her home. About a year ago, Josephine noticed significant swelling in her face and neck as well as a "tightness in her chest"

cont.

Case 10H *cont.*

that had never been there before. Initially, she brushed these off as possible side effects from the new medication she was taking for her arthritis. Soon after, though, she began coughing up blood, which prompted her to visit her primary care physician. After extensive testing, it was determined that Josephine had non-small cell lung cancer (NSCLC) with lymph node metastases (N3), which made her ineligible for surgical resection. The consulting oncologist suggested, nonetheless, that she undergo chemotherapy to combat the spread of the disease and possibly induce a remission. After considerable reflection and talking with her pastor, Josephine consented to the chemotherapy.

Nine months of on-again, off-again chemotherapy did little to deter the NSCLC and after talking with her physicians, Josephine decided hospice was the best option for her. She told her oncologist "her time had come" and it "made no sense to keep fighting when God was calling." The hospice nurse was notified and the next day came to visit Josephine to discuss plans for leaving the hospital and being enrolled in hospice. During the visit the hospice nurse made it clear that all curative treatments would be forgone and that this included artificial nutrition and hydration. Josephine informed the nurse that she understood and made it clear she did not want a feeding tube if and when the time came. To the astonishment of the hospice nurse, though, Josephine asked if she could also have her pacemaker turned off. Her reason was she did not want to have her life prolonged "any more than it needed to be." The hospice nurse consulted with Josephine's primary care physician, who did not like the idea of turning off the pacemaker. She thought this was "tantamount to euthanasia" and called for an ethics consult to help her work through the conflict.

Case 10I

Mr. Kind is a 71-year-old man with multisystem organ failure. Presently, his kidneys are not functioning appropriately. However, his underlying problem is non-small cell lung cancer with metastases to the liver. He has been unconscious in this most

cont.

Case 10I *cont.*

recent hospitalization for more than five days. Fluid is accumulating around his heart, and within the last 24 hours he was placed on mechanical ventilation. This is the third hospitalization for Mr. Kind. His first resulted in physician requests to make him a "no code" or do-not-resuscitate and to limit the extent of aggressive technological interventions and instead focus solely on comfort care. Mr. Kind's three daughters, all of whom are single and have quit work to live with and care for their father, refuse to believe their father is dying and think that if appropriate medical interventions are given, he will go home and live peacefully for some months, if not years.

After Mr. Kind's daughters took him home following his first hospitalization, Mr. Kind seemed to stabilize for a short time, but was then hospitalized again with similar complications. Physicians and hospital staff took the same course of action and again requested a DNR order and minimal technological and intensive care use, only to have all of these requests denied by the daughters. The daughters have learned how to provide excellent home care and despite their father's limited mobility, he is free from infection, bedsores, and any other medical difficulties. The third and most recent hospitalization was caused by an increase in respiratory difficulty and an increasing lethargy and unresponsiveness. Again, physicians are requesting that Mr. Kind be made a "no code" and that he be removed from the intensive care unit and be given only comfort measures. The daughters see these requests as financially motivated and as disrespectful to the dignity of their father. They said if their father were not resuscitated upon arresting, they would bring a wrongful death suit against the hospital, as well as the participating physicians and nurses. Periodically, they invoke faith in support of their requests but never elaborate on the dictates of their faith.

Case 10J

Mrs. Y, an 89-year-old woman, was a resident of a skilled nursing facility (SNF), living in the same room since admission eight

cont.

Case 10J *cont.*

years ago. During this time, she was diagnosed with a dementia that was now fairly advanced. She was alert and able to recognize individual members of the nursing home staff. Her daughter was her closest relative and was quite involved in her care. Mrs. Y spoke only Greek despite living in the United States for many years. Apparently she had spent most of her time at home and had depended on her late husband for all communication and interaction with the non-Greek community. After suffering pneumonia a few weeks previously, her appetite diminished. She experienced a significant decline in her body weight and developed a painful decubitus ulcer. Her daughter reluctantly agreed to the placement of a nasogastric tube, voicing concerns over her mother's possible discomfort with the tube. Mrs. Y regained much of the lost weight. However, the tube repeatedly became dislodged and was finally removed altogether.

Mrs. Y again began to lose weight. The care team recommended placement of a percutaneous endoscopic gastrostomy tube. However, the nursing facility would require Mrs. Y be transferred to a different unit for residents with greater care needs. Mrs. Y's daughter said she would rather have her mother die than be moved from her "home." However, she agreed to the gastrostomy on the condition that they not change her residence. Mrs. Y never executed a formal advance directive and the daughter admitted to no direct knowledge of her mother's preference regarding artificial nutrition. She recalled her mother stating she "never wanted to become a burden" to her children and "when the time comes, God will take me." She also recalled that the patient's cousin had throat cancer and lived for many years at home with a feeding tube. Mrs. Y had remarked she was thankful the tube had allowed him to have a decent life despite the cancer.

The SNF complied with the daughter's request. The PEG was placed. During the next six months, Mrs. Y suffered from cellulitis at the PEG site and was sent to the hospital for endoscopic replacement of the tube after it fractured. She gradually became nonverbal and did not recognize her family but was alert and apparently comfortable. The tube became clogged and nonfunctional. The SNF contacted the daughter to have the

cont.

Case 10J *cont.*

tube replaced, but the daughter refused, stating that her mother "had no life" and that she should be left in peace. Her caregivers told the daughter that you "can't starve her to death."

Case 10K

Ms. Jones, a 79-year-old widow, had been a resident of a nursing home for several years. In the past she had experienced repeated transient ischemic attacks (brief neurological disturbances due to decreased cerebral blood flow). Because of progressive dementia, Ms. Jones had lost some of her cognitive abilities and had become somewhat disoriented. She also had episodes of thrombophlebitis, as well as congestive heart failure. Her daughter visited often and obviously loved her deeply. One day Ms. Jones was found unconscious on her bathroom floor. She was hospitalized and diagnosed with a severe cerebrovascular accident (stroke). She recovered minimally, remaining mostly nonverbal, but continuing to manifest a withdrawal from noxious stimuli and exhibiting some purposeful behaviors. Ms. Jones refused to allow the temporary placement of the nasogastric (NG) tube. At each attempt she thrashed about violently and pushed the NG tube away. After the tube was finally placed, Ms. Jones pulled off her restraints and managed to remove it. After several days, her sites for intravenous infusion were exhausted and the caregivers approached Ms. Jones' daughter about inserting a PEG tube, which would offer long-term fluid and nutritional support. Though the daughter was legally designated as Ms. Jones' health care agent, she did not know what her mom would want in this situation because her mom would always say, "God will take me when it is my time to go."

SUGGESTED READINGS

Brody, Howard et al. "Withdrawing Intensive Life-Sustaining Treatment." *New England Journal of Medicine* 336 (February 27, 1997): 652–7.

Hamel, Ronald, and Michael R. Panicola. "Must We Preserve Life?" *America* 190 (April 19, 2004): 6–13.

Hamel, Ronald P., and James J. Walter, eds., *Artificial Nutrition and Hydration and the Permanently Unconscious Patient: The Catholic Debate.* Washington, DC: Georgetown University Press, 2007.

Kelly, David F. *Medical Care at the End of Life: A Catholic Perspective.* Washington, DC: Georgetown University Press, 2006.

McCormick, Richard A. *The Critical Calling: Reflections on Moral Dilemmas Since Vatican II.* Washington, DC: Georgetown University Press, 1989.

Miles, Stephen H. "Informed Demand for 'Non-Beneficial' Medical Treatment." *New England Journal of Medicine* 325 (August 15, 1991): 512–5.

Panicola, Michael R. "A Catholic Guide to Medically Administered Nutrition and Hydration." In *A Catholic Guide to Health Care Ethics,* edited by Ronald Hamel, 109–26. Saint Louis: Liguori Publications, 2006.

Schneiderman, Lawrence J. *Embracing Our Mortality: Hard Choices in an Age of Medical Miracles.* New York: Oxford University Press, 2008.

Schneiderman, Lawrence J., and Nancy S. Jecker. *Wrong Medicine: Doctors, Patients, and Futile Treatment.* Baltimore: Johns Hopkins University Press, 1995.

MULTIMEDIA AIDS FOR TEACHERS

The Death of Nancy Cruzan. PBS *Frontline.* 1992. For information see *www. pbs.org/wgbh/pages/frontline/programs/info/1014.html.* This 90-minute video documenting the case of Nancy Cruzan may be hard to obtain, but many university libraries, especially those with medical or law schools, have copies.

Persistent Vegetative State: To Live . . . or Let Die. DIA Learning. 2006. For information see *http://fac.ethicsprograms.com/.* This 30-minute video can be purchased separately or together with other videos on select issues in health care ethics.

The Terri Schiavo Story. Franklin Springs Family Media. 2009. For information see *http://www.amazon.com/Terri-Schiavo-Story-Schaivos-family/ dp/B001REMSHG.*

ABC News Nightline Terri Schiavo. ABC News. 2008. For information see *http://www.amazon.com/ABC-News-Nightline-Terri-Schiavo/dp/ B0012JHX1W/ref=pd_cp_d_1.*

The Cost of Dying. CBS *60 Minutes.* 2009. For information see *http://www. amazon.com/60-Minutes-Cost-Dying-November/dp/B002XZMJZY/ref= sr_1_8?s=dvd&ie=UTF8&qid=1293495920&sr=1-8.*

ENDNOTES

1. Much of what follows is adapted from Michael R. Panicola, "A Catholic Guide to Medically Administered Nutrition and Hydration," in *A Catholic Guide to Health Care Ethics,* ed. Ronald Hamel (Liguori, 2006), 109–26; and Ronald Hamel and Michael R. Panicola, "Must We Preserve Life?" America 190 (April 19, 2004): 6–13.

2. Daniel A. Cronin, *Conserving Human Life,* ed. Russell E. Smith (Braintree, MA: Pope John Center, 1989), 92. This work is a republication of Cronin's doctrinal dissertation *The Moral Law in Regard to the Ordinary and Extraordinary Means of Conserving Life* (Rome: Gregorianum, 1958).

3. Congregation for the Doctrine of the Faith, "Declaration on Euthanasia," May 5, 1980, accessible at *http://www.vatican.va/roman_curia/congregations/cfaith/documents/rc_con_cfaith_doc_19800505_euthanasia_en.html.*

4. John Paul II, *Evangelium vitae,* March 25, 1995, accessible at *http://www.vatican.va/holy_father/john_paul_ii/encyclicals/documents/hf_jp-ii_enc_25031995_evangelium-vitae_en.html.*

5. See, for example, the Hastings Center, *Guidelines on the Termination of Life-Sustaining Treatment and Care of the Dying* (Briar Cliff Manor, NY: Hastings Center, 1987); Cynthia B. Cohen, ed., *Casebook on the Termination of Life-Sustaining Treatment and the Care of the Dying* (Briar Cliff Manor, NY: Hastings Center, 1988).

6. The medical information in this section comes from Myles Sheehan, "Feeding Tubes: Sorting Out the Issues," *Health Progress* 82 (November–December 2001): 22–7.

7. Cronin, *Conserving Human Life,* 90.

8. John Paul II, "Address to the Participants in the International Congress on 'Life-Sustaining Treatments and Vegetative State: Scientific Advances and Ethical Dilemmas,'" March 20, 2004, accessible at *http://www.vatican.va/holy_father/john_paul_ii/speeches/2004/march/documents/hf_jp-ii_spe_20040320_congress-fiamc_en.html.*

9. U.S. Conference of Catholic Bishops, *Ethical and Religious Directives for Catholic Health Care Services,* 5th ed., November 17, 2009, accessible at *http://www.usccb.org/meetings/2009Fall/docs/ERDs_5th_ed_091118_FINAL.pdf.*

10. Thomas E. Finucane, "Tube Feeding in Patients with Advanced Dementia: A Review of the Evidence," *JAMA* 282 (1999): 1365–70.

11. Francisco de Vittoria, *Comentarios a la Secunda Secundae de Santo Tomas,* in II:II, q. 147, art. 1 (trans. as in Cronin, *Conserving Human Life,* 37).

12. Lawrence J. Schneiderman and Nancy S. Jecker, "Is the Treatment Beneficial, Experimental, or Futile?" *Cambridge Quarterly of Healthcare Ethics* 5 (1996): 248–56, at 249–50.

13. Lawrence J. Schneiderman and Nancy S. Jecker, *Wrong Medicine: Doctors, Patients, and Futile Treatment* (Baltimore, MD: Johns Hopkins University Press, 1995), esp. chapters 1–3.

14. Mark J. Hanson and Daniel Callahan, eds. *The Goals of Medicine: The Forgotten Issues in Health Care Reform* (Washington, DC: Georgetown University Press, 1999).

15. Ina Li, "Feeding Tubes in Patients with Severe Dementia," *American Family Physician* 65 (April 15, 2002): 1605–10.

16. J. P. Burns and R. D. Truog, "Futility: A Concept in Evolution," *Chest* 132, no. 6 (December 2007): 1987–93.

17. D.J. Murphy and T. E. Finucane, "New Do-Not-Resuscitate Policies: A First Step in Cost Control," *Archives of Internal Medicine* 153, no. 14 (July 26, 1993): 1641–8.

18. L. J. Schneiderman, N. S. Jecker, and A. R. Jonsen, "Medical Futility: Its Meaning and Ethical Implications," *Annals of Internal Medicine*, 112, no.12 (June 15, 1990): 949–54.

19. R. D. Truog, A.S. Brett, and J. Frader, "The Problem with Futility," *New England Journal of Medicine* 326, no. 23 (June 4, 1992): 1560–64.

20. A. Halevy and B. A. Brody, "A Multi-Institution Collaborative Policy on Medical Futility," *Journal of the American Medical Association* 276, no. 7 (August 21, 1996): 571–4.

21. C. W. Plows et al., "Medical Futility in End-of-Life Care: Report of the Council on Ethical and Judicial Affairs," *Journal of the American Medical Association* 281, no. 10 (March 10, 1999): 937–41.

22. R. L. Fine and T. W. Mayo, "Resolution of Futility by Due Process: Early Experience with Texas Advance Directives," *Annals of Internal Medicine* 138, no. 9 (May 6, 2003): 743–6. See also, M. L. Smith et al., "Texas Hospitals' Experience with the Texas Advance Directives Act," *Critical Care Medicine* 35, no. 5 (May 2007): 1271–6.

23. Burns and Truog, "Futility: A Concept in Evolution," 1991.

24. Burns and Truog, "Futility: A Concept in Evolution," 1991–92.

25. Burns and Truog, "Futility: A Concept in Evolution," 1992.

CHAPTER 11

Rethinking End-of-Life Care

David Belde

Introduction

In January 1988, the *Journal of the American Medical Association* (AMA) published a terse article recounting the experience of an anonymous medical resident at a large private hospital who, for only a few minutes, took care of a patient named Debbie. Debbie was 20 years old and painfully dying from ovarian cancer. Debbie's only words to the medical resident were, "Let's get this over with." In response, the medical resident proceeded to inject the patient with morphine. Within four minutes, Debbie died.[1]

The article prompted a series of responses in a subsequent edition of the same journal. Some declared that euthanasia and assisted suicide should be available options to patients, especially in those rare cases where modern medicine cannot relieve intractable pain and suffering.[2] Others warned that euthanasia threatens the moral fabric of medicine to its core and that, even in response to a specific patient's request or demand, euthanasia has no rightful place in the medical profession.[3] Some wondered whether patient requests for direct aid from physicians in facilitating death were not simply a response from patients and the public to the increased medicalization of the dying process—a process many believe is controlled by clinicians and the medical establishment and not patients. As a result, end-of-life (EoL) care, at least at that time, was inadequately meeting the myriad needs of dying patients and their families.[4]

Three years later, Dr. Timothy Quill, a renowned advocate for better EoL care and an outspoken supporter of physician-assisted suicide, published the now-famous article "Death and Dignity: A Case of Individualized Decision Making," in the *New England Journal of Medicine.*[5] In the article, Quill recounts his experience caring for one of his patients, Diane. A patient of Quill's for more than eight years, Diane was diagnosed with leukemia and decided not to pursue aggressive, curative treatment. Moreover, when it was no longer possible for Diane to maintain "control of herself and her own dignity," she sought assistance from her doctor in taking her life. Quill's article soon took a central place in the debate over what precisely counts as good EoL care. Even though EoL care does not solely concern whether physician-assisted suicide and euthanasia should be legal, two states, Oregon and Washington, have legalized physician-assisted suicide. A third state, Montana, subsequent to its December 2009 supreme court ruling in favor of the constitutionality of physician-assisted suicide, is now debating whether to legalize physician-assisted suicide. Countries across Western Europe are debating similar policies. Other countries, like the Netherlands, have long held that physician-assisted suicide and euthanasia are ethically permissible.

Though we have made significant strides in EoL care in the years since the *JAMA* and Quill articles were published, clinicians, patients, and families continue to report that symptoms associated with illness near the EoL are not often adequately controlled,[6] that patient wishes and values regarding their personal preferences for EoL care are often unknown, are underappreciated, or insufficiently inform decision making in the EoL context,[7] and that the processes health care institutions use to help patients and families prepare for the dying process—such as assistance with completing an advance directive—are unhelpful.[8]

Getting EoL care right is extremely important. Though much of the "public" conversation around EoL care is often dominated by debates over the permissibility of physician-assisted suicide and euthanasia, there is much about EoL that gets overlooked. Given the normative basis and ethical priorities we argue for in this book (see also chapter 10, "Forgoing Treatment at the End of Life"), we argue that physician-assisted suicide and euthanasia are unnecessary for meeting the care demands of dying patients. Often, requests for physician-assisted suicide or euthanasia are a cry for help or an indication that one's physical, emotional, social, or spiritual needs are not being met.

Most people who die each year in the United States do so as a result of a chronic illness. Most have experienced many hospitalizations over the course of their illness, especially during the last six months of life. In fact, more than 33 percent of persons who die each year in the United States see ten different physicians in the last six months of life.[9] Much can be made of this overwhelming statistic, but for the chronically ill, and the dying person in particular, it means that one of the primary elements in rethinking EoL care must be to create better processes for planning and preparing for death. Dying persons have one chance to tailor their dying process in a way that is consistent with their particular understanding of what brings meaning and purpose to their life. The failure to meet the needs of dying persons during such a time of utter dependence and vulnerability should concern us all. The death of a loved one is memory making for those left behind, who will need to form a new way of living in the aftermath of their loss. To leave grieving loved ones with final memories and images of the one they lost in pain or suffering only compounds their grief. This is especially true if this pain and suffering could have been prevented.

In chapter 1, we framed health care ethics as having three over-lapping levels of inquiry. We referred to these as the macro, middle, and micro levels of health care ethics. Macro issues in health care ethics center on health policy issues such as health care reform. Middle issues in health care ethics center on organizational concerns such as patient rights and responsibilities and strategic planning. Micro issues center on clinically oriented ethical issues such as forgoing life-sustaining treatment. EoL care spans all three levels, giving it a degree of significance that other ethical issues in health care may not have. From a macro ethical perspective, the focus is on ethical issues at the health policy level. From this standpoint, health care reform stands front and center. End-of-life care is expensive, especially EoL care that is delivered in acute care hospitals. Rethinking how EoL care is understood and delivered can promote a more efficient and humane use of resources for individuals and for society as a whole. From a middle ethical perspective, the focus is on ethical issues at the organizational level. From this standpoint, EoL care has become one of many priorities for health care organizations. As a result, our focus on getting it right has diminished. In rethinking EoL care, given its overall importance for promoting human well-being, giving EoL care a more central priority in organizational life is warranted. From a micro ethical perspective, the focus is on ethical issues that arise in the context of clinical care. This book is testament to the many ethical issues that arise at this level. Suffice it say, on balance and historically, many of these very issues emerge from within EoL care.

In this chapter EoL care is examined in more detail, specifically, with a view toward improving it for all those involved. In the light of our normative basis of ethics, which provides a foundation for judging how the structure and delivery of health care can best enhance human flourishing, we believe that EoL care in the United States requires rethinking. Though we believe the ethical issues associated with EoL care are relatively well known, not enough progress has been made in meeting basic and key goals including managing physical symptoms associated with the dying process, enhancing communication around the values and preferences that patients, families, and caregivers bring to EoL decision making, and coordinating care so that the needs of dying patients are met seamlessly as they experience EoL care at various settings in the community.[10]

In what follows, we present five specific strategies that we believe will enhance EoL care in the United States. We recognize that EoL care takes place in many institutions and settings, from hospitals to nursing homes to long-term care centers to the home. Also, EoL care applies to both pediatric and adult populations. While our strategies emerge from evidence-based studies primarily in the adult population, there is no apparent reason why these strategies could not also be applied in the pediatric population. Before examining these strategies, how and where people die is addressed in order to create a better understanding of health care delivery in the EoL context.

Setting the Context: Health Care at the End of Life

EoL care is the care of persons who have been diagnosed with a terminal illness, those who are actively dying and near death, and those who have made a conscious choice to shift the goals of their care from curative and aggressive to comfort-oriented. EoL care ideally takes account of the holistic needs and concerns of patients, not just their physical needs and concerns. Evidence for the progress we have made in caring for the dying includes the creation of advanced training programs for clinical professionals. The best example of this is the growth of the hospice and palliative medicine specialty. Though by no means the only clinical professionals who attend to dying persons, the emergence and growth of palliative and hospice care are indications that care for dying persons is complex and multifactorial.

More and more hospitals are integrating palliative medicine into their specialty referral services. Palliative care, as we discuss in more detail below, focuses on treating the symptoms—most notably physical pain and existential suffering—that inevitably arise when working with patients who have a life-limiting illness. From this standpoint, palliative care is principally designed to keep patients informed about their illness, to discuss the goals of care as their disease progresses, to respect that their life plan and set of experiences will shape their values and wishes in the EoL context, and to promote as much quality of life as possible, given one's overall medical condition.[11] Most people will experience their death over time and as a process. It is the role of palliative care specialists—working in collaboration with other clinicians in the various settings in which dying persons seek care—to coordinate care along the progression of a life-limiting illness.

Aside from accidents, most deaths result from a chronic illness that will require one or even many hospitalizations over the course of the illness.[12] A chronic illness is one that lasts three or more months, generally cannot be prevented by vaccines or cured by medication, and does not disappear. A chronic illness, like congestive heart failure or chronic obstructive pulmonary disease, may last several years. More than 90 million Americans have at least one chronic illness and 70 percent of all deaths are due to complications associated with a chronic disease.[13] EoL care can be expensive, especially for persons with a chronic illness.[14] Many persons with a chronic illness will have two to six visits to an intensive care unit (ICU) in the final six months of life. This adds stress to patients and families and raises questions about whether such care even benefits the patient. EoL care in an ICU is challenging for patients, often marked by inadequate control of pain and other symptoms, poor communication about patient values and the goals of care, and ethical conflict among patients, families, and clinicians.[15]

Where people die is an important factor in good EoL care. For those who die in the hospital setting, it is common for their deaths to be preceded by removing some form—often many forms—of life-sustaining treatment. Most of these treatments are removed in a stepwise fashion, as opposed to being removed all at once. Their removal is often influenced by clinician bias. For instance, some clinicians are predisposed to allow the removal of blood products but not artificial nutrition and hydration.[16] This can affect patient well-being through the unnecessary prolongation of pain and suffering. A better approach would be to understand that all life-sustaining treatments have attendant side effects. Such side effects can be amplified in dying persons. The patient is the best person to judge whether these side effects are burdensome or beneficial. As noted in chapter 10, forgoing life-sustaining treatment is a commonly accepted practice by many in the clinical, ethical, and legal communities. It should not impede good EoL care, as it often appears to in the health care ethics literature. In fact, when done appropriately, given the particular circumstances of each situation, removing life-sustaining treatment with skill and compassion is an essential element of good EoL care for dying patients who may need or choose this route of medical management.[17]

In surveys, most Americans report they want to die at home.[18] Patients who experience their EoL care at home—as well as their families—report increased satisfaction with the entire process as compared to patients (and their families) who do not have their EoL in the home.[19] Even though hospital deaths are declining while home deaths are on the rise, more people continue to die in some form of institution (hospital, long-term care facility, nursing home) than at home.[20]

Many individuals choose hospice services when they have entered into the terminal phase of their illness. By *terminal*, we mean the phase of the dying process in which only the symptoms of illness are being treated, not the underlying disease itself. During this phase, curative treatments cease because they are no longer beneficial from the patient's perspective, or because the patient has chosen to modify the goals of care. This typically occurs in the last weeks to months of life. Hospice services cover a wide array of interventions aimed toward the holistic treatment of patients. These typically include pain and symptom management, spiritual and psychosocial needs of the patient, and family bereavement services. Hospice services are usually provided in the home but can be delivered in other care settings, including hospitals, nursing homes, and long-term care centers. In 2009, more than 1 million people died under the care of a hospice organization. This amounts to approximately 41 percent of all deaths in the United States.[21]

The median length of service in hospice is twenty-one days—meaning that half of all hospice patients received care in hospice for less than three weeks and the other half received care in hospice for more than three weeks. Patients and families tend to report high satisfaction with hospice. Contrary to popular belief, hospice services can actually prolong the lives of some terminally patients. This is principally due to better management of symptoms, which helps stabilize patients.[22] If patients and families perceive that hospice referrals are unnecessarily delayed for some reason, they tend to report decreased satisfaction with hospice as whole. For this reason, many people are advocating for better standardization around the practices and processes that manage the timely identification of hospice patients and referrals to hospice.

An Inadequate System

Clinicians report that systems in place for EoL care often do not sufficiently meet the needs of patients. Inadequacies include the lack of coordination of patient care from the inpatient setting (hospital) to the outpatient setting (doctor's office). Clinicians have different knowledge and skill sets, and many lack technical and interpersonal skill in the oversight of good EoL care. As a result, many medical organizations such as the American Medical Association, the American Academy of Hospice and Palliative Medicine, and the Center to Advance Palliative Care have justifiably created evidence-based practice guidelines for EoL care, drafted consensus statements, and dedicated clinical research to issues related to improving EoL care.

Given that people receiving EoL care experience unnecessary burdens due to the lack of adequate control of their symptoms; that poor communication between and among clinicians, patients, and families continues to exist; that more persons want to die at home than currently are doing so; that EoL care across various settings tends to be poorly coordinated; and that many clinicians are not adequately trained in technical or interpersonal aspects of EoL care, we need to focus on making systemic changes to remedy these issues. In the next section, strategies for rethinking how EoL care is approached in the United States are examined.

Discussion: Ethical Issues and Analysis

Strategies for Rethinking End-of-Life Care

We argue that EoL care requires a systematic approach to promote better outcomes for dying patients. A systematic approach is one that takes into account all aspects of high-quality EoL care and then creates a rational and humane process for aligning these aspects toward the best outcomes for dying persons. Providing care for persons facing life-limiting illness in the hospital setting is a complex enterprise. It is not unusual for one patient to have several doctors involved in his or her care. For instance, it is common for ICU patients to have a "hospitalist" physician whose role is to oversee and coordinate all aspects of care. ICU patients often also have an "intensivist" to manage the dimensions of critical care, especially the pulmonary aspects of care. In addition to these physicians, ICU patients commonly have other specialists to monitor their heart, kidneys, and neurological state. There is likely to be an infectious disease specialist to prevent and manage the multitude of infections that often beset a critically ill person. Other providers may include dieticians, pharmacists, respiratory therapists, or wound-control specialists. This is complexity at its height. All of this is well intended and directed toward the overall good of the patient with life-limiting illness. However, without significant attention to how these specialists communicate with one another and how they and other care providers communicate with patients (at least those who are able) and families, it can be all too easy to lose sight of the big-picture plan for care of critically ill patients.

At least five basic steps can be taken to make EoL care systems work better for patients: (1) reinforce the core values and goals of medicine, (2) establish parameters and consensus around the primary attributes of a "good death," (3) incorporate narrative competence into EoL care, (4) promote a systematic approach to advance care planning, and (5) use palliative and hospice care appropriately across the continuum of care. Each is addressed in turn.

Reinforce the Core Values and Goals of Medicine

The goals of medicine stem from the normative values of medicine. Over the centuries, a core set of goals for medicine has been offered as a means to shape its ethical basis. These goals have developed as a guide to better understand why medicine exists in the first place. Daniel Callahan, a noted bioethicist, who, along with colleagues across the world, conducted a five-year international study dedicated to gaining consensus around the goals of medicine,[23] argues that medicine has four primary goals:[24]

1. the prevention of disease and injury and the promotion and maintenance of health
2. the relief of pain and suffering caused by maladies
3. the care or cure of those with a malady and the care of those who cannot be cured
4. the avoidance of a premature death and the pursuit of a peaceful death

These goals require a holistic view of the person. They have a "both-and" character that requires broad focus and a commitment to balance. For example, in caring for the dying, one is mindful of disease and maintaining the patient's overall health. In relieving physical pain, one must also be mindful of existential suffering. For dying persons, a general and underlying philosophy of care must balance one's desire to cure specific problems. Finally, one cannot allow a general aversion regarding a premature death to drown out the importance of a peaceful death. Dying persons often experience significant physical and psychosocial distress that can result in the disintegration of the self. EoL care is an ideal domain in which to incorporate these medical goals precisely because, we believe, there is no other context in medicine in which treating a person holistically and with due proportion is more vital.

Although these goals may appear straightforward and basic, there is much that can impede their integration into EoL care. For instance, there could be disagreement about which goals of medicine

relate to EoL care. There could be turf battles over who has ultimate authority and responsibility for incorporating these goals into
EoL care structures and processes. Often, as the section on futility
in chapter 10 indicates, patient values are not aligned with the goals
of medicine. This can inhibit the peaceful death that Callahan uses
to anchor one of his goals of medicine. As Callahan argues, different
patients have different needs. A curing mentality is not helpful when
a patient is dying. Knowing when to shift from curing and caring to
caring only is a judgment that can be difficult to make. These goals
alone cannot solve disagreements among stakeholders. Only persons
working together and in relationship can do this. These goals do offer
an organizing humanistic basis for the practice of medicine.

Establish Parameters and Consensus around the Primary Attributes of a "Good Death"

To be sure, a "good death" is an elusive concept and notions of a good
death are far from univocal. Even in a clinical setting in which there is
relative agreement on professional norms such as the goals of medicine,
there may not be consensus on contentious issues such as whether physician-assisted suicide or euthanasia fall within the parameters of good
EoL care. What we believe to be credible, however, is what appears to
be the shared consensus among caregivers, patients, and families about
EoL care. This consensus, though it may be fragile in individual cases,
is reflected in evidence-based studies in the health care profession that
report the experiences of dying persons, their loved ones, and clinicians.[25] For instance, Steinhauser et al. report that patients, families, and
clinicians agree on the importance of five key elements in preparing for
the dying process: (1) identifying clear decision makers if the patient
cannot make decisions, (2) understanding how the dying process will
proceed, (3) having one's financial affairs in order, (4) controlling the
place and timing of one's death, and (5) resolving unfinished personal
business in one's relationships. The question for EoL care providers
and those institutions providing EoL care is, How can adequate care
be "institutionalized" into EoL care processes? The short answer is
through collaborative teamwork, system monitoring, and evaluation.[26]

  In their research on EoL care for those with life-limiting illness, Judith Nelson and colleagues report on the factors that present

obstacles to good EoL care.[27] They divide their findings into three categories: patient/family factors, institutional/ICU factors, and clinician factors. For the sake of simplicity, only the top five issues identified as requiring systemic attention in each category are listed in figure 1.

- **Patient/Family Factors**
    - unrealistic patient and/or family expectations for prognosis or effectiveness of ICU treatment
    - inability of many patients to participate in treatment decisions
    - lack of advance directives
    - disagreements within families on care goals
    - absence of a surrogate decision maker for patients lacking this capacity

- **Institutional/ICU Factors**
    - suboptimal space for meeting with families of ICU patients
    - lack of palliative care service to which a dying patient can be transferred
    - the "technological imperative" of the ICU[28]
    - ICU admission of patients not predicted to survive critical illness
    - insufficient recognition by colleagues or institutional leadership of the importance of optimal EoL care

- **Clinician Factors**
    - insufficient clinician training in communication about EoL care issues
    - competing demands for clinicians' time
    - inadequate communication between the ICU team and patient/families about appropriate goals of care
    - fear of legal liability for forgoing life-sustaining treatment
    - unrealistic expectations by clinicians for patient prognosis or effectiveness of ICU treatment

FIGURE 11A Factors Affecting EoL Care

Based on the results of this research, if one were to set out only to mitigate how open, frank, and ongoing communication about the goals of treatment are inhibited within the care system, the resulting system changes would most likely enhance EoL care.[29]

Steinhauser and colleagues examined the observations of patients, families, and clinical providers regarding what a good death actually looks like.[30] Where Nelson and colleagues state the barriers to good EoL care, Steinhauser and colleagues aim to identify what constitutes good EoL care. In their research, six themes emerged that can help ground a rethinking of EoL care: (1) pain and symptom management, (2) clear decision making, (3) preparation for death, (4) completion/spiritual meaning, (5) contributing to others, and (6) affirmation of the whole person.[31]

Pain and symptom management is straightforward. Dying persons fear they will die in pain. This fear, in turn, can cause existential distress. Clear decision making refers to the degree to which communication flows freely and in both directions between patients and their clinicians. Dying persons not only want a voice in their treatment plan, they also want opportunities to express their values and wishes about life's meaning as it comes to an end. Perhaps most important in Steinhauser's research, dying persons want their preferences known. Emotional reserves can be low in the death and dying context and knowing a dying person's preferences can prevent crisis-driven decision making.

In terms of preparing for death, Steinhauser and colleagues found dying persons want to know what to expect as the dying process progresses—emotionally, physically, rationally, and spiritually. In addition, this aspect includes finding opportunities to gain a sense of closure—economically and relationally. Spiritually, dying persons hope to achieve completion in life. They want their death process to be meaningful. They seek this completion through life review, conflict resolution, being in the presence of loved ones, and saying their good-byes. Ira Byock, a physician with more than twenty-five years of experience in caring for dying persons, believes that dying persons can find completion by saying, and experiencing, four things: please forgive me, I forgive you, thank you, and I love you.[32] This may be viewed as a spiritual practice that speaks to the importance of seeing persons as more than skin and bones.

In their discussion of the study, the authors report that the first four domains are standard in the EoL care literature,[33] although the final two are "unexpected" findings and therefore advance the understanding of what enhances patient well-being in the dying. Steinhauser and colleagues claim that the fifth domain, contributing to others, posits the view that as "death approaches, many patients reflect on their successes and failures and discover that personal relationships outweigh professional or monetary gains."[34] Though they expected to find that dying persons need good health care, they "did not consider the extent to which they also need to reciprocate. . . . Dying patients need to participate in the same human interactions that are important throughout all of life."[35] The sixth domain, affirmation of the whole person, reflects the view that dying persons are more than "diseased" patients and that they have a desire to be "understood . . . in the context of their lives, values, and preferences."[36] The "very personal language of this theme"[37] indicates a simple, though strong "desire to simply be known"[38] as a person first and not merely as another medical case. In the study, the authors report how one physician remembers a dying patient:

> That last day I saw him in the emergency room, he was looking at me with those roving eyes and gasping for breath. I leaned over him and stroked his hair. He looked at me and said, "How's that new house of yours?" "I'm not really moved in." And he said, "You make sure you decorate it nicely." It was a very personal interchange. He was dying, and his last interaction with me was as a person, not as a doctor.[39]

Steinhauser and colleagues suggest that their study points to one of the failures of modern medicine, particularly as it relates to EoL care, and this is the failure to see the dying process as more than a simply biomedical, physical event. This failure, they claim, has implications for medical education and clinical practice. Cultural attitudes around death, they rightly maintain, changed significantly in the twentieth century:

> When people died primarily at home, family, community, and clergy assumed responsibility for EoL decision making in ways that modern, high-tech rescue medicine often

impedes. As the location of death shifted to the hospital, physicians became the gatekeepers. As a result, death is viewed through the lens of biomedical explanation and is primarily defined as a physical event. Most medical education programs and training regimens reinforce that framework.[40]

At the end of life, such a strict biomedical view is shortsighted, for "psychosocial and spiritual issues are as important as physiologic concerns," and "patients and families want relationships with health-care providers that affirm this more encompassing view."[41] Modern medicine excels at separating parts from the whole. In the current medical model, each part of the body receives close attention. Medical specialists have an opportunity to treat the patient with their best set of tools. In the separation of the body part from the whole body, however, a tendency emerges to lose sight of the big picture and its significance for the overall well-being of the person. One answer to this need for a more comprehensive and holistic approach to EoL care comes from the growing trend in medicine to incorporate narrative competence in clinical and ethical decision making.

Incorporate Narrative Competence into EoL Care

Narrative competence refers to a caregiver's ability to enter into the worldview of a patient to get to know the patient as a person. All persons have a unique story. The role of EoL caregivers is to elicit that story so that it can be integrated respectfully into the care process. All too often, a patient is viewed only as a patient with a specific malady. The important decisions, experiences, and values that all persons have often remain unknown. To incorporate a patient's personal narrative or life story into the shared decision-making processes of EoL care requires skills that many clinical providers do not learn in their training.[42] To understand, rather than simply assume, what individual dying persons consider important in their notions of human flourishing, concerted efforts to recognize, absorb, interpret, and be moved by particular, individual narratives are increasingly being embraced in the medical community.[43]

Though it may appear that narrative competence is a recent addition to holistic health care delivery, Sir William Osler (1849–1919), one of the most influential physician educators in the modern era, understood quite well the importance of coming to know the patient well in order to properly attend to the patient's needs: "For the junior student in medicine and surgery it is a safe rule to have no teaching without a patient for a text, and the best teaching is that taught by the patient himself."[44] To Osler's point, good medicine requires good relationships that, in turn, promote a deeper understanding of a person's needs. In the end, all individuals will succumb to death. This reality does not have to mean that care cannot be tailored to meet the specific notions of value, meaning, and purpose held by individual dying persons.

Narrative competence represents a "move beyond rational objectivity in ethics" and considers the "uniqueness of individuals" from a "particular perspective as a situated self."[45] This is a challenge to clinical reasoning, for clinical reasoning is largely a rational, objective effort: elicit symptoms, conduct an exam, infer what could be the problem, diagnose the patient, recommend a course of treatment, and follow up with the patient. This process is largely rational and objective. Though critically important, purely objective approaches to reasoning alone are not sufficient to effect holistic healing for dying persons.

Narrative reasoning, in contrast, is less about linear and logical analysis and more about emotional connection and intuitive judgment. In the EoL setting, this approach is helpful in illuminating, as well as understanding and appreciating, the particular values of the dying person, for these are the values that emerge within the context of one's life plan. If intuitive ethical reasoning is to have any value in promoting human flourishing for dying persons, a significant investment must be made in relating with patients in ways that are often unfamiliar in today's rescue-oriented, technologically driven mode of caregiving. Narrative reasoning begins with engaging another's experience. This beginning is other-centered, not medicine-centered. Such a point of departure for EoL care validates the importance that particular notions of flourishing can have in making each patient feel recognized as uniquely original and therefore valued.

Promote a Systemic Approach to Advance Care Planning

Advance care planning refers to the process by which individuals—no matter where they are on the health–sickness continuum—plan their future health care decisions. One method by which individuals make future plans for their treatment is by completing advance directives. There are many kinds of advance directives, including oral declarations of one's future wishes, living-will documents that state a person's wishes should certain conditions be met, and durable power of attorney documents in which a patient appoints someone to make decisions on his or her behalf should the patient lose that capacity. After years of experience with such processes, many have concluded that attempts to promote advance directives have largely failed.[46] Completing an advance directive is one thing, but working through a formal process of advance care planning dynamically and systematically over the course of a life-limiting illness is altogether different.[47]

Advance care planning is best understood as a process, not a single event in the life of a perfectly healthy or severely chronically ill person. Advance care planning is, in its simplest form, best understood as care coordination across what clinicians call the continuum of care. Chronically ill persons with life-limiting illnesses will receive care in many different settings across a wide span of time: their doctor's office, ambulatory surgery centers, dialysis centers, hospitals, and rehabilitation facilities. It is likely that such chronically ill persons will receive care multiple times within these various facilities throughout the course of their illness. Not only are these separate care sites, they are most likely separate agencies operating independently from each other. Throughout all these points of care, especially within the practice of one's primary care doctor, one would think that opportunities abound for discussions about patient beliefs, preferences, priorities, and values that inform one's views about decision making in the EoL context when one's underlying illness progresses to its terminal and more final stages. Yet, such discussions do not appear to be happening enough. To date, aside from some pockets of success across the country,[48] there has not been a broad, sustained success in developing processes that promote advance care planning.

Where advance care planning has been successful, the process has included the following broad steps: "(1) Ensure that patients and families clearly understand the health condition, (2) design a plan around the patient's beliefs and values, (3) store the plan in a rapidly retrievable format through the health system, and (4) have system-wide commitment in honoring the plan."[49] Perhaps the best evidence for this comes from the advance care planning process in La Crosse, Wisconsin. The advance care planning process in this Midwestern community is named "Respecting Choices" and provides proof that coordinated processes can help promote advance care planning that works when it is needed most—throughout the entire phase in which a chronic illness advances. This program is a collaborative one in which each health care organization in the area promotes a structured process for advance care planning. Their results are staggeringly successful compared with those that only encourage the completion of an advance directive. According to Hammes et al., the health care organizations in La Crosse work together to create a routine system of care involving six interrelated parts:

(1) Adult patients are invited to understand, to reflect on, and to discuss plans for future health care relevant to their stage of illness; (2) adult patients are provided competent assistance by trained nonphysicians in the planning process; (3) written plans (however documented) are accurate, as specific as possible, and understandable to all stakeholders; (4) written plans are stored, transferred, and retrievable where the patient is being treated; (5) plans are updated and become more specific as illnesses progress; and (6) plans are reviewed and honored at the right time.[50]

Because this process is approached systematically at every stage of its implementation and evaluation, the program's outcomes are impressive. Ninety percent of all persons in their study died with an advance directive in the chart, and 99 percent of these had their advance directive in the medical record before they died.[51] In the end, these persons died in ways that were consistent with their plans and in ways that made sense given their diagnosis and prognosis. According to Hammes et al., there are many reasons for their sustained success, primary among them that the health care organizations in the community collaborate to identify an important need, deploy resources to meet that need, and redesign their care systems and processes to meet that need.[52]

Use Palliative and Hospice Care Appropriately across the Continuum of Care

Diane Meier, physician and leading advocate for the appropriate use of palliative and hospice care, defines palliative care as follows:

> Palliative care focuses on relieving suffering and achieving the best possible quality of life for patients and their family caregivers. It involves the assessment and treatment of symptoms; support for decision making and assistance in matching treatments to informed patient and family goals; practical aid for patients and their family caregivers; mobilization of community resources to ensure a secure and safe living environment; and collaborative and seamless models of care across a range of care settings (i.e., hospital, home, nursing home, and hospice). Palliative care is provided both within the Medicare hospice benefit (hospice palliative care) and outside it (nonhospice palliative care). Nonhospice palliative care is offered simultaneously with life-prolonging and curative therapies for persons living with serious, complex, and life-threatening illness. Hospice palliative care becomes appropriate when curative treatments are no longer beneficial, when the burdens of these treatments exceed their benefits, or when patients are entering the last weeks to months of life.[53]

In this definition, Meier makes an important distinction between palliative care that is offered with treatment aimed at curing a life-limiting illness and palliative care that is offered with hospice care. This is important because for many years—and even today—people have not accurately distinguished palliative care from hospice care. Given Meier's definition, it can safely be concluded that all hospice care is palliative care but not all palliative care is hospice care.

Also important in this definition is the purpose of palliative care: "it involves the assessment and treatment of symptoms; support for decision making and assistance in matching treatments to informed patient and family goals; practical aid for patients and their family caregivers; mobilization of community resources to ensure a secure and safe living environment; and collaborative and seamless models of care across a range of care settings (i.e., hospital, home, nursing home, and hospice)." This sounds much different than other medical specialties. That's because it is different. From the outset and at its core, palliative care is holistic care. It is not simply a specialty of medicine that is aimed at fixing certain body parts. Part and parcel of palliative care, regardless of the setting in which it takes place, is that it promotes quality of life, interpersonal relationships, and the importance of communication among patients, caregivers, and families so that plans of care match patient values and wishes.

One of the challenges for palliative care is the degree to which it can work collaboratively with other clinical disciplines to facilitate a coordinated care plan for persons facing chronic, life-limiting illness. By implication and necessity, then, palliative care professionals have a special role to play in advance care planning. Early in its evolution, palliative care began inside the hospital, functioning as a specialty consult service. Although this model is still in place, many programs have increased their palliative care offerings to promote better access to palliative care across the continuum. Many programs, for example, have opened outpatient palliative clinics designed to promote the values and purposes of palliative care outside of the institutional setting.[54]

Palliative care must perform a delicate balancing act to stay clear of some its less-informed critics. For example, many people misinterpret palliative care, suggesting its mere presence confirms that health care reform is more about saving money than improving care. Some facts can help dispel this myth. Palliative care can reduce length of stay in the hospital, prevent hospital readmissions, and decrease expensive, ineffective, and burdensome treatments (all of which are, by and large, helpful from an economic perspective).[55] But this is only part of the story. Palliative care also increases the quality of life, lowers the rates of depression associated with advanced illness, and prolongs life without the use of aggressive and often burdensome treatment (all of which is good from a holistic care perspective).[56]

Conclusion

We have examined how five strategies can help us rethink, and eventually redesign, the way in which EoL care is conducted in the United States. These strategies are to (1) reinforce the core values and goals of medicine, (2) establish parameters and consensus around the primary attributes of a "good death," (3) incorporate narrative competence into EoL care, (4) promote a systematic approach to advance care planning, and (5) use palliative care appropriately across the continuum of care. These strategies are specific, practical, and accessible to any care system that is committed to doing the work required to create processes and structures aimed at improving the outcomes of EoL care.

These strategies do not exist in an ethical vacuum. That is, they are meant to promote a normative ethical grounding for human existence. The reason we care about rethinking and reshaping EoL care in the first place is precisely because people matter. Good EoL of life care is a practical demonstration of our social commitment to dignity and human flourishing. Striving for excellence in EoL care indicates a collective vow to transform pain and suffering into hope even—indeed especially—when one's life is close to an end.

Case Studies

Case 11A

Mr. Toms is 58 years old. He has had chronic obstructive pulmonary disease (COPD) for eight years. He smokes about 100 packs of cigarettes per year and chews tobacco on a regular basis. About nine months ago, he noticed a circular and grayish discoloration on his tongue. Because it did not hurt, he left it alone and continued with his activities. About three months ago, he noticed that this discoloration was growing larger and had become painful. He went to the doctor to have it examined. Further testing revealed it was cancer. This testing also

cont.

Case 11A *cont.*

revealed the cancer had spread to his lymph nodes. The area on his tongue was treated surgically, requiring the removal of parts of his tongue. Despite further treatment, the cancer grew in his mouth and continued to spread throughout his body. Because of the illness, he began to lose teeth, experienced facial disfigurement and mouth pain, lost his ability to speak intelligibly, and had difficulty swallowing. Mr. Toms refused further treatment; all he requested was to be pain free. Initially Mr. Toms's pain was well controlled. Over time, however, he was admitted to the hospital to manage his symptoms. While in the hospital, Mr. Toms's care team arranged a "goals of care" conversation with Mr. Toms and his immediate family. After being presented the current medical facts of the situation and treatment options, Mr. Toms refused further curative treatments and elected not to use any life-sustaining treatments, such as mechanical ventilation or artificial nutrition and hydration, to prolong his life. All he wanted was comfort care. At this point in his disease, the best and probably only option for Mr. Toms was something his doctor referred to as "palliative sedation." Palliative sedation is the intentional lowering of consciousness for the purpose of treating pain that cannot be controlled by other measures. In palliative sedation, the means by which pain is treated is to intentionally lower the patient's consciousness to the degree needed to treat pain and suffering. The patient is sedated to a point of being unable to experience any pain or discomfort. Under the palliative sedation protocol, Mr. Toms died three days later in the hospital. His death was peaceful. He was accompanied by his family and close friends. Mr. Toms's physician was approached by a physician colleague with concerns about the manner in which Mr. Toms died. He thought it was simply an effort to euthanize the patient.

Discussion questions. Do you believe Mr. Toms's goals were met? Why or why not? Do you believe that palliative sedation is the same as euthanasia? Why or why not? How does Mr. Toms's death conform to the goals of medicine?

Case 11B

Matt is 71 years old. He is a retired high school teacher and baseball coach. He has recently been diagnosed with congestive heart failure (CHF). This diagnosis puts him at risk for heart attack, stroke, and general poor health. He is regularly experiencing shortness of breath, and the edema (swelling in his lower legs, ankles, and feet) appears to be getting worse each day. His primary care doctor believes that his particular case will progress quickly, and so aggressive treatment is recommended. With three grandchildren who live close by, Matt is eager to begin treatment. Though his CHF will not go away, and particularly severe bouts of it could kill him, he complies with his doctor's treatment recommendations. One of these recommendations is, as his doctor puts it, "to get his affairs in order." Matt understands perfectly well what his doctor means. So, as part of getting his affairs in order, Matt goes to his attorney to execute an advance directive. He completes the advance directive, appointing his son, not his wife, as his authorized decision maker. Under this arrangement his son is to decide as his father instructs should the time come when Matt cannot make health care decisions for himself. Matt does not tell his son that he has chosen him for this special role. Matt does not share his wishes about end-of-life treatment with his son or anyone else, including his wife of forty-nine years. He does not share the document with his son either. In fact, he puts the original in his desk drawer at home and a copy in his safety deposit box at his bank. Two years after his diagnosis of CHF, Matt suffers a debilitating stroke. After four weeks of aggressive treatment in the intensive care unit in the hospital, Matt's doctors ask the family for help in discerning Matt's wishes. Matt's prognosis for a meaningful recovery is very low. His family, including his wife, does not know what Matt would have wanted. His family contacts Matt's primary care physician for any assistance she can give with understanding Matt's wishes. She informs the family that she does not know Matt's wishes; they had never discussed them over the course of their fifteen-year relationship.

cont.

Case 11B *cont.*

Discussion questions. What is wrong with this picture? What consequences could this confusion have on how Matt is treated in the hospital? What could have occurred differently so that Matt's wishes could be better known?

Case 11C

Sophie is 72 years old. She has had diabetes for 10 years. Due to her own hard work and collaborative partnership with her doctor's office, her diabetes is well controlled. One of the most important reasons for this, she believes, is due to her regular participation in the local hospital's diabetes treatment center program. This is a comprehensive program that provides education by experts in the field, group counseling support, and nutritional therapy to assist persons with diabetes with their total health needs. Recently, Sophie was trained as a volunteer life coach in the program. In this role, she helps others with diabetes cope with their illness. She now feels that she is able to give back to the diabetes treatment center for all she has received.

Sophie sees her doctor every four months for a checkup. At the most recent one, her doctor noticed changes in Sophie's health. After further testing, she is diagnosed with another chronic illness, congestive heart failure (CHF). Because she goes to the doctor regularly, her doctor believes her CHF was diagnosed at an early stage. This could help manage the disease. On diagnosis, her doctor schedules a follow-up appointment with a licensed clinical social worker to further discuss the disease, learn about support systems in the community that can help Sophie live well even with CHF, and begin to discuss her particular wishes, values, and goals in life, which CHF may affect.

On her initial diagnosis, Sophie was feeling a bit depressed. After her appointment with the social worker three weeks later, she feels differently: she now knows more about the disease, understands there are support systems in the community, and has information to help her in discussing her values, wishes, and goals in life, which will help her complete an advance care plan

cont.

Case 11C *cont.*

---

that is consistent with her views about living a high-quality life. Four months later, at her next doctor's visit, Sophie brings her written advance care plan, which includes her advance directive. Her doctor then sends an electronic copy to the medical records office at the local hospital where Sophie is treated. Her doctor also sends an electronic copy to Sophie's cardiologist so she will be aware of Sophie's wishes. Last her doctor schedules an appointment for Sophie to attend a program at her hospital similar to the one in which she participates for her diabetes. The community where Sophie lives also has an electronic retrieval system for advance directives, which all health care providers can access should they need to see a copy. With the help of her licensed clinical social worker, Sophie submits her advance directive to the registry. Two weeks later, Sophie receives three letters in the mail: one from her hospital, another from her cardiologist, and a third from the advance directive registry program. All three letters inform Sophie that they received her advance directive and have it on electronic file and readily accessible should it be needed in the future. Sophie feels satisfied that her wishes will be honored when it comes to make any kind of EoL decisions in which she cannot participate.

Discussion questions. What is right with this picture? What processes, structures, and practices does this community have that will benefit Sophie in the future? What barriers prevent other communities from instituting the same kind of advance care planning structure and services Sophie enjoys?

SUGGESTED READINGS

Cassell, Eric J. *The Nature of Suffering and the Goals of Medicine,* 2nd ed. New York: Oxford University Press, 2004.

Charon, Rita, and Martha Montello, eds. *Stories Matter: The Role of Narrative in Bioethics.* New York: Routledge, 2002.

Nelson, Hilde Lindemann, ed. *Stories and Their Limits: Narrative Approaches to Bioethics.* New York: Routledge, 1997.

Weissman, David E., and Diane E. Meier. "Identifying Patients in Need of a Palliative Care Assessment in the Hospital Setting." *Journal of Palliative Medicine* 14 (2011): 17–22.

Wilmes, D. M. *Seven Days of Hospice: A Memoir*. Bloomington, IN: iUniverse Publishing, 2007.

MULTIMEDIA AIDS

"Pain and Palliative Care: What the Future Holds." William Otterson Memorial Lecture, University of California San Diego Cancer Center. 2008. *http://www.youtube.com/watch?v=Ai-MbsANxHY&feature=relmfu*. Kathleen Foley, MD., an international expert on pain and palliative care, examines the future of palliative care.

Facing Death: How Far Would You Go to Sustain the Life of Someone You Love or Your Own? PBS *Frontline*. 2011. *http://www.pbs.org/wgbh/pages/frontline/facing-death/*. This video explores current approaches to managing critically ill patients in the U.S. health care delivery system.

Palliative Care: Improving the Quality of Life for People with Serious Illness. Produced by Chaplain Debra Jarvis, M. Div. 2010. *http://www.amazon.com/Palliative-Care-Improving-Quality-Illnesses/dp/B003JBI4LY/ref=sr_1_1?ie=UTF8&qid=1298999279&sr=8-1*. This video explores the meaning and significance of palliative care from the patient and caregiver perspectives.

ENDNOTES

1. Anonymous, "It's Over, Debbie," *Journal of the American Medical Association* 259 (1988): 272.

2. Kenneth L. Vaux, "Debbie's Dying: Mercy Killing and the Good Death," *Journal of the American Medical Association* 259 (1988): 2140–41.

3. Willard Gaylin et al., *Journal of the American Medical Association* 259 (1988): 2139–40.

4. David Thomasma, "It's Over Debbie," *Journal of the American Medical Association* 259 (1988): 2098.

5. Timothy E. Quill, "Death and Dignity: A Case of Individualized Decision Making," *New England Journal of Medicine* 324 (1991): 691–4.

6. Joan M. Teno et al., "Family Perspectives on End-of-Life Care at the Last Place of Death," *Journal of the American Medical Association* 291 (2004): 88–93.

7. Karen Steinhauser et al., "In Search of a Good Death: Observations of Patients, Families, and Providers," *Annals of Internal Medicine* 132 (2000): 825–32.

8. Karen Steinhauser et al., "Preparing for the End of Life: Preferences of Patients, Families, Physicians, and Other Care Providers," *Journal of Pain and Symptom Management* 22 (2001): 727–37.

9. Dartmouth Atlas, *Trends and Variation in End-of-Life Care for Medicare Beneficiaries with Severe Chronic Illness*, April 12, 2011. The full report is available at *http://www.dartmouthatlas.org/downloads/reports/EOL_Trend_Report_0411.pdf. See also* The Dartmouth Atlas, *http://www.dartmouthatlas.org/data/table.aspx?ind=17*.

10. David E. Weissman and Diane E. Meier, "Identifying Patients in Need of a Palliative Care Assessment in the Hospital Setting," *Journal of Palliative Medicine* 14 (2011): 17–22.

11. Diane E. Meier, "Palliative Care—A Shifting Paradigm," *New England Journal of Medicine* 363 (2010): 1533.

12. *http://www.cdc.gov/nchs/fastats/lcod.htm* (accessed February 28, 2011).

13. Dartmouth Atlas, *Tracking the Care of Patients with Severe Chronic Illness*, 2008. The full report is available at *http://www.dartmouthatlas.org/downloads/atlases/2008_Chronic_Care_Atlas.pdf* (accessed February 28, 2011).

14. Dartmouth Atlas, *Tracking the Care of Patients*.

15. J. Stein-Barbury, and S. McKinley, "Patients' Experience of Being in an Intensive Care Unit: A Select Literature Review," *American Journal of Critical Care* 9 (2000): 20–27.

16. David A. Asch et al., "The Sequence of Withdrawing Life-Sustaining Treatment from Patients," *American Journal of Medicine* 107 (1999): 153–6.

17. Nicholas Christakis and David A. Asch, "Biases in How Physicians Choose to Withdraw Life Support," *Lancet* 342 (1993): 642–6.

18. Andrea Grunier et al., "Where People Die: A Multilevel Approach to Understanding Influences on Site of Death in America," *Medical Care Research and Review* 64 (2007): 351–78.

19. Teno et al., "Family Perspectives."

20. Centers for Disease Control, *Health, United States, 2010*, 43; see *http://www.cdc.gov/nchs/data/hus/hus10.pdf#specialfeature* (accessed February 28, 2011).

21. National Hospice and Palliative Care Organization, "NHPCO Facts and Figures: Hospice Care in America," 2010, 4, *http://www.nhpco.org/files/public/Statistics_Research/Hospice_Facts_Figures_Oct-2010.pdf* (accessed February 28, 2011).

22. National Hospice and Palliative Care Organization, "NHPCO Facts and Figures," 2010, 5.

23. Hastings Center, "The Goals of Medicine: Setting New Priorities," *The Hastings Center Report* 26 (November–December 1996): S1–27 (special supplement).

24. Daniel Callahan, "Remembering the Goals of Medicine," *Journal of Evaluation in Clinical Practice* 5 (1999): 103–6.

25. Teno et al., "Family Perspectives."

26. Steinhauser et al., "Preparing for the End-of-Life."

27. Judith Nelson, et al., "End of Life Care for the Critically Ill: A National Intensive Care Unit Survey," *Critical Care Medicine* 34 (October 2006): table 2, 2550.

28. The "technological imperative" in medicine refers to the view that if an institution has a technology, it will use the technology first for its original intent and, in some cases, for innovative treatments. The technological imperative can also refer to what appears to be the insatiable desire of health care organizations to use the most technologically advanced machines. Either way, each view assumes that technology, in and of itself, is necessary for healing.

29. Robert D. Truog et al., "Recommendations for End-of-Life Care in the Intensive Care Unit: A Consensus Statement by the American Academy of Critical Care Medicine," *Critical Care Medicine* 36 (2008): 953–63.

30. Steinhauser et al., "In Search of a Good Death, 825–32.

31. Ibid., 825.

32. Ira Byock, *The Four Things That Matter Most: A Book about Living* (New York: Free Press, 2004).

33. See, for example, Sean R. Morrison and Diane E. Meier "Palliative Care," *New England Journal of Medicine* 350 (2004): 2582–90.

34. Steinhauser et al., "In Search of a Good Death," 828.

35. Ibid., 829.

36. Ibid., 828.

37. Ibid., 829.

38. Ibid., 829.

39. Ibid., 828.

40. Ibid., 829.

41. Ibid., 830.

42. Truog et al., "Recommendations for End of Life Care in the Intensive Care Unit," 954–5.

43. Rita Charon, "Narrative and Medicine," *New England Journal of Medicine* 350 (2004): 862.

44. William Osler, "On the Need of Radical Reform in Our Methods of Teaching Medical Students," *Medical News* 82 (1903): 50.

45. Sally Gadow, "Relational Narrative: The Postmodern Turn in Philosophical Ethics," *Scholarly Inquiry for Nursing Practice* 13 (1999): 62.

46. Bernard J. Hammes et al., "A Comparative, Retrospective, Observational Study of the Prevalence, Availability, and Specificity of Advance Care Plans in a County that Implemented an Advance Care Planning Microsystem," *Journal of the American Geriatrics Society* 58 (2010): 1249–55.

47. Ibid., 1249.

48. Bernard J. Hammes et al., "Death and End-of-Life Planning in One Midwestern Community," *Archives of Internal Medicine* 158 (1998): 383–90.

49. Gerlyn Brasic and Bernard J. Hammes, "Letter to the Editor," *Annals of Internal Medicine* 148 (2008): 406.

50. Hammes, "Observational Study of Advance Care Plans," 1249–50.

51. Ibid., 1249–50, 1252.

52. Ibid., 1249–50, 1254.

53. Meier, "Palliative Care—A Shifting Paradigm," 1533.

54. See, for example, the Mount Sinai Medical Center's palliative care program. A leading center across the country, it has been committed to increasing access to palliative care: *http://www.mountsinai.org/patient-care/service-areas/palliative-care/areas-of-care* (accessed March 1, 2011).

55. R. Sean Morrison et al., "Cost Savings Associated with U.S. Hospital Palliative Care Consultation Programs," *Archives of Internal Medicine* 168 (2008): 1783–90.

56. Jennifer S. Temel, "Early Palliative Care in Patients with Metastatic Non-Small Cell Lung Cancer," *New England Journal of Medicine* 363 (2010): 733–42.

CHAPTER 12

Health Care Reform

David Belde

Health Care Reform and Human Well-Being

If health care ethics is the study of how the structure, organization, delivery, and relationships within health care should promote human well-being, there is perhaps no more important subject than how health care could be reformed so that the goal of human well-being can be achieved. Traditionally, health care reform has been organized around three structural elements: increasing access to health care, increasing the quality of health care services, and lowering the costs of health care. By implication, this means our current health care system has not adequately delivered on these three elements. The goal of health care reform, then, is to restructure how health care is delivered so as to address these inadequacies.

Health care reform is not simply a question of economics. Nor is it simply a matter of spending our dollars differently—though that is one element of health care reform. It is about ethics, as well. Health care reform centers on two practical and interrelated ethical questions: how can health care be reformed in a way that better demonstrates (1) our commitment to the inherent value of individual persons and their flourishing and (2) our commitment toward building a just society in which all persons receive their fair share of health care resources so that life can be lived abundantly?

According to the Center for Medicare and Medicaid Services (CMS), the government agency that oversees federal health insurance programs, $2.5 trillion was spent on health care services in 2009.[1] This represents a total of 17.4 percent of the nation's gross domestic product, which is defined as the total value of all goods and services produced within a country in a given year. This amounts to $8,086 of spending per person. Comparatively, although the United States annually spends more than twice as much as other industrialized nations per person on health care, it ranks only thirty-seventh in terms of overall population health and health system efficiency.[2] This means Americans are not getting the best value for their dollar on health care. Moreover, according to the most recent Census Bureau data, more than 15 percent of all American citizens—more than 50 million people—do not have health insurance.[3] In terms of the overall quality of health care delivered and access to health care, the American system is falling short.

To promote a system that more adequately and efficiently integrates access, quality, and cost, President Barack Obama signed into law the Patient Protection and Affordable Care Act (PPACA) on March 23, 2010. Though many U.S. presidents have attempted to overhaul the health system in the last century, this act comprises the first comprehensive health care reform package passed by the U.S. Congress. No matter where one stands on the necessity, value, and political appropriateness of PPACA, no one can deny its social significance. This is the most significant piece of social legislation since the civil rights legislation of the 1960s. As the bill moves through the legislative process, it will be modified. However, its central intent and reforms will likely stand the test of time. Among other reforms, the act expands access to health care and changes how clinicians and health care organizations will be paid so that the quality of care provided becomes the organizing payment principle as opposed to the quantity of care. In addition, the bill advances scientific research known as "comparative effectiveness research," which compares "gold standard" treatments against other treatments to determine the least costly and most effective treatments, and also promotes significant changes in health care delivery so that more attention is given to the way in which access, quality, and cost can be improved. Although it comes with a hefty price tag—$938 billion over ten years—the bill promotes an entirely new kind of discussion and social practice around health care delivery, which many believe is long overdue.[4]

Setting the Context: Why Health Care Reform Is Vital

From an ethical perspective, health care reform is vital precisely because health care is crucial for human flourishing. Health is a precondition for human flourishing. Health enables and promotes personal and social well-being. Reforming health care demonstrates both a tangible response to promoting the inherent value of persons and an explicit appreciation that justice requires all of us to work toward creating a more humane world.

This chapter discusses two ethical principles that ground health care reform: human dignity and justice. These principles guide our decision making, conscience formation, and discernment in the concrete task of reforming health care. After explaining these principles and identifying their importance for health care reform, we address three key assumptions that should govern the attitudes, perspectives, and conclusions drawn about how health care and its reform affect human flourishing. From this point, we can better understand the current conditions giving rise to health care reform and the role that delivering high-quality health care plays in reforming this important social good.

Discussion: Ethical Issues and Analysis

Consistent with the normative basis of ethics put forth in this book, two important notions should guide ethical analysis and decision making as they relate to health care reform: (1) who ought we to become as persons and (2) how ought we to act in relation to people, God, and creation? The first is a question about how we develop as humans over the course of a lifetime (Being) and the second is a question of acting in a way that promotes right relationships and a just social order (Doing). Given this normative basis, human dignity and justice can form the foundational ethical principles for health care reform. Human dignity places the value of the person at the center of health care decision making, and justice provides a basis for developing health care delivery processes and structures so that health care resources can be used in a way that benefits all persons. Moreover, both human dignity and justice tie directly to the notion that ethics generally and health care ethics specifically are grounded in a normative basis geared toward the promotion of human flourishing and just social relations.

Human Dignity

Human dignity is a foundational ethical principle that stems from the view that humans have inherent worth as members of the human family. It commits us to promoting practices, building structures, and creating conditions within society that promote individual and social well-being. It is a principle that reflects the long-held view that humans, precisely because they are humans, have special worth. This inherent worth exists irrespective of one's social rank, utility, achievements, and intellect. Theologically, human dignity has been grounded in the view that (1) persons are made in the image and likeness of God, the *imago dei*, as described in Genesis 1:27; (2) rationality—what has historically been understood as a distinctively human capacity—represents the spark of the divine in humanity; and (3) human dignity is realized in community. Such a view of human dignity creates individual and communal obligations of respect, provides individuals and communities with the conditions for positive development, and promotes the view that human dignity is as much about social advancement as it is about individual progress.

Any important social reform must have a moral foundation, for reform is often grounded in moral indignation about social experiences that demean persons and groups. Consider the civil rights movement in the United States. The movement itself grew out of the experience of marginalization—the opposite of what a robust and healthy sense of human dignity should promote. Such experiences sparked the need for change. Human dignity plays an essential role in any social reform that aims to promote the quality and value of life of individuals and the community.

It is important to distinguish between universal and particular human dignity. Taken together, both dimensions operate dynamically to give human dignity its proper significance for individuals and societies. With respect to health care reform, each dimension has a role to play.

In its universal dimension, human dignity applies to all individuals precisely because they are in the human family; it respects the basic equality of persons. On the other hand, human dignity has a deep-seated particular dimension, in that individual persons—but also individual countries, regions, states or provinces, and municipalities—have distinguishable interests, needs, and views regarding what brings meaning and purpose to life. In this dimension, human dignity is more contextual and empirical. As such, particular human dignity is a notion that respects the essential uniqueness of human persons. Both conceptions should be held in creative tension and relation with each other when considering social reform in general, and health care reform in particular. The universal aspect of human dignity needs the particular so that real-life issues can be incorporated into ethical discourse on important social matters. The particular notion of human dignity needs the universal to provide a foundational starting point and common platform for ethical discourse.

In health care reform, both notions of human dignity work in tandem. Human dignity in the universal sense offers the conceptual and rhetorical framework required to justify health care reform. This framework should not be particularly controversial, but having seen recently and historically how debates over health care reform have proceeded in this country raises the question of whether, and to what extent, human dignity has the moral priority it deserves. All persons should be able to accept that because people matter, they deserve some form of universal access to health care. Yet, this explicit appeal to human dignity is not often stated in social discourse. Human dignity in the particular sense inspires the concrete and specific work required for design, implementation, assessment, and so forth. Whereas universal human dignity grounds the premise that humans, by virtue of their inherent worth, should be guaranteed some minimal level of health care, particular human dignity grounds conversations in whether, and to what extent, specific regions of the country will devise health care systems tailored to their specific health needs and demographic realties, such as cultural composition and educational levels.

Human dignity does not commit us to a one-size-fits-all notion of health care reform. The work grounded in particular human dignity is complex and controversial, especially in a pluralistic society in which agreement on complex matters is often difficult and driven by self-interest instead of the common good. Whether in the universal sense or the particular sense, human dignity provides an important ground for the moral justification of health care reform. This moral ground includes a number of commitments: to the value of persons and human well-being, to the normative values that frame the meaning and limits of social policies, to the political-historical movements for human rights, to the creation of institutions designed to move society forward in positive ways, and to the psychological dimensions of personal growth, virtue, and quality of life.

Justice

Justice concerns persons getting their due.[5] This means that justice centers on fairness and "recognizing the difference between legitimate and illegitimate claims, . . . recognizing priorities among different values, [and] . . . determining who should get what when all cannot get everything they seek."[6] Given these goals of justice, one can conclude that justice is the "consistent determination to respect the rights of others"[7] through recognizing, appreciating, and advocating that people, especially those on the margins of society, receive their fair share of society's goods so that all people can realize their full potential.

Although justice generally concerns giving people what they deserve and creating a society that distributes benefits and burdens fairly, how a society should go about accomplishing these goals demands careful discernment. What follows is a brief description of five competing views of justice. These notions operate in our ethical, political, and social systems. As a result, and as a practical reality, each will have proponents and opponents as the debate over health care reform continues to unfold. In a morally diverse society such as in the United States, the challenge will be how people, as a society, agree on which views of justice—or which combination of the views of justice presented above—will be integrated into social policy on health care. Elements of each type of justice can be found in current U.S. health policy. This is partly due to the fact that health care reform is a political process that will include diverse voices. This is precisely why one's moral foundations matter. Moral foundations ground decision making. They offer insight into the way in which—and the degree to which—societies value persons. They offer a glimpse into the priorities, interests, and needs of a country. They reveal deep-seated moral insights and perspectives around important issues.

Though there is danger in pigeonholing any one view or its proponents, the following presentation attempts to offer a panoramic view of justice at work. Health care reform is then briefly examined in the light of each view of justice.

1. Utilitarian Justice

The best-known modern defense of utilitarian justice comes from John Stuart Mill, whose views are described in his 1861 text *Utilitarianism*. Mill was interested in maximizing the well-being of citizens at a time of industrial expansion and economic growth. Mill's idea of utilitarian justice is simple: the best thing to do, given the circumstances of the time, is to produce the greatest good for the most people. This is referred to as his principle of utility. Practically, this means that justice-based decision making will require the analysis of empirical realities—statistics, numbers, economic and population data, and so on—so that utility can be demonstrated through evidence. A common application of this view is the cost-benefit analysis. In a health care reform context, this justice might begin by asking which health care reform proposal promotes the best outcome for the most people most of the time. As you might imagine, there is no single answer to this question. So, utilitarian decision making would be concerned primarily with weighing the financial costs and benefits against the human costs and benefits of not moving forward with a given approach to health care reform.

2. Contractarian Justice

John Rawls, in his influential text *A Theory of Justice*, provides the best-known contemporary defense of contractarian justice. Assuming that in a pluralistic society there will be disagreement regarding the acceptability of particular ethical principles, some have proposed the only way to work through this moral pluralism is to devise a contractual strategy to promote agreement on various issues pertaining to justice and equal opportunity. Such a strategy could, then, provide a universal and common source of agreement around ethical principles and their application. In such a view, justice requires that each person's welfare should be equally and impartially considered—apart from, say, their talents, skills, intellect, and so on. This means all those agreeing to enter into a social contract must be willing to abandon their self-interests to take equal and impartial account of the general welfare. This view has been called the "original position." This position may not exist in reality, but it is a device necessary for creating impartiality and promoting everyone's interests equally. From this position, a set of standards could be devised and agreed on that give each person his or her due. These principles may not be universal, but they could ideally work for those within a particular society. In the health care context, this process could work through bringing a cross-section of society together and creating an impartial and deliberative process intended to produce a health care system that would divide resources equally among the population. Such a process would, for example, help create the boundaries around what treatments would be covered under a universal health care insurance benefit and how much individuals would contribute out of pocket to pay for each treatment.

3. Libertarian Justice

Although libertarian justice may not be Robert Nozick's primary concern, his view of the minimal state as outlined in *Anarchy, State, and Utopia* provides grounding for libertarian thinking, particularly as it relates to the importance of individual liberty, free-market development and exchange, and lack of state control over the daily life of people. The state has a duty to intervene only when certain basic rights are at risk: the right against injury from others, the right to individual liberty, the right to own private property. Libertarian justice is not concerned with schemes that seek to redistribute social goods such as health care. Justice in this view is relegated primarily to individual exchange—what has traditionally been referred to as "commutative" justice. Moreover, libertarian justice is neither organized by seeking the greatest good for the largest number of people most of the time nor by providing for the least-well-off among society. Assuming the rules for free and open exchange are just, although it may be unfortunate that some are disadvantaged, it cannot be said that it is unfair that some are disadvantaged. It will be the responsibility of those disadvantaged to change their circumstances. In the health care reform context, this notion of justice would tend to stay clear of reform that requires government expansion, raising of taxes, or the redistribution of taxpayer money to pay for health care services, even if such redistribution helped the least-well-off in society. Additionally, libertarian justice would tend to rely on free-market mechanisms to keep costs down and to promote high-quality health care. Such free-market approaches could include processes like allowing individuals to use individual and tax-free spending accounts. It would allow for free and open competition to help drive supply and demand and health care resources.

4. Socialist Justice

The best-known modern defense of socialist justice can be found in the work of Karl Marx and Friedrich Engels, and particularly Marx's *Communist Manifesto*. In their view, equality is the ultimate political and social ideal. Marx elaborated more positively on the socialist ideal in his 1891 text, *Critique of the Gotha Programme*. An immature society based on the socialist idea of distribution would conform to the following principle: from each according to one's ability, to each according to one's contribution. A mature society based on the socialist idea of distribution would conform to the following principle: from each according to one's ability and to each according to one's need. The general theme in this concept of justice is to attain equal opportunity to an equally satisfying way of life in society. Although some goods may be more important than others as they relate to individual and social flourishing, all goods are shared and distributed equally. In the health care reform context, such a view of justice would endorse the view that health care resources should be redistributed to all persons on the grounds that, as a social good, profit and ownership of the means of production could get in the way of the just distribution of resources. Moreover, the ownership of such goods would be public. Private ownership of the means of production creates conditions of inequality.

5. Communitarian Justice

The best-known classical defense of communitarian justice is in the work of Aristotle. His view is described in his *Nicomachean Ethics*. Thomas Aquinas, the medieval Catholic scholar and Dominican priest, embraced this concept of justice and provided a moral foundation for the Catholic body of work most resembling it, what is known as Catholic social teaching. Catholic social teaching has endorsed communitarian justice, which views human development in the context of a set of common goods that will, when properly aligned and equally distributed, provide for a just social existence in which all persons will be liberated from that which thwarts their development. The approach has less patience with debates on issues like the proper role of the state in a political system or the freedom to be left alone and focuses more on solving concrete social problems such as crime, famine, poverty, racism, and war. It is grounded in the view that humans have dignity, that humans are by nature social, and that life in abundance is an important goal that social systems should promote. In this concept of justice, social justice and distributive justice are critical. Where distributive justice promotes the equal and proper distribution of goods, social justice requires that all persons have a voice and role in creating the common good. In the health care reform context, this view of justice would endorse reforms that, precisely because of the value that health care has for human and social flourishing, support comprehensive changes without limits or variations to care based on age, race, ethnicity, financial means, or citizenship. Health care reform under this concept of justice would create conditions that can promote each person's full participation in society.

Application of Concepts of Justice

Having examined some of the foundational elements and varying views of justice, we now move to a case study that requires application of these foundational concepts.

Case 12A

Mrs. Johns is 92 years old. For her age, she is in relatively good health. She has a heart condition that is treated medically. Two years ago, she declined a surgical fix to her heart blockage, citing concerns and risks about how surgery could affect her overall

cont.

Case 12A *cont.*

quality of health. She is now wheelchair bound and lives in an assisted-living facility where she requires moderate to full assistance with her activities of daily living. Though in relatively good health compared to others her age, she has told her children and caregivers that she knows her health is steadily declining and that she does not have long to live. She can communicate effectively and participates in her health care decision making. For the past year, she has lived with a rare blood disorder that requires frequent blood transfusions (three–five times per week) and regular doses (two–four per day) of an additional synthetic blood product that helps her blood to clot properly. This blood product is manufactured in California, shipped to the East Coast where Mrs. Johns lives, and costs $5,000 per dose. This treatment regimen has gone on for one year and, given the nature of the blood disorder, it is likely that she will require this synthetic blood product more frequently over time. The company that produces the product called the hospital where Mrs. Johns gets her treatment to let it know that the entire Southeastern region of the country where Mrs. Johns lives is facing a dire shortage in the supply of this product, which is the only one that has demonstrated any benefit for Mrs. Johns. The company makes it clear that many other patients in the region who could benefit from the blood product are going without it and that the short supply for the entire region is at risk for as long as Mrs. Johns will require the therapy. The company is limited in how much of the product it can produce because, though synthetic, it requires natural blood properties to make it—the supply of the natural blood properties rise and fall depending on the overall supply of blood.

Discussion questions. Examine the ethical implications, particularly as they relate to human dignity and justice, of limiting Mrs. Johns's beneficial treatment. What process would you develop to ensure that the short supply of this resource could be balanced fairly? How would you apply this process in Mrs. Johns's case? How would the five different views of justice address the conflicts raised by this case?

Three Assumptions That Can Guide Health Care Reform

Given the foundational importance human dignity and justice ought to have in guiding health care reform, three important assumptions follow that could inform particular perspectives and conclusions around what health care reform should look like so that health care delivery can promote human flourishing. These assumptions flow from the views of human dignity and justice presented above. Health care reform is about many things. Principally, however, it is meant to promote the better use of resources so the community as a whole achieves and experiences health and well-being. The assumptions that follow, then, can best be viewed as a kind of practical application of human dignity and justice in a health care reform context.

1. Health care is a unique type of business activity. Given this, it should be understood differently from other commercial enterprises.

2. As a finite and social good, health care delivery should be designed to benefit society as a whole. Given this, the burdens and benefits of health care reform should be shared equitably by all.

3. Individual and social health is more than a matter of access to health care services. More attention needs to be given to understanding how physical environment, cultural norms, and social interactions impact individual and community health.

Health Care Is a Unique Kind of Business Activity

Though many argue otherwise, health care is a different sort of business activity. The organizing ethical purpose of health care is centered on the traditional notion that health care is meant to be a service to humanity precisely because such service promotes human flourishing. Such goals as saving and prolonging life, preventing illness, promoting wellness, and researching the cause of and treatments for disease combine well with the generally accepted Western view that persons have inherent value. This combination of medicine's traditional goals and Western ethical values give health care inherent moral ends and a proud moral tradition.[8] To allow health care to be dominated solely by commercial ends and wealth generation is shortsighted and morally corrupt given its important ethical and social roots.

One prevailing ethical assumption regarding the business activity of health care organizations is that their work is rooted in service to the community.[9] As such, the "basic purpose of health care organizations is to meet the health care needs of individuals and to promote the health of the community."[10] This is another way of saying that an original intent of health care delivery is to promote human flourishing. Although health care organizations are businesses—and thus designed in part to make money—they must not lose sight of their historically foundational ethical mandate: to provide an important social service to individuals and the community. Health care ought to be more intentionally designed to promote the health of individuals and the community rather than the generation of wealth for individuals and organizations.

Commercial interests can have a corruptive influence on health care delivery. For instance, it can benefit health care providers financially if members of local communities are sick. Sickness increases the volume of health care services and interventions. Volume produces financial well-being for clinicians and health care organizations. The more people who catch the flu or need cardiac surgery in a community, the more health care organizations will benefit financially in that community. Sickness provides business. Business generates wealth. Wealth provides growth. Growth means more jobs. More jobs generate more money for consumption. Consumption produces tax revenue. For some, it is precisely this kind of economic cycle that makes the world a better place, for it promotes the maximization of individual preference, which for many is *the* normative basis of ethics. The current payment system in U.S. health care supports health care delivery that promotes doing more because doing more is currently financially advantageous. The current system, called fee for service, pays health care providers for treating sick people, not for keeping people well. At present, there is little financial incentive to design a system more aligned with promoting wellness and preventing illness.

The business of health care ought to be directed toward human flourishing, and health care delivery warrants a normative basis to match. Recognizing this, health care reform efforts must promote the service-oriented ideals of health care organizations. Health care reform should establish incentives for health care providers and organizations to keep individuals and societies well while recognizing and accepting that doing so may put a dent in an organization's financial bottom line and a country's economic engine.

Health Care Is a Social Good Intended to Benefit Society

On August 10, 2010, the World Health Organization (WHO) declared an end to the global H1N1 (swine flu) pandemic. The virus was first detected in the United States in April 2009. Just two months after that first U.S. case was detected, the WHO announced that a global flu pandemic was under way. By that time, seventy countries had confirmed cases of H1N1.[11] According to the U.S. Centers for Disease Control and Prevention, there were about 60 million cases and 12,270 deaths in the United States alone.[12]

For the better part of eighteen months, daily reports informed the country of the magnitude of the pandemic. Governmental agencies responsible for the public's health issued regular communications and held frequent press conferences to educate the public, including health care providers, on the development, characteristics, and treatments of the disease. Local and national media told endless stories about individuals who had died from H1N1. Ethicists, public health professionals, and policy makers debated the ethical issues involved in determining the allocation of limited resources, such as mechanical ventilators and immunizations, which were needed to treat the disease.[13]

In situations like this, we are reminded that life is precarious, medicine is imperfect, and health and health care delivery are crucial social goods; that is, they are necessary for the community to flourish. Unlike personal property such as a car or bicycle, a social good is collectively owned—all persons within society have a stake in society's well-being. Education is another such social good. No single person—or corporation—owns the educational system. However, all of us own it in the sense that we depend on it—and therefore care for it—for the overall well-being of society. Health care is similar. Whether health care is more important than other social goods is not the point. Also, just because it happens to be financially profitable does not mean that business and corporate interests should dictate how it is reformed to benefit the whole.

Intrinsic to the view that health care is a social good are rational, deliberate, and just efforts to allocate health care services so that everyone within the social system can benefit equitably.[14] Ethically, this means that health care reform is a practical application of the various forms of justice described above. Yet, in a pluralistic society, diverse concepts of justice exist, making agreement—both regarding the meaning of justice and its practical implementation—challenging.[15] Regardless of these challenges, health care reform must go forward in a way that respects the importance of how health care can promote the well-being of all persons, not just those fortunate to have access to health care services.

Viewing health care as a social good raises some important ethical challenges. Daniel Callahan, the noted bioethicist and social critic of the U.S. health care system, raises the allocation and limits challenge—perhaps the most important and vexing of all.[16] There are at least two ways in which the need for allocation enters into health care reform. First, a number of social goods compete with health care at the social level of existence, among them education, national defense, transportation, emergency relief, and more. The national budget allocates only so much for social goods. Health care's portion of that expenditure has steadily increased, a trend that shows no signs of abating—hence the need to bring justice concerns into our social debate about health care reform.

Second, within the health care delivery system itself, a number of allocation questions must be addressed. We dealt with some of those in the case study above. One way some have divided the allocation question within health care delivery is to distinguish between public health initiatives and individual health initiatives.[17] Public health initiatives focus on basic public health needs such as sanitation processes that create clean drinking water, safe foods, and the development of vaccines, antibiotic treatments, and immunizations, as well as access to emergency care in times of national disasters. Individual health initiatives focus on treatments for individuals. They extend beyond primary care for common illnesses and enter into the world of genetic treatment and other high-tech and low-touch treatments that address such concerns as back and joint pain and male and female fertility. Such treatments are more tailored to the individual and also more expensive than public health-oriented activities.

The challenge will be to find ways to balance public and individual health initiatives and still maintain the socially conscious view that regardless of one's social merit, gender, ethnicity, age, or ability to pay, we can provide health care for the well-being of society as a whole precisely because health care is a social good.

Individual and Social Health Involve More than Access to Care

We have long known that even if health care reform efforts succeed in offering all persons affordable access to a basic level of health care, there is still more to think about regarding individual and social health. Consider the following:

- A baby born to a mother who has completed fewer than 12 years of education is almost twice as likely to die before her first birthday as a baby born to a mother with 16 or more years of education.[18]
- Adults with family incomes below the federal poverty level are more than twice as likely to have diabetes and nearly 1.5 times as likely to have coronary heart disease.[19]
- Even when important variables such as insurance status, age, income, and the presence of other poor health conditions are accounted for, African Americans and Hispanics are less likely than whites to receive appropriate cardiac medication or undergo necessary cardiac surgery.[20]
- African American patients with congestive heart failure or pneumonia receive inferior care compared with whites.[21]

Such statistics are chilling. They refer to what are called the "social determinants" of health. This means regardless of whether one has access to health care, there exist implicit attitudes and sensitivities within a culture that can bias treatment decisions and affect health outcomes. If lack of access does not drive such phenomena, then what does? Deeply ingrained in our social dynamics are complex realities that significantly affect the health status of individuals and communities, regardless of whether one has health insurance. Individual and community health is affected by one's culture, ethnicity, physical environment, personal behavior, economic and educational level, and other social realities.

Conditions Creating the Need for Health Care Reform

Economically speaking, our health care system is at a crossroads. Our current health care system is economically stressed in ways that make it unsustainable. Costs of health care continue to rise, both in the amount of money spent annually on health care and the rate of growth of that spending. More people are living longer. With greater longevity comes more chronic illness, which creates the need for more health care. Demographically, there will be fewer people to support the number of people who will begin receiving government-sponsored social insurance programs such as Medicare and Social Security. Although all of these factors may be the immediate economic stressors on our health care system, how that system is currently structured will not significantly reduce these economic pressures. Hence, change is necessary.

In health care, there are providers (individuals and organizations such as doctors and hospitals), payers, patients, manufacturers, and many others who interact to deliver health care services. Providers consist of health care professionals and organizations that are paid by third-party payers (either private or government-run insurance companies) for their service. Patients visit providers to seek help for health problems. There is a charge for each office visit, as well for other services (for example, immunizations, surgery, X-rays, physical therapy, etc.) that may be needed to address a particular health problem. Ideally, health care professionals recommend treatments they believe are helpful based on professional experience, sound clinical reasoning, and scientific evidence demonstrating the efficacy of particular treatments.

Health care professionals and organizations are paid for the work they do on an item-by-item basis. For example, if a physician resets a broken bone, she is paid to reset the bone. She then submits a claim to a third-party insurer using a numerical code that corresponds to resetting a broken bone. This form of payment, called fee for service, is the most common in the U.S. health care system. According to some, this payment system turns physicians and other health care providers into "pieceworkers"[22] who are paid for their interventions but not for how well their interventions work. The important ethical implication here is that some providers, either intentionally or unintentionally, do more to be paid more. Doing more does not always translate into better clinical care. In fact, doing more in many cases harms patients and contributes to rising costs and unnecessary spending. This is especially true for medical procedures that are not strongly supported by scientific evidence as beneficial.

One such example is platelet-rich plasma injections for healing injuries to tendons and other parts of the body. In this procedure, the patient is injected with her own blood—which is concentrated so that it is primarily her blood platelets—designed to heal injured tissues.[23] Many professional athletes, including Tiger Woods, have claimed this procedure—which can cost more than $1,000 per treatment—has healed them of their orthopedic injuries. According to one leading orthopedic surgeon, of all surgical specialties, orthopedic surgery is perhaps among the least grounded in strong evidence of long-term benefit to the patient.[24] This does not necessarily mean orthopedic surgeons or orthopedic surgery are ethically suspect. It simply means some forms of orthopedic surgery—and this extends to other medical specialties as well—may not always be as well grounded in strong scientific evidence regarding their necessity and long-term value. Such surgeries, therefore, could lead to unnecessary procedures and increased costs in health care without proportionate benefits to patients or society.

Many hospitals and organizations invest significant capital in health care services that have larger fee-for-service reimbursement associated with them, irrespective of whether there is a significant demonstrable community benefit from the services. In major U.S. cities, there are many duplicate and expensive technologies. More than anything else, hospital competition drives excess capacity. Excess capacity refers to the overabundance of health care services, principally technology and number of hospital beds, such that they exceed what a community justifiably needs to provide adequate service to the population. This marks a major intersection for the ethics and economics of health care delivery. Hospital competition could mean, as Shannon Brownlee, freelance science writer, points out in her evocative book *Overtreated*, much of the health care delivered in our country is motivated more by the economic interests of individuals and organizations than the health needs of patients and communities. Brownlee concludes this is the nexus that could be making the United States sicker and poorer—sicker because of the potentially problematical health side effects that unnecessary treatment may have and poorer because there is unnecessary spending and waste of resources that could be used for those who truly need it.[25]

One way scholars and health care writers demonstrate that overtreatment could be making our country sicker and poorer is by considering how the supply of health care services stimulates demand. In the health care industry it appears that supply drives demand—an "if you build it they will come" equation.[26] In virtually every other industry, demand creates supply. If people are buying fewer cars, then car manufacturers begin making fewer cars because there is less demand. In health care, regions with high health care supply tend to have higher demand for health care services.[27] The economic reality behind this phenomenon is that in the health care industry more is better—at least financially. This dovetails nicely with the entrepreneurial spirit.[28] Ethics notwithstanding, there are economic pressures on all health care organizations to increase market share, employ more providers, dominate referral patterns, and have more imaging machines. More is better, or so the economic assumption goes. One way to get more is to increase supply—even when the community may not need it and even when lower-cost interventions (for example, counseling, diet, and exercise as opposed to weight reduction surgery) could do the job just as well without the real risks of costly and complicated interventions.

While it is true that many uninsured and underinsured Americans receive too little care, it is also true many Americans—whether in public or private insurance programs—receive too much care.[29] As it turns out, long-term and consistent evidence demonstrates overspending and overtreatment in health care is related primarily to where one lives and the practice patterns of clinicians and the number of specialist providers in that region.[30] There is evidence that different parts of the country—both metropolitan and rural—have

significantly different patterns of health care spending, a phenomenon termed *regional variation*. Interestingly, in those regions where
health care spending is far less, outcomes are as good, and often
better.[31] (Note to readers: for a visual representation of "regional
variation" across a myriad of health care indicators consult the various data and charts presented by the Dartmouth Atlas. This data can
be accessed online at: *http://www.dartmouth.org/data/region/.*)

The causes of regional variation are difficult to explain. Even so,
many health care experts, policy scholars, and practitioners have drawn
conclusions. Two possible explanations are the different practice patterns of physicians and the lack of clarity and agreement about the
best evidence regarding various interventions. Maggie Mahar, health
care business writer and fellow at the Century Foundation, notes in
her book *Money-Driven Medicine*, that one medical study, comparing
how patients were treated for a six-month period after hip replacement surgery, found patients receiving care in a high-treatment
region at prestigious academic medical centers received 82 percent
more physician visits, 26 percent more imaging studies, 90 percent
more diagnostic procedures and tests, and 46 percent more minor
surgeries than patients in low-spending regions at equally prestigious
academic medical centers.[32] The delivery of high-quality, low-cost
health care is an attainable goal. But, it requires moderating the supply of health care resources. The Mayo Clinic, internationally recognized for excellence, provides low-cost, high-quality care in all three
of its locations in Arizona, Florida, and Minnesota. Mayo practices
protocol-driven and evidence-based medicine with attention to the
patient's needs—not the clinic's bottom line—as their central concern.[33] This has proved a successful business and clinical strategy for
the Mayo Clinic and similar health care facilities.

Given that health care is a social good and health care spending is an ethical, as well as an economic, issue, as well as the overuse
of medical services without a proportionate increase in health outcomes in some regions of the country, attention must be directed
toward spending health care resources more wisely and with greater
scientific rigor.[34] This means we must set reasonable limits on
health care spending—a controversial issue for many Americans.
Setting reasonable limits assumes there is a commitment, in general
and across the board, from all those with an academic, economic,

personal, and social interest in health care delivery to developing an ethos of cost consciousness.

Waste, Fraud, and Abuse in Health Care

In March 1863, the False Claims Act was signed into law by President Abraham Lincoln. The law was designed to hold dishonest contractors accountable for wrongdoing in their business with the federal government. At that time during America's Civil War, some contractors had sold the government deficient goods, such as poorly functioning weapons, ill horses, and rotten food rations. This act is used today to prosecute persons and organizations making fraudulent claims to government-run health insurance plans such as Medicare and Medicaid. The act helps the federal government steward its resources and prevent waste, fraud, and abuse of health care resources.

In May 2009, the Department of Justice (DOJ) and the Department of Health and Human Services (DHS) announced the creation of the Health Care Fraud Prevention and Enforcement Action Team. Granted cabinet-level authority, this team is charged with coordinating national efforts to prevent waste, fraud, and abuse of government resources.[35] This particular initiative also played a part in the announcement regarding a $22 million suit that was settled between the DOJ and Saint Joseph Medical Center (SJMC) in Towson, Maryland. The hospital agreed to pay the amount in recompense for violations falling under the False Claims Act. Although the hospital did not admit to any wrongdoing as part of the settlement, the allegations included the following:

1. paying kickbacks to MidAtlantic Cardiovascular Associates "under the guise of professional service agreements, in return for MACVA's referrals to the medical center for lucrative cardiovascular procedures, including cardiac surgery and interventional cardiology procedures"

2. accepting payments from federal health care programs "for medically unnecessary stents performed by Dr. Mark Midei, MD., a one time partner in MACVA who was later employed by SJMC"

An oversight committee of the U.S. Senate is investigating whether Midei may have implanted hundreds of medically unnecessary stents at SJMC. The review is examining whether the case of Midei is isolated or indicates a larger national problem.[36]

To offer a sense of the magnitude of fraudulent activity in federal health care programs, consider that in fiscal year 2010, the government recovered more than $4 billion in taxpayer dollars from fraud.[37] Above and beyond the cost of such fraudulent activity lies a well-accepted body of evidence demonstrating that up to one third of our nation's health care dollars are spent on ineffective, unproven, and unwanted medical procedures.[38] By some reports, this amounts to nearly $700 billion per year spent on unnecessary and ineffective treatments,[39] an amount that would go a long way toward subsidizing the cost of universal, high-quality health care in the Unites States.

Rationing

The mere mention of rationing is often a deal breaker for health care reform. Rationing involves the deliberate reduction or outright denial—whether temporary or permanent—of health care services that could benefit an individual or group of persons. There is little dispute that implicit forms of such rationing already occur in our health system. Examples include waiting lists for organ transplants, locations of health care services (some services are offered only in metropolitan areas), and decisions by employers to exclude certain procedures from employer-financed health insurance programs. Such implicit rationing extends further, such as when access is limited through inconvenient hours of operation or locations that are not adequately accessible with public transportation.

More explicit forms of rationing take place as well. Two examples are the cost to patients of copayments or out-of-pocket fees payable at the doctor's office and the cost of deductibles. (The deductible is the cost payable by the patient for a particular service after their health insurance has paid its portion.) Finally, one of the most explicit forms of rationing is the lack of affordable health care for people who are underinsured or uninsured. A significant form of rationing is the lack of universal access to affordable health care for all U.S. citizens.

Before critics of health care reform raise their voices against rationing, it should be acknowledged that our current system not only has rationing, but employs rationing intentionally to keep costs down through decreasing potentially beneficial use. In this sense, rationing is actually a tool employed to moderate consumer use. Rationing means different things to those with different interests in health care. For instance, for insurance companies, rationing procedures—such as those that make use of high deductible plans in which consumers pay a high share of costs out-of-pocket—give consumers pause before undertaking a particular service. For the insurance company, the intended beneficial outcome is that they will not have to pay a claim, thereby saving them money. Such savings contributes to their financial bottom line, but it might also mean a patient goes without a necessary treatment.

The word *rationing* raises fears, many of which are not grounded in a factual understanding of either our current system or how the shared benefits and burdens of a more universal coverage system would work in terms of cost-containment and resource allocation. In any health care system comprised of finite goods, some rational limits to treatments are necessary and unavoidable. We simply cannot cover every form of treatment for every person in every instance. Given this, our orientation needs to have greater focus on fair allocation.

In allocating health care resources, a distinction is drawn between *macroallocation* and *microallocation*. According to John Kilner, professor of bioethics at Trinity International University, macroallocation concerns the distribution of health care resources at the "broad institutional or societal" levels;[40] it covers the "way a hospital budgets its spending, as well as the amount of resources a nation devotes to primary or preventive care compared with high technology curative medicine and nonmedical activities such as education and defense."[41] Microallocation refers to "treatment decisions regarding particular persons" and may include "deciding which of several potentially beneficial treatments to provide an individual patient, particularly when only a limited time of treatment is available."[42] Each type of allocation has its own set of ethical issues and degree of complexity. Because macroallocation occurs at such a broad level, it can be overly abstract and seemingly merit less attention from the masses. Microallocation occurs at a low level and affects persons intimately, thus earning more public attention. Given that microallocation seems to evoke this more visceral response, it is prudent to briefly address four criteria for microallocation decisions,[43] all of which raise ethical issues.

1. Social Criteria[44]

These criteria give treatment preferences to persons judged to be of most value to society. These criteria are characterized by the assumption that, all things being equal, health care resources should be provided within society with a concern for the best return on the social investment of resources. Hence, under such criteria, some would argue persons of greater merit should, all things considered, receive health care resources that are in short supply. What does greater merit mean? For many, it centers on the economic and social contribution that individuals bring to society. This means that social criteria for rationing would give a greater share of beneficial treatments to those who have a greater economic and social effect on society.

Given our normative ethical basis, what are some ethical concerns with this approach?

2. Sociomedical Criteria

These criteria are similar to social criteria in that they attempt to produce an overall social good. They have the added characteristic of combining a set of medical justifications for microallocation. The first of the sociomedical criteria is age-based decision making. Given one's age, assuming the elderly may be less likely to benefit from health care resources because of their age, some advocate limiting care to certain elderly populations. Another criterion some employ is psychosocial, with treatment "rationed" if a patient cannot manage the treatment emotionally or intellectually, or if weak coping capacities might limit the efficacy of treatment. The assumption is that for treatment to be beneficial, one must possess the capacity to be engaged in the treatment and healing process. Another dimension to such sociomedical criteria favors those who have a supportive environment before, during, and after treatment, allocating scarce resources to those with adequate social supports.

Given our normative ethical basis, what are some ethical concerns with this approach?

3. Medical Criteria

Allocation decisions made using medical criteria may limit resource use by those for whom benefit is less likely. *Benefit* in this sense is broad—it centers on the length and quality of overall benefit that a particular medical treatment might provide. Treatments that do not confer benefit in this broad sense are considered futile and, based on medical criteria, are often limited. These criteria arise frequently in the end-of-life context in which life-sustaining measures are demanded but may not, other than prolonging the inevitability of death, benefit the patient holistically. The potential for imminent death is another kind of medical criteria that might be a determining factor in allocation decisions. Those who may die imminently without medical intervention could take priority in allocation decisions if they could benefit from medical interventions.

Given our normative ethics basis, what are some ethical concerns with this approach?

4. Personal Criteria

These criteria give personal values and choices a primary place in allocation decisions. For example, based on one's values, one may decide that further life-sustaining interventions do not meet one's goals or purpose in life. As a result, the patient may choose to discontinue life-prolonging therapy that is providing some benefit. Another aspect of these criteria involves responsibility and accountability. For example, those who have smoked their entire lives may not receive priority in allocation decisions regarding cardiac surgery. Another example of these criteria could be the patient's ability to pay. One who cannot afford services could, even if one's life is at stake, be passed over in some allocation decisions. On the other hand, one who can pay could, in the end, benefit first in allocation decisions precisely because they can pay for the service out-of-pocket—this could happen irrespective of one's overall medical condition and potential benefit from treatment.

Given our normative ethical basis, what are some ethical concerns with this approach?

Transparency in the Costs of Health Care

Have you ever been to your medical doctor and seen a pricelist behind the front desk? Have you gone to the hospital emergency department and seen a listing of the services and their costs? Do you know what an X-ray will cost you out-of-pocket? What does it cost a doctor's office or hospital to do an X-ray? What is the difference between hospital charges and the amount the hospital receives for reimbursement from third-party payers? What would your prescriptions cost if you had to pay them out-of-pocket versus through your prescription benefit? You get the point. The costs of health care are not transparent in this country. Those lucky enough to have health insurance and prescription coverage tend not to ask what something costs. Gaining more transparency for health care costs and creating a system that delivers more effective care at less cost could help patients become better stewards of a finite social good.

Effective Community Oversight and Planning Measures

Originally conceived under the 1974 National Health Act, certificate of need (CON) laws were intended to achieve three goals: to curb escalating health care costs, to avoid duplication of resources in local communities, and to help provide equal access to high-quality health care. In states with CON laws, health care organizations must file an application with the state for a particular activity—for example, the construction of a new hospital or the intent to purchase new technologies like magnetic resonance imaging. Among other things, community need must be demonstrated for projects to proceed. Competitors often oppose one another's CON applications, citing lack of community need and other concerns; typically, such objections are a stall tactic to preserve market share. Health care is an important part of community planning, and the CON process can ensure health care resources are used effectively and equitably. CON laws explicitly connect the just distribution of health care resources with community need. Some states do not have CON laws, arguing that free-market forces will sufficiently limit oversupply. Others argue that state and federal public agencies have significant oversight responsibility, and that because health care resources are precious, any use of them should consider the community's need in a regulated manner.

Personal Responsibility

In health care reform, all too often it appears individuals believe health care delivery is a one-way transaction. That is, many view health care as though it exists for individuals only. Many fail to see the importance personal choices have in keeping health care costs down, promoting wellness, and preventing illness. We all know many benefits are associated with, for example, a good diet and regular exercise. We all know excessive drinking and smoking are harmful to one's health. Personal responsibility also extends to the type of medical services one wants. Some medical services are directed toward personal enhancement and are not necessary for the treatment of a specific condition. Should cosmetic surgery be covered by insurance? Should assisted reproductive technologies be covered by insurance? Should human growth hormone therapy in children be covered by insurance?

Seeking Excellence in Health Care: New Rules for the Twenty-First-Century Health System

Seeking excellence in health care explicitly relates to the ethical foundations of health care reform. From the perspective of human dignity and justice, health care systems, processes, and relationships should be organized in ways that demonstrate respect for persons and the just use of resources. This will, in the end, promote individual and social well-being. Seeking excellence in the quality of health care we deliver, then, is one way our society can demonstrate its commitment to the belief that people are valuable and that human flourishing should be an organizing value for health care delivery.

One significant barrier to health care reform is the public's concern that lower-cost health care will equate to lower-quality. This fear is misplaced, for we have long known more treatment does not necessarily equate to better outcomes. In fact, it can create poorer health outcomes. Also we have known that in many regions across the country, health care organizations and providers are delivering high-quality care at comparatively lower costs than their counterparts. The challenge seems to be in replicating the success of such organizations and providers. Although there may not be a specific formula for achieving these results, there are specific, important steps the best providers and organizations take to promote higher quality and lower costs.

In its important 2001 book, *Crossing the Quality Chasm*, the Institute of Medicine (IOM) advances ways in which U.S. health care can reform to allow the best possible health outcomes at the lowest costs, while also making health care a rewarding profession for those who choose it.[45] In this book, the IOM offers ten simple rules for health care in the twenty-first century. These rules are presented next to the way in which health care is now organized (see figure 12A).[46]

Several themes emerge from these "new rules." The first, and perhaps most important, is that the value of health care should be gauged first by the outcomes it produces, not the money it generates. Yet, most health systems and physician practices, whether for profit or not for profit, are organized around a financial business model that chases money. In our current system, clinicians are paid for the volume of work conducted—more tests, more procedures, more everything. To put it differently, clinicians are paid for doing more health care, not for doing health care well. This encourages waste and overconsumption and, as we have seen, can produce poor outcomes for patients precisely because complications arise from doing more things to patients.

Many health care organizations known for their high quality take a different approach. They have organized their business model around providing high-quality, patient-centered care. Instead of simply doing more, they are doing what is appropriate for the patient's overall well-being and healing. Moreover, they do this in a way that respects patient values and goals, in a shared decision-making context. In such patient-centered health care, the patient's needs drive health care relationships and delivery. With this approach, it is no longer simply "doctor knows best" but a shared decision-making approach in which patients and their clinicians work together to produce better health outcomes.

This notion has flowered into a philosophy of health care delivery often referred to as the "patient-centered medical home" (PCMH).[47] This approach seeks to redesign how care is offered so that it is delivered by a team of providers led by one's physician that provides coordinated care for patients throughout their lives. One hallmark of a PCMH is the use of electronic health records. Electronic records include evidence-based decision-making software that is built within the computer program, thereby allowing the best and

HEALTH CARE	
Current Approach	New Rule for Twenty-first Century
Care is based primarily on visits	Care is based on continuing healing relationships
Professional autonomy drives variability	Care is customized by patient needs and values
Professionals control care	Patients control care
Information is a private record	Knowledge is shared and information flows freely
Decision making is based on training and experience	Decision making is based on evidence
"Do no harm" is an individual responsibility	"Do no harm" is a system responsibility
Secrecy is common	Transparency is endorsed
The system reacts to needs	The system anticipates needs
Cost reduction is sought	Waste is continually decreased
Professional competition runs the system	Cooperation among clinicians is a priority

FIGURE 12A Ten Rules for Health Care

most current evidence to guide the recommendations that clinicians make for patients. This means decision trees describing treatments and potential outcomes are available to clinicians electronically. They have the information they need to make quick and sound recommendations to patients. Electronic records also allow an entirely new mode of communication among health care professionals and between health care professionals and their patients. This promotes a different kind of access and develops more engaged patients who have more tools to help them increase their level of accountability for their own well-being. Using these systems, patients can more easily communicate with their doctor's office through e-mail and enter and track critical health data such as daily or weekly weights, blood pressures, and blood glucose levels that give caregivers real-time information critical for monitoring patients and tailoring treatment recommendations.

With electronic health records, there is less need to rerun common, often expensive, tests—test results are visible in the electronic medical record and ideally available for referring and consulting physicians to see. All a consulting physician needs to do is to see a patient in the office or hospital setting, write an electronic (instead of an often indecipherable handwritten) note in the electronic chart and as soon as that note is entered into the record, it will be in the patient's record for all his or her providers to see. Imagine: a single, central location for a complete electronic health record that is accessible to a patient's full panel of clinicians. The beauty of this scenario is that it is no longer imaginary. It is already happening in health systems across the country. Moreover, it is happening in health systems known for their high-quality, low-cost, patient-centered health care, because they understand its value for health outcomes.

The downside to electronic health record software systems is that they are costly, they vary in their degree of sophistication and customization, and many do not "talk" to one another or have the capacity to link with one another to share patient information. This means many patients will not be able to benefit from the real-time data, evidence-based decision-making tools, and enhanced communication and health-promotion features these systems offer. The challenge for us now and in the future is to find ways to provide secure information exchanges so that the masses can benefit from electronic health records. One important feature of the new health care reform law is that it provides financial incentives for providers to purchase electronic health-record systems. It also promotes the creation of information exchanges that will allow different electronic health records to "talk" with one another more effectively.

A number of ethical issues are raised by electronic health records, however. Security questions must be addressed to safeguard private information. Questions of access, such as who should have access to medical records and how much access is needed must also be addressed. All of these issues must be considered fully so that the interests of privacy are balanced by the vital health benefits that electronic health records offer.

Another important feature of PCMH is the seamless coordination of patient care. Providing such care requires a shift in thinking and practice for health care providers and physician practices. Primarily, it means physicians will not be solely responsible for the health needs of their patients. Under this movement, care is team-based, grounded in preventive and comprehensive care, and more efficient. As discussed, the electronic health record can assist with such coordination. However, it also requires redesigning how work is done in the clinic and hospital. In fact, it means doctor appointments become just one way in which patients interact with their providers, not the only or even the primary way.

Under this way of thinking, traditional views of the physician as the primary clinical decision maker will be challenged. All health care professionals will be asked to operate at the highest level of their license. This will challenge traditional roles. Care coordinators, nurses primarily, will regularly follow up with chronically ill and unstable patients by phone to keep the lines of health communication open between patients and medical practices. This will help prevent unnecessary emergency department visits where costs are highest. This will also help prevent rehospitalizations that drive up costs. When transitions take place that require a move from curative to comfort care (for example, between aggressive medical care aimed at reversing an illness versus symptom management aimed at treating the symptoms of the illness), they will be approached with the understanding that patient wishes and values will be considered in treatment decisions.

The PCMH concept is quickly making its way throughout the primary care setting. In fact, the concept is nearly forty years old. Today, more systematic projects are under way to deepen its benefit for patients. Pilot projects are seeking to transform how care is delivered. Early reports show a high degree of satisfaction from clinic staff. However, these reports are also noting that patients seem a bit confused by the PCMH changes.[48] This brings home one of the most important elements in the PCMH process and in health care reform generally: until individuals take responsibility for their health, and until the health system actively partners with them to help them take responsibility for their health, successful reform of health care delivery will be difficult to attain. This means, in part, that those in the health care profession, as well as all others with an interest in health care reform, must do the work required to empower individuals to take charge of their health.

This is health care delivery in the twenty-first century: electronic, patient-centered, collaborative, coordinated, and grounded in science. All too often, health care reform focuses solely on debates over access, cost, and quality. These are key considerations, but equally key is reforming how care is delivered. As these reforms continue to take shape, new ethical issues will emerge that will call for new, creative thinking in ethical discourse.

In this new era of health care delivery, new ethical issues will arise. They will call for creative solutions and approaches. Regardless of how new, however, health care issues will continue to raise age-old ethical questions. The case below is intended to spark new thinking while at the same time incorporating age-old ethical frameworks to help address the issues the case raises.

Case 12B

With the installation of its electronic medical record, Southside Pediatrics and Family Practice can now offer patients electronic access to their medical record via a patient portal system. The patients can see all lab results, progress notes, immunizations,

cont.

Case 12B *cont.*

patient "problem" lists, and so forth. There is emerging evidence suggesting that such access enhances patient satisfaction, as well as participation in clinical decision making. Additionally, patients become more active participants in their health and well-being.

In determining how patients should use the portal, the leadership team confronts a series of interrelated ethical questions. They wonder whether pediatric patients should have access to their electronic medical record. If yes, at what age should electronic access be granted? What should pediatric patients be able to see on their electronic medical record? Should pediatric patients be able to decide whether they have access? Or should their parents or guardians decide? The leadership team also discusses whether parents should have access to their child's electronic medical record. Should parents have full access to their child's record? There are sometimes sensitive conversations that doctors have with young children. Such conversations, if public and accessible to their parents—such as sexual activity—could be harmful to children. At what age should parental access be limited or restricted altogether? What rights do pediatric patients have in limiting parental access to their own medical chart? Though the members of the practice are convinced an electronic medical record will improve the quality of patient care, they are concerned it may have some downsides as well.

Discussion questions. What ethical issues and implications do the practice leaders' questions raise? What ethical principles and values are important in approaching these questions? Whose voice should be heard when answering these questions? What creative options and measures can the team take to accommodate the competing interests raised by the practice leaders' questions? What would you advise the team to do? Defend your approach.

Conclusion

For any person, organization, or society, reform is necessary. Reform is simply committing to a rational process that can make "things" better for individuals, organizations, and society. Though complex and often costly, both financially and socially, reform seeks to enhance well-being. What makes health care reform ethically vital is the degree to which health care promotes human flourishing. Without access to affordable, high-quality health care services, total well-being is difficult to attain. Financially, the health care system in the United States is compromised—many are increasingly arguing it is in crisis mode. The United States spends far more per person and as a nation on health care than any other country in the world. Yet, for all that money, U.S. citizens and communities are far less healthy than those of many other industrialized countries.[49] Health care in the United States is largely viewed as just another industry. As a result, it is measured primarily by its economic effect and potential to build wealth as opposed to its ability to improve the health of the community. Efforts to achieve comprehensive reform have long been undermined by partisan politics, not the lack of effort or desire. U.S. health care in the twenty-first century should be grounded in important social and professional ethical norms, the economic realities facing the system, and a systematic commitment to change the delivery system to increase the quality of care.

SUGGESTED READINGS

Brownlee, Shannon. *Overtreated: Why Too Much Medicine Is Making Us Sicker and Poorer.* New York: Bloomsbury, 2007.

Callahan, Daniel. *Taming the Beloved Beast: How Medical Technology Costs Are Destroying Our Health Care System.* Princeton: Princeton University Press, 2009.

Mahar, Maggie. *Money-Driven Medicine: The Real Reason Health Care Costs So Much.* New York: Collins Books, 2006.

Reid, T. R. *The Healing of America: The Global Quest for Better, Fairer, and Cheaper Health Care.* New York: Penguin, 2009.

MULTIMEDIA AIDS FOR TEACHERS

Important Web sites

http://www.dartmouthatlas.org/
"For more than 20 years, the Dartmouth Atlas Project has documented glaring variations in how medical resources are distributed and used in the United States. The project uses Medicare data to provide information and analysis about national, regional, and local markets, as well as hospitals and their affiliated physicians. This research has helped policymakers, the media, health care analysts and others improve their understanding of the U.S. health care system and forms the foundation for many of the ongoing efforts to improve health and health systems across America" (text from Web site).

http://www.commonwealthfund.org/
"The Commonwealth Fund is a private foundation that promotes a high performing health care system that achieves better access, improved quality, and greater efficiency, particularly for society's most vulnerable, including low-income people, the uninsured, minority Americans, young children, and elderly adults" (text from website).

http://www.moneydrivenmedicine.org/
Money-Driven Medicine. Directed by Andy Fredericks. 2009. This film examines how medicine is organized around the pursuit of money. Contains commentary from the nation's leading health care policy experts, ethicists, and clinicians.

http://www.pbs.org/wgbh/pages/frontline/sickaroundtheworld/
Sick around the World. Produced and directed by Jon Palfreman. Aired April 15, 2008. This PBS *Frontline* documentary provides a comparative analysis of how health care is delivered in five capitalist democracies. The film provides a platform for learning about health care systems around the world and offers an analysis of different approaches to health care delivery.

http://www.pbs.org/wgbh/pages/frontline/sickaroundamerica/view/
Sick around America. Written, produced, and directed by Jon Palfreman. Aired March 31, 2009. This PBS *Frontline* film inspects the U.S. health care system and considers factors contributing to the need for fundamental health care reform.

ENDNOTES

1. *http://www.cms.gov/NationalHealthExpendData/downloads/highlights.pdf* (accessed January 19, 2011).

2. *http://www.pbs.org/newshour/indepth_coverage/health/healthreform/july-dec09/chart_08-18.html* (accessed January 19, 2011).

3. *http://www.cbpp.org/cms/?fa=view&id=628* (accessed February 27, 2011).

4. For a comprehensive summary of reforms in the original legislation and timelines for implementation, see *http://www.commonwealthfund.org/Health-Reform/Health-Reform-Resource.aspx.* See also *http://www.kff.org/healthreform/upload/housebill_final.pdf* (accessed January 19, 2011).

5. For an accessible introductory review of justice, see Karen Lebacqz, *Six Theories of Justice* (Minneapolis: Augsburg, 1986).

6. Leonard Weber, *Business Ethics in Healthcare* (Bloomington: Indiana University Press, 2001), 9.

7. Benedict M. Ashley, Jean DeBlois, and Kevin D. O'Rourke, *Health Care Ethics: A Theological Analysis,* 5th ed. (Washington, DC: Georgetown University Press, 2006), 45.

8. For a critique on the relationship between medicine's moral ends and Western beliefs on the sanctity of life, see Daniel Callahan, *The Troubled Dream of Life: In Search of a Peaceful Death* (Washington, DC: Georgetown University Press, 2000), esp. 23–90.

9. Weber, *Business Ethics in Healthcare,* 4–6.

10. Ibid., 4.

11. *http://www.cdc.gov/H1n1flu/update.htm* (accessed January 19, 2011).

12. *http://www.cdc.gov/h1n1flu/pdf/graph_March%202010.pdf* (accessed January 19, 2011).

13. For a final draft of the ventilator guidance document prepared for the Ventilator Workgroup for the Ethics Subcommittee of the Advisory Committee to the Director of the CDC, see *http://s3.amazonaws.com/propublica/assets/docs/Vent_Guidance_.draftoc2008pdf.pdf* (accessed January 19, 2011).

14. See, for example, Leonard M. Fleck, *Just Caring: Health Care Rationing and Democratic Deliberation* (New York: Oxford University Press, 2009). See also Mary J. McDonough, *Can Health Care Market Be Moral: A Catholic Vision* (Washington, DC: Georgetown University Press, 2007).

15. See, for example, Norman Daniels, *Just Health: Meeting Health Needs Fairly* (New York: Cambridge University Press, 2007).

16. Daniel Callahan, *What Kind of Life: The Limits of Medical Progress* (Washington, DC: Georgetown University Press, 1990), 123ff.

17. Ibid., 136–49.

18. Paula A. Braverman, Susan A. Egerter, and Robin E. Mockenhaupt, "Broadening the Focus: The Need to Address the Social Determinants of Health," *American Journal of Preventive Medicine* 40, Supplement 1 (2011): S6.

19. Braverman et al., "Broadening the Focus," S6.

20. Institute of Medicine, *Unequal Treatment: Confronting Racial and Ethnic Disparities in Health Care* (Washington, DC: National Academies Press, 2003), 29.

21. Institute of Medicine, *Unequal Treatment*, 30.

22. Shannon Brownlee, *Overtreated: Why Too Much Medicine Is Making Us Sicker and Poorer* (New York: Bloomsbury, 2007), 40.

23. Gina Kolata, "Popular Blood Therapy May Not Work," *New York Times*, January 12, 2010. See article online at *http://www.nytimes.com/2010/01/13/health/13tendon.html?adxnnl=1&adxnnlx=1306757739-mmRIDE09BN7jS-ToVzzuSOA* (accessed May 30, 2011).

24. Shepard Hurwitz, "Evidence-Based Medicine in Orthopaedic Surgery: A Way for the Future," *Iowa Orthopaedic Journal* 23 (2003): 61–5.

25. See Atual Gawande, "The Cost Conundrum," *The New Yorker*, June 1, 2009.

26. Brownlee, *Overtreated*, 109–16.

27. See, for example, the Dartmouth Atlas, *http://www.dartmouthatlas.org/keyissues/issue.aspx?con=2937* (accessed February 27, 2011).

28. Maggie Mahar, *Money-Driven Medicine: The Real Reason Healthcare Costs So Much* (New York: Collins Books, 2006), esp. 159–73.

29. Mahar, *Money-Driven Medicine*, 159–73.

30. Elliott Fisher et al., "The Implications of Regional Variations in Medicare Spending, Part 1: The Content, Quality, and Accessibility of Care," *Annals of Internal Medicine* 138 (February 18, 2003): 273–87.

31. See, for example, the Dartmouth Atlas, *http://www.dartmouthatlas.org/downloads/reports/Joint_Replacement_0410.pdf* (accessed February 27, 2011).

32. Mahar, *Money-Driven Medicine*, 164. For the primary source, see John Wennberg, "Variation in Use of Medicare Services among Regions and Selected Academic Medical Centers," Duncan W. Clarke Lecture, New York Academy of Medicine, New York City, January 24, 2005.

33. Gawande, "The Cost Conundrum."

34. See, for example, the experience of Grand Junction, Colorado. Relatively speaking, health care delivery in this city is cheaper and better than other places around the country: *http://newamerica.net/files/GrandJunctionCO-HealthCommunityWorks.pdf* (accessed February 26, 2011).

35. For more information, see *http://www.stopmedicarefraud.gov/heatsuccess/index.html* (accessed January 21, 2011).

36. For more information on this case, see *www.justice.gov/opa/pr/2010/November/10-civ-1271.html* (accessed January 21, 2011).

37. See *http://www.hhs.gov/news/press/2011pres/01/20110124a.html* (accessed January 21, 2011).

38. According to Dr. Jack Wennberg of the Center for the Evaluative Clinical Sciences at Dartmouth Medical School, quoted in Mahar, *Money-Driven Medicine*, 159.

39. *http://www.ppionline.org/ppi_ci.cfm?contentid=254814&knlgAreaID=111&subsecid=900033#item1* (accessed January 21, 2011).

40. John Kilner, "Health-Care Resources, Allocation of," in *Encyclopedia of Bioethics*, vol. 2, ed. Warren Thomas Reich (New York: MacMillan Library Reference, 2005, 1067.

41. Ibid., 1067.

42. Ibid., 1075.

43. Ibid., 1076–82.

44. For this section, I have relied heavily on Ibid., 1076–82.

45. Institute of Medicine, *Crossing the Quality Chasm: A New Health System for the 21st Century* (Washington, DC: National Academy Press, 2001), 66–83.

46. Institute of Medicine, 67, table 3-1.

47. See *http://www.acponline.org/running_practice/pcmh/understanding/what.htm* (accessed February 7, 2011).

48. Pauline Chen, "Putting Patients at the Center of the Medical Home," *New York Times*, July 15, 2010. See full article at *http://www.nytimes.com/2010/07/15/health/15chen.html* (accessed February 7, 2011).

49. *http://www.oecd.org/dataoecd/46/2/38980580.pdf* (accessed February 9, 2011).

GLOSSARY

abortion, induced The medical or surgical termination of pregnancy before the time of fetal viability.

abortion, surgical Any method of manually removing an unborn fetus from the womb using either manual or electric vacuum aspiration (suction curettage), dilation and evacuation (D&E), or dilation and extraction (D&E) using surgical instruments.

advance care planning The process by which individuals—no matter where they are on the health-sickness continuum—proactively plan for their future health care decisions. One method by which individuals make future plans for their treatment is by completing advance directives. There are many kinds of advance directives, including oral declarations of one's future wishes, living-will documents that state a person's wishes should certain conditions be met, and durable power of attorney documents in which a patient appoints someone to make decisions on the patient's behalf should the patient lose that capacity.

allele Two or more variants of a gene responsible for causing certain physical characteristics or traits.

allowing to die In the Catholic tradition, allowing to die involves the withholding or withdrawing of life-sustaining treatment that is judged by the patient or the patient's family or surrogate to be excessively burdensome, of little or no benefit, or both. It involves a decision to no longer prevent the underlying disease process or pathology to run its course.

artificial insemination (AI) Collecting sperm from a male (usually by means of masturbation) and injecting the sperm directly into the woman's uterus.

artificial nutrition and hydration (ANH) A technological method or medical means of getting nutrients to individuals whose nutritional needs cannot otherwise be met, temporarily or permanently, due to a medical condition.

autonomy The capacity for rational thought, self-determination, and the ability to determine for oneself what is right and wrong, good and bad.

Belmont Report A report from the Department of Health, Education, and Welfare, Office of the Secretary, concerning Ethical Principles and Guidelines for the Protection of Human Subjects of Research, issued in 1979.

benefit As a moral norm or criterion for treatment decisions, it refers to positive effects of treatment that result in improvements in one's condition such that one is able to pursue goods bound up with human flourishing, especially human relationships and other personal goods one finds important, at least at a minimal level.

best-interests standard An ethical standard used in treatment decisions when a patient's wishes are not known that bases such decisions on what is perceived to promote maximally the overall good of the patient in question.

blastocyst A very early embryo consisting of approximately 150 to 300 cells. The blastocyst is a spherical cell mass produced after approximately five to seven days of cell divisions. It contains a microscopic cluster of cells called the inner cell mass (from which embryonic stem cells are derived) and an outer layer of cells called the trophoblast (that forms the placenta).

burden As a moral norm or criterion for treatment decisions, it refers to negative effects of treatment that result in pain, suffering, or other hardships such that one is profoundly frustrated in the pursuit of goods bound up with human flourishing, especially human relationships, and other personal goods one finds important.

cardiopulmonary resuscitation (CPR) Various methods for reversing cardiac or respiratory arrest that include chest compressions, assisted ventilation, defibrillation, and the use of drugs.

carrier A person who has an abnormal copy of a gene and can pass an inherited genetic disease on to his or her offspring.

cell line Cells of a particular type that have been grown and proliferated in culture, outside the body, in a petri dish.

chromosome A threadlike structure of nucleic acids and protein found in the nucleus of most living cells, carrying genetic information in the form of genes.

chronic illness A disease state that typically lasts at least three months, generally cannot be cured by medications or vaccines, and does not disappear. Many chronic illnesses such as diabetes or chronic obstructive pulmonary disease (COPD) will last many years.

circumstances The factual and contextual features that surround concrete situations and have a bearing on ethical decision making.

cloning The process of replicating genetic material and even whole organisms. It is an asexual method of reproduction in which offspring are created from a single "parent." Reproductive cloning refers to implanting a cloned embryo in the uterus of a female so that she will later give birth to the cloned offspring. Therapeutic cloning creates embryos that are then allowed to develop to the blastocyst stage (three to five days), at which time they will be destroyed for the purpose of obtaining their stem cells for research that might one day lead to actual therapies.

Code of Federal Regulations (45 CFR 46)—Human Subjects Research Issued by the Office of Human Subjects Research in the Department of Health and Human Services of the federal government that provides the basis for the protection of human subjects enrolled in research.

comparative effectiveness research Clinical research designed to determine the effectiveness of one treatment versus another.

conflict of interest A divergence between an individual's or institution's private interests and the professional obligations to administer or monitor clinical research in an objective manner.

congenital malformations A physical defect in an infant present at birth caused either by a genetic factor or by prenatal events that are not genetic in nature (e.g., toxic exposure or birth injury).

Congregation for the Doctrine of the Faith (CDF) The oldest of nine congregations of the Roman Curia responsible for overseeing Catholic Church doctrine.

consequences The result or outcome of one's actions.

consequentialist theories Rooted in modern thought, these theories focus on the consequences of our actions, in light of the good we are trying to promote through our actions.

continuum of care Also commonly referred to as continuity of care. The degree to which care for a patient is coherent and linked over the course of the many transitions from place to place and from professional to professional that the patient will experience (for example, doctor's office, outpatient surgery, hospital, rehab therapy).

critically ill newborn Newborns who are extremely sick or suffering from serious medical complications due to, among other things, prematurity, severe brain damage, or congenital malformations.

cryopreservation A process that involves freezing the "excess" or "spare" embryos at appropriate temperatures so they can be used later if needed.

culture (cell) The propagation of microorganisms or cells in a petri dish or other medium.

curative treatment Medical treatment aimed at curing a specific disease. Throughout the course of a chronic illness (for example, cancer), decisions are often made to transition from medical therapies directed to curing a disease toward treating only the symptoms of the disease as a means of maintaining patient comfort and holistic well-being.

Declaration of Helsinki A document issued by the World Medical Association in 1964, and most recently revised in 2000, addressing ethical principles for the medical community regarding human experimentation.

deontological theories Rooted in the legal traditions of Judaic and later Roman thought, these theories focus mainly on our actions, what we choose to do as the means to an end.

deoxyribonucleic acid (DNA)   Two long strands of nucleotides twisted in the shape of a double helix and responsible for carrying genetic information in the cell.

disability   A physical or mental condition that limits a person's functions, senses, or activities.

discernment   The skill or virtue that enables one to perceive and distinguish degrees of value among diverse factors, differentiate among possible options, and come to the most loving and virtuous response in concrete moral situations.

dominant gene   A gene that results in the manifestation of a trait associated with it whether or not it is matched with an identical allele.

do-not-resuscitate (DNR)   A medical order not to employ various measures to restore heartbeat and respiration after a patient's heart has stopped beating.

double effect   A methodological principle in Catholic moral theology that helps guide decisions related to actions that have two effects—one good and the other bad. The principle holds that one may perform such actions if (1) the action is good or neutral in itself; (2) one intends the good effect and not the bad; (3) the good and bad effects occur together so that the evil effect does not become a means to the good effect, and (4) there is a proportionately serious reason for allowing the unintended bad effect to occur.

egg harvesting   A process in which a woman receives fertility drugs so that her ovaries produce an abnormally large number of eggs. The woman undergoing this process must have her blood tested every other day to measure hormone levels, and she must have periodic ultrasounds. Before egg retrieval, the woman must receive a hormone shot of human chorionic gonadotropin (HCG) to prepare the eggs for release. The actual retrieval is done under anesthesia, using a long needle to obtain ten to twenty eggs.

ELSI   Part of the Human Genome Project dedicated to studying the ethical, legal, and social implications (ELSI) of genetic research and manipulation.

embryo   An unborn human baby in the first eight weeks from conception, after implantation but before all the organs are developed.

embryo transfer (ET)   The transferring of one or more of the resulting embryos from some sort of reproductive technology, after they have incubated for three to five days in a culture medium, into a woman's uterus.

Ethical and Religious Directives for Catholic Health Care Services   An official document published and approved by the United States Conference of Catholic Bishops that provides moral guidance and direction on various aspects of health care delivery and to which all U.S. Catholic health care organizations must adhere.

ethical relativism   The view that morally right and wrong actions are relative to a particular group of people or an individual.

ethics   In its broadest sense, any behavior or decision that affects human well-being (dignity, character, quality of life) and the good of the community. The basic task of ethics is to ask and seek answers to two related questions: "Who ought we to become as persons?" (Being) and "How ought we to act in relation to people, God, and creation?" (Doing).

ethics committee   A multidisciplinary group composed of a broad spectrum of personnel—physicians, nurses, social workers, chaplains, ethicists, and others—that addresses the ethical issues within a health care organization. Typical functions include education, policy writing and review, and consultation.

eugenics   The manipulation of genetic inheritance to promote desirable traits (positive eugenics) or minimize the occurrence of undesirable traits (negative eugenics) in the general population.

euthanasia   An action or an omission that directly and intentionally brings about a terminally ill patient's death in order to relieve suffering.

evidence-based medicine   Also known as evidence-based practice, the process of grounding clinical decisions, to the extent possible, in the best and most current available science and research.

extraordinary or disproportionate means   Medical treatment that either fails to offer a proportionate hope of benefit or imposes an excessive burden on the patient or an excessive expense on the patient's family or the community.

extremely low birth weight Infants born weighing less than 1000 grams (2 pounds, 3.27 ounces).

fertility drugs Medication prescribed to a woman participating in reproductive technology to hyperstimulate the woman's ovaries for the purposes of egg production.

fetus An unborn human baby more than eight weeks after conception.

forgoing treatment Either withholding (not starting) or withdrawing (removing after starting) a treatment for a patient, typically at the end of life.

freedom Refers to freedom of self-determination and freedom of choice. Freedom of self-determination relates to being; it is the basic freedom to shape our lives and become the person we want and are called to be. Freedom of choice relates to doing; it is simply our ability to make our own choices.

gene A unit of heredity that is transferred from a parent to offspring and is held to determine some characteristic of the offspring.

gene mutation A permanent change or abnormality in the DNA sequence. Most gene mutations do not cause any problems, but some lead to genetic disorders, result in the inheritance of a genetic disorder, or increase one's risk of being affected by a genetic disorder.

gene therapy A technique of correcting defective genes to reverse, reduce, or eliminate diseases that have a genetic basis. When performed on genes in nonreproductive cells, this is known as somatic cell gene therapy. When performed in reproductive cells and the corrected genes will be passed on to offspring, this is known as germ-line gene therapy.

genetic enhancement The intentional alteration of human genes to improve traits that without intervention would otherwise be within the range of what is commonly regarded as normal, or improving them beyond what is needed to maintain or restore good health.

genetic testing The examination of a person's chromosomes to predict the risk of disease (predictive), screen newborn babies for genetic disease (newborn screening), identify carriers of genetic disease (carrier testing), and confirm the diagnosis of a genetic disease (diagnostic testing).

genomics The branch of molecular biology concerned with the structure, function, evolution, and mapping of genomes.

gestation The period of development in the uterus from conception to birth.

health care ethics A specialty of ethics, generally, is the study of how health care, in its structure, organization, delivery, relationships, and means, affects human well-being (dignity, character, quality of life) and the good of the community.

hospitalist physician A physician who treats patients solely in the hospital. Hospitalists do not see patients in the clinic or an office-based setting. Their role within the hospital setting is designed to oversee and coordinate the care of hospitalized patients.

human flourishing The goal to which all other goals should be directed. For Christians, human flourishing is understood as love of God, which is pursued most tangibly within the context of relationships. From an ethical perspective, we cannot love God and flourish as human beings without loving our neighbor as we love ourselves. Love of God and love of neighbor are thus inextricably bound together in ethics.

Human Genome Project A collaborative project among the government and private research organizations to identify and map the entire human genome, or complete set of genes and genetic instructions that make up the biologic basis of human life.

human subjects Human persons who enroll in human subjects research. Use of the term *subject* instead of *patient* denotes the distinction between rights and protections accorded a subject as compared with those accorded a patient.

Imago Dei The theological view that all human life is made in the image and likeness of God and destined for eternal union with God and, therefore, is endowed with an inherent and inalienable dignity or moral value.

induced pluripotent stem cells Adult cells that have been genetically reprogrammed to an embryonic stem cell-like state by being forced to express genes and factors important for maintaining the defining properties of embryonic stem cells.

induction of labor and delivery The use of synthetic hormones at sixteen weeks of pregnancy or beyond to cause contractions and the delivery of the fetus.

infant mortality Death of an infant within the first year of life.

informed consent A process whereby an individual is provided adequate information about a treatment option, its risks and benefits, alternatives and their risks and benefits, and makes a free choice about a particular option.

isolation (cell) In microbiology, separation of an organism or cell from others, usually by making serial cultures.

institutional review board (IRB) A specific group that is charged with protecting the rights and welfare of people involved in research. The IRB reviews plans for research involving human subjects. Institutions that accept research funding from the federal government must have an IRB to review all research involving human subjects (even if a given research project does not involve federal funds). The Food and Drug Administration and the Office of Protection from Research Risks (part of the National Institutes of Health) set the guidelines and regulations governing human subjects research and IRBs.

intensivist physician A physician who is specially trained in critical care medicine. Intensivists work in a hospital's critical care unit overseeing and coordinating the care of the sickest patients within the hospital.

intention The aim or end one is seeking to achieve through one's actions.

in vitro fertilization (IVF) A medical intervention that entails (1) harvesting eggs from a woman's ovaries (this could be either the woman seeking to have a baby or a donor); (2) collecting sperm from a male (husband, partner, or donor), usually obtained through masturbation, though other procedures offer options for such collection; (3) bringing the eggs and sperm together in a small laboratory dish (i.e., in vitro); and (4) facilitating fertilization of the eggs outside the body.

knowledge In ethics, the information we have to make decisions in concrete situations. This knowledge can be personal, moral, or circumstantial. Personal knowledge has to do with the level of insight we have into ourselves in terms of who we are and are called to become as persons. Moral knowledge deals with the sources of morality or ethics that guide us in making a decision. Circumstantial knowledge encompasses the facts surrounding the decisions with which we are faced.

life-sustaining treatment   A treatment, or set of treatments, designed to maintain the life of a critically ill person. Without such treatments, the person will die. Life-sustaining treatments can be highly technical, such as ventilator support to assist in the breathing process, or they can be nontechnical, such as antibiotic treatment for an infection or oral fluids for hydration.

medical futility   Any effort to initiate or continue a treatment when it is highly unlikely to succeed in achieving its desired ends or when its rare beneficial exceptions cannot be systematically explained or reproduced.

medical indications standard   An ethical standard used in treatment decisions that bases such decisions on objective medical information (e.g., physiological or clinical data) as opposed to quality of life considerations.

mind-body dualism   The idea that a human being is essentially a body that is inhabited by a mind.

morbidity   An illness or abnormal condition or quality.

multipotent (cells)   Stem cells that are believed to be limited to becoming only the type of cell of the tissue in which they are found.

narrative ethics   As used in the medical context, seeks to incorporate the lived experience of persons into ethical and clinical decision making. *Narrative competence* refers to a caregiver's ability to enter into the worldview of a patient to understand the person in all her entirety. In so doing, patient choice becomes an expression of one's life story or narrative. Narrative ethical reasoning is designed to promote shared decision making between patients and their caregivers.

neonatal intensive care unit (NICU)   A unit of a hospital specializing in the care of ill or premature newborn infants.

neonatal mortality   Death of a live-born infant within the first twenty-eight days of life.

nonpersonal view   A moral perspective that holds that the fetus does not deserve the same respect and protection as other members of the moral community because it has not yet actualized the capacities normally associated with fully functional persons.

normative basis A framework, point of reference, or backdrop against which we make ethical decisions and evaluate who we are as persons, the morality of our actions, and the effect of our actions on others. A normative basis gives us insight into the goals of human life, the virtues and characteristics that should define us as persons, and the principles that should guide our actions in concrete situations.

Nuremberg Code A set of research ethics principles for human experimentation set as a result of the subsequent Nuremberg Trials at the end of the Second World War.

ordinary or proportionate means Medical treatment that offers a proportionate hope of benefit without imposing an excessive burden on the patient or an excessive expense on the patient's family or the community.

palliative care A particular kind of medical care that focuses on the relief of suffering and the best possible quality of life for a patient (and the patient's caregivers) living with a life-limiting illness. Palliative care focuses on the continual assessment and treatment of the symptoms of a disease. It is important to distinguish between non-hospice palliative care and hospice palliative care. Non-hospice palliative care is offered in conjunction with life-prolonging and curative treatments for persons living with (but not yet dying from) life-limiting illnesses. Hospice palliative care begins when curative treatments are no longer effective and the decision has been made to transition care in a way that focuses solely on treating the symptoms of a disease that has progressed toward its final and more terminal phase.

patient-centered medical home (PCMH) The process of redesigning health care delivery in the clinic setting that is team oriented and coordinated across the life span of the patient. The idea is that the clinic, as opposed to the patient alone, will coordinate and manage patient care across the continuum of care. In so doing, patients take more ownership in their overall health, and decision making is more shared versus unilateral.

Patient Protection and Affordable Care Act (PPACA) A federal statute signed into law by President Barack Obama on March 23, 2010.

The law reforms many facets of health care access, delivery, and financing.

persistent vegetative state (PVS)   A medical condition resulting from severe brain damage that is characterized by the loss of all higher brain functions, with either complete or partial preservation of hypothalamic and brain-stem autonomic functions.

personal position   The view that human life, even at its earliest stage of existence, from the time the process of fertilization is complete, deserves the same moral respect and protection as any human person regardless of whether it ever actually becomes capable of conscious, autonomous, and rational thought.

physician-assisted suicide   The assistance of a physician in bringing about a patient's death when the patient is terminal.

placebo   A substance that has no therapeutic effect, used as a control in testing new drugs.

plasticity   The ability of stem cells to cross over from being the type belonging to one tissue or organ to a differentiated cell of another tissue or organ.

pluripotent (cells)   Stem cells that can become all the cell types that are found in an organism, but not the embryonic components of the trophoblast and placenta.

preimplantation genetic diagnosis (PGD)   A process that involves removing and testing a polar body (a small cell that is the by-product of meiosis) from an egg cell or, more commonly, a single cell from an early embryo before implantation, for identification of genetic mutations associated with disorders.

prenatal screening   A type of genetic testing performed during pregnancy to determine whether the unborn baby has or is at risk of having certain types of genetic abnormality.

pre-personal view   According to this view, the embryo deserves the respect and protection due to other human beings at a stage of development long before it has developed the capability to function in ways commonly associated with fully functional, autonomous individuals. However, according to this view, the embryo is not in fact due such respect and protection from the moment it comes into existence. Rather, the human embryo deserves respect and protection only once it reaches the biological point of development in which twinning is no longer possible.

pre-term or premature birth Birth of an infant before 37 completed weeks of gestation.

principal investigator (PI) The individual responsible for conducting the human subjects research protocol.

principles Moral norms that guide our decision making, conscience formation, and discernment in concrete situations (e.g., human dignity, justice, solidarity).

professional Specialized expert in a particular field, in the case of the physician, medical expertise and the particular moral commitments associated with physician practice.

proliferation Growth and reproduction of cells of the same type.

protocol Written detailed procedures for conducting the research study and collecting data.

rationing The deliberate reduction or outright denial—whether temporary or permanent—of health care services that could be beneficial for an individual or group.

recessive gene A gene that does not result in the manifestation of the trait with which it is associated unless matched with an identical allele.

regenerative medicine Medical interventions that aim to repair damaged organs, most often by using stem cells to replace cells and tissues damaged by aging and by disease.

regional variation in health care spending The phenomenon demonstrating that different parts of the country have different utilization habits, and therefore spending and cost trends, for the same medical procedure.

relational quality of life standard An ethical standard used in treatment decisions that bases such decisions on the perceived relationship between the patient's overall medical condition and the patient's ability to pursue the goals of life, understood as material, emotional, moral, intellectual, social, and spiritual values that transcend physical life itself.

reproductive technology (RT) A classification of medical interventions that separate human reproduction from the act of sexual intercourse in order to unite sperm to egg.

RU486 A combination of two drugs, mifespristone and misopristol, used to induce a medical abortion.

social determinants of health The view that individual and community health is determined by factors other than access to health care services. For instance, one's age, race, gender, educational level, socioeconomic status, and personal lifestyle choices all have affect one's overall health.

somatic cell nuclear transfer (SCNT) A cloning technique in which a nonreproductive (somatic) cell, such as a skin cell, is taken from an individual. The nucleus (the part of the cell containing the person's entire genetic code) is then extracted from that cell. That nucleus is then inserted into an ovum (egg) that has had its own nucleus and DNA removed. The egg with the nucleus from the somatic cell is then mixed with chemicals and given a small electric shock to start it growing.

stem cells Cells that have not yet developed a specialized function within the body or have not yet become a specific type of cell. Adult stem cells are found in the placenta and cord blood and different tissues of developed organisms. Embryonic stem cells are derived from the inner cell mass of a blastocyst and can differentiate into any cell or tissue type in the body, or potentially in a laboratory dish. These cells are obtained from five- to seven-day-old embryos.

supply-driven demand In health care spending, the view that the supply of resources (e.g., beds, operating rooms, MRI machines) as opposed to the underlying health needs of individuals and communities drives demand for service.

survival-to-discharge Refers to patients who are alive upon leaving the hospital.

teratoma A type of germ cell tumor, usually benign, composed of multiple tissues, including tissues not normally found in the organ in which it arises.

terminal illness A disease state that cannot be cured by current medical interventions and that has reached its final phase of progression.

transdifferentiation The conversion of stem cells derived from one tissue into cells normally found in another tissue.

Trisomy A genetic mutation in which an individual has an extra chromosome. The most common Trisomies include an extra chromosome at the twenty-first, eighteenth, and thirteenth pairs of chromosomes. Trisomy 21, the most common form, is known as Down syndrome. Trisomy 18, also known as Edwards syndrome, is often life threatening and results in kidney malformations, structural heart defects, intestines protruding outside the body, and esophageal obstructions. Trisomy 13, also known as Patau syndrome, results in muscular and skeletal malformations, as well as conditions affecting the nervous system and results in neonatal death within one month of birth in 80 percent of cases.

trophoblast The outermost layer of the developing blastocyst of a mammal.

twinning The process by which a single embryo divides into two distinct but genetically identical embryos.

undifferentiated (cells) Cells that have not yet developed a specialized function within the body or have not yet become a specific type of cell.

virtues Habits, character traits, feelings, and intuitions that comprise who we are as human beings and that are necessary for being a good person and living a moral life.

virtue theories Rooted in ancient philosophy, virtue theories focus on who the person is and who they are becoming in light of a particular notion of the ideal human person and the moral (or good) life.

vulnerability Risk of not being seen as a person deserving of respect and loving concern.

INDEX

Page numbers followed by "c," "f" or "n" indicate a case study, figure or note, respectively.

eudaemonia, 47, 49
eugenics, 179, 223–226, 235, 238
Eunice Kennedy Shriver National
  Institute of Child Health and
  Human Development Neonatal
  Research Network (NRN), 131,
  132, 145
euthanasia
  basics, 20
  cases, 35, 38, 316, 323–324, 343
  Christian views, 14, 280, 282
  end-of-life care and, 323–325,
    343
  ethical theories and, 35
  food and water and, 294
  "good death" and, 332
  intentions and, 279
  legal context, 324
Evangelium vitae (Gospel of Life)
  (John Paul II), 282
evidence-based decisions, 378, 380
evil, 266
excuses, 7
executive case, 2–3, 22, 47
expectations, 333
experimental design, 258, 260
experimentation on humans. *see*
  research (experimentation) on
  humans
experts, 83, 91
exploitation, 168, 209, 256, 260,
  265, 266. *see also* vulnerability
external criteria, 71–72, 73f, 77c
extraordinary means, 281–282
eyes, 195

F

fairness. *see also* equitable distribu-
    tion; justice
  basics, 8
  capital punishment and, 34

cases, 361
conflicts of interest and, 87
egg and sperm donors, 168
gene technologies and, 230, 232,
  237
health care reform and, 351, 356,
  373
hospitals and, 13, 19
libertarian justice and, 358
medical indications standard
  and, 139
reproductive technologies and,
  169–170
faith, 54, 59, 64, 317
fallibility, 70–71
False (1863) Claims Act, 371
families
  burdens, 145–146, 147, 329
  home settings and, 328
  medical futility and, 300–301
family-physician relationships,
  301–310, 311–319c
Fanconi anemia, 231
FDA, 231, 245
Federal Regulations, Code of (45
  CFR 46), 253, 254, 255, 257,
  267, 272
feeble-minded, the, 224–225
feeding tubes. *see* artificial nutrition
  and hydration (ANH)
fee for service, 363, 367–368, 378.
  see also reimbursements
feelings. *see* emotions
feminist views, 189n29
Fernald, Massachusetts, school
  experiment, 250
fertility, 366
fertility clinics, 194, 200, 204
fetuses. *see* persons; viability
fidelity, 52
financial considerations. *see*
  commercialization; conflicts of
  interest; cost-benefit analyses;